Radiation Medicine Rounds

Charles R. Thomas, Jr., MD

Editor-in-Chief

Professor and Chair
Department of Radiation Medicine
Professor, Division of Hematology/Oncology
Department of Medicine
Knight Cancer Institute
Oregon Health Sciences University
Portland, Oregon

Editorial Board

Forthcoming Volumes

Lower Gastrointestinal Malignancies
Edgar Ben-Josef, MD and Albert Koong, MD, PhD
Guest Editors

Proton Therapy
James M. Metz, MD
Guest Editor

Radiation Medicine Rounds

VOLUME 1, ISSUE 1

Thoracic Malignancies

Steven E. Schild, MD
Guest Editor

Professor and Chairman
Department of Radiation Oncology
Mayo Clinic
Scottsdale, Arizona

demosMEDICAL
New York

Acquisitions Editor: Richard Winters
Cover Design: Joe Tenerelli
Compositor: NewGen North America
Printer: Hamilton

Visit our website at www.demosmedpub.com

Radiation Medicine Rounds is published three times a year by Demos Medical Publishing.

Business Office. All business correspondence including subscriptions, renewals, and address changes should be sent to Demos Medical Publishing, 11 West 42nd Street, 15th Floor, New York, NY, 10036.

Subscription Rates. Volume 1, 2010. For Institutions: $275, For Individuals $225, Single Copy Price: $85. Outside the United States: For Institutions $315, For Individuals $255. Individuals residing outside the United States wishing to purchase individual issues of *Radiation Medicine Rounds* should contact their local reseller/agents for pricing and shipping details. Payment must be made in advance by check (in U.S. Dollars drawn on a U.S. bank) or international money order made payable to Demos Medical Publishing, or MasterCard, Visa, or America Express.

ISSN: 2151-4208
ISBN: 978-1-933864-89-1

Library of Congress Cataloging-in-Publication Data

Thoracic malignancies / Steven E. Schild, guest editor.
p. ; cm. — (Radiation medicine rounds ; v. 1, issue 1)
Includes bibliographical references and index.
ISBN 978-1-933864-89-1
1. Lungs—Cancer—Radiotherapy. I. Schild, Steven E. II. Series: Radiation medicine rounds ; v. 1, issue 1.
[DNLM: 1. Lung Neoplasms—radiotherapy. 2. Esophageal Neoplasms—radiotherapy. 3. Esophageal Neoplasms—surgery. 4. Lung Neoplasms—surgery. WF 658 T487 2010]

RC280.L8T49 2010
616.99'42406—dc22

2009048985

Reprints. For copies of 100 or more of articles in this publication, please contact Reina Santana, Special Sales Manager.

Special discounts on bulk quantities of Demos Medical Publishing books are available to corporations, professional associations, pharmaceutical companies, health care organizations, and other qualifying groups. For details, please contact:

Reina Santana, Special Sales Manager
Demos Medical Publishing
11 W. 42nd Street
New York, NY 10036
Phone: 800–532–8663 or 212–683–0072
Fax: 212–941–7842
E-mail: rsantana@demosmedpub.com

Made in the United States of America
10 11 12 13 14 5 4 3 2 1

Contents

Foreword

FROM THE EDITOR-IN-CHIEF

Radiation Medicine Rounds is a hard cover periodical published three times a year that is designed to provide an up-to-date review of a dedicated radiation medicine topics of interest to clinicians and scientists who are involved in the care of patients receiving radiotherapy. It is intended to serve as both a reference and instructional tool by students, housestaff, fellows, practicing clinicians, medical physicists, cancer biologists, radiobiologists, and interdisciplinary colleagues throughout the oncology spectrum.

For the current issue, *Thoracic Malignancies*, Guest Editor, Dr. Steven Schild has assembled a dedicated group of investigators who have written a compilation of succinct and timely reviews on the most important aspects of radiotherapy for the most common solid tumors that originate in the thorax. On behalf of the editorial board, I congratulate Dr. Schild for putting together a state-of-the-art product of superior quality that will serve as a valuable resource in the field of thoracic radiation medicine.

Charles R. Thomas, Jr.

Preface

This first issue of *Radiation Medicine Rounds* focuses on thoracic malignancies. It is most appropriate to start here because these tumors take more lives than any others. In addition, they are amongst the most preventable adding to the huge human tragedy associated with them. Smoking is a huge problem that has fortunately been decreasing in the United States. This is in large part due to education regarding the risks, increases in taxes, and prohibition of smoking in many public places.

This book includes the multidisciplinary nature of the care of these tumors. There is representation from radiation oncology, medical oncology, and surgery. This provides a well-rounded summarization of the current practices. This book also reflects the practice and insights of a group of caregivers who work primarily at Mayo Clinic. This institution has provided incredible opportunities for the authors, many of whom were trained and practice there. The clinic emphasizes the importance of putting the patient's needs above all others.

Included are chapters on lung cancer, esophageal cancer, and thymomas. These include the bulk of thoracic tumors. Most of the authors are relatively young and, thus, potentially less biased and likely to be more aware of current findings. The basic organization for each chapter is

1. Pathology and Natural History
2. Clinical Behavior, Evaluation, and Staging
3. Therapy
4. Algorithm
5. Future Research and Future Therapy

The multidisciplinary nature of the authors provides an up-to-date summary giving readers a well-rounded education regarding these tumors and their care.

Steven E. Schild, MD

Contributors

Jonathan B. Ashman, MD, PhD
Senior Associate Consultant
Department of Radiation Oncology
Mayo Clinic
Assistant Professor of Radiation Oncology
Mayo College of Medicine
Phoenix, AZ

Jason A. Call, MD
Resident Physician
Department of Radiation Oncology
Rochester, MN

Matthew D. Callister, MD
Assistant Professor of Oncology Consultant
Department of Radiation Oncology
Mayo Clinic
Scottsdale, AZ

Walter J. Curran, Jr., MD, FACR
Professor and Chairman
Department of Radiation Oncology
Emory University School of Medicine
Atlanta, GA

Kelly K. Curtis, MD
Division of Hematology/Oncology
Mayo Clinic
Scottsdale, AZ

Yolanda I. Garces, MD
Department of Radiation Oncology
Mayo Clinic
Rochester, MN

Dawn E. Jaroszewski, MD, MBA
Division of Thoracic Surgery
Mayo Clinic
Scottsdale, AZ

O. Kenneth Macdonald, MD
Assistant Professor of Radiation Oncology
Department of Radiation Oncology
Rochester, MN

Kenneth R. Olivier, MD
Department of Radiation Oncology
Mayo Clinic
Rochester, MN

Harshita R. Paripati, MD
Division of Medical Oncology
Mayo Clinic
Scottsdale, AZ

Helen J. Ross, MD
Division of Hematology/Oncology
Mayo Clinic
Scottsdale, AZ

Steven E. Schild, MD
Professor and Chairman
Department of Radiation Oncology
Mayo Clinic
Scottsdale, AZ

Sandra C. Tomaszek, MD
Division of General Thoracic Surgery
Mayo Clinic
Rochester, MN

Sujay A. Vora, MD
Assistant Professor
Department of Radiation Oncology
Mayo Clinic
Phoenix, AZ

Dennis A. Wigle, MD, PhD
Division of General Thoracic Surgery
Mayo Clinic
Rochester, MN

JoDee Winter, PA-C, MS
Division of Thoracic Surgery
Mayo Clinic
Scottsdale, AZ

demos
MEDICAL

RADIATION
MEDICINE ROUNDS

Radiotherapy for Early-Stage Non–Small Cell Carcinoma of the Lung

Jason A. Call and O. Kenneth Macdonald*
Mayo Clinic, Rochester, MN

■ ABSTRACT

Pathology: Lung cancer is the most common cause of death from cancer in the United States and is divided into small cell lung cancer and non–small cell lung cancer (NSCLC). NSCLC includes adenocarcinomas, squamous cell carcinomas, and large cell carcinomas. Smoking is the most likely cause of many cases of NSCLC.

Evaluation and Staging: For early-stage NSCLC, evaluation begins with a computed tomography (CT) scan of the chest and upper abdomen, history and physical, and basic laboratory work. Once the diagnosis has been confirmed, further evaluation with positron emission tomography (PET)/CT scan, pulmonary function tests (PFTs), and bronchoscopy may be in order. Some patients may require mediastinoscopy or brain magnetic resonance imaging. Staging relates to the primary tumor (T), nodal status (N), and presence of distant disease (M).

Therapy: Standard therapy for early-stage NSCLC involves surgery with an anatomic resection. Long-term survival of up to 60% to 80% can be achieved in some patients after surgery. Radiotherapy with or without chemotherapy has been offered to patients who either cannot tolerate surgery or refuse surgery. Results of local control with conventional radiotherapy in early-stage NSCLC are poor compared with the results of surgery. Some patients achieve high rates of local control (80%–95%) using high-dose-per-fraction stereotactic body radiotherapy (SBRT).

Algorithm: Patients should undergo surgical resection when no contraindications exist. For medically inoperable lung cancer, radiotherapy with or without chemotherapy should be offered to patients with adequate performance status and life expectancy. For conventional radiotherapy alone, a dose of up to 77.4 Gy in fractions of 2 to 2.15 Gy can be used. When used with chemotherapy, doses of up to 74 Gy in 2-Gy fractions are recommended. SBRT may be used in some patients with peripheral T1–2 or T3 (by chest wall invasion) tumors ≤5 cm without nodal or distant metastasis.

■ EPIDEMIOLOGY

Lung cancer remains the most common cause of cancer-related death in North America. A total of 219,440 new cases with 159,390 deaths related to cancer of the lung or bronchus were predicted in the United States in 2009 (1). Although prostate cancer is more common in men and breast cancer more common in women, cancer of the lung and bronchus remains the leading cancer type in terms of mortality in either sex (1). Smoking is most likely the major cause of these statistics as it has been shown to increase the risk of all major histologic types of lung cancer (2).

*Corresponding author, Department of Radiation Oncology, 200 1st St. SW, Rochester, MN 55905
E-mail address: macdonald.orlan@mayo.edu

Radiation Medicine Rounds 1 (2010) 1–20.

DOI: 10.5003/2151–4208.1.1.1

TABLE 1 Published results of resection for early-stage non–small cell lung cancer

Study	Stage	*n*	Surgery	Size	Locoregional Failure (%)	5-Year Survival (%)	5-Year Cancer-Specific Survival (%)
Okada et al. (6)	Stage I	778	Various	<20 mm 21 to <30 mm ≥31 mm			92.4, 96.7, 85.7[a] 87.4, 84.6, 39.4[a] 81.3, 62.9, 0[a]
Ginsberg and Rubinstein (7)	T1 N0	247	Limited lobectomy		17 6	~45 ~65	
Gajra et al. (8)	T1 N0	246	Anatomic resection	≤ 1.5 cm 1.6–3.0 cm		85.5 78.6	
Port et al. (9)	T1 N0	244	Mostly lobectomy	≤ 2 cm > 2 cm		77.2 60.3	81.4 63.4

[a]Lobectomy, segmentectomy, and wedge resection, respectively.

Current preoperative staging techniques may be able to identify a subgroup of patients with favorable tumors for whom more limited surgery may be suitable. This issue is being addressed in an ongoing phase 3 randomized trial being conducted by the Cancer and Leukemia Group B (CALGB).

Observation

For some patients with early-stage NSCLC surgery may not be feasible because of poor pulmonary reserve or other comorbidities. When a patient has medical contraindications to surgery, radiation is often given, and some patients are observed. At the Richard L. Roudebush VA Medical Center, 128 patients were found with stage I to IIA NSCLC from 1994 to 1999 (13). These patients were treated with surgery or radiotherapy or underwent observation only. The median OS was 14.2, 16.0, 20.8, and 46.2 months for observation, radiotherapy with palliative intent, radiotherapy with curative intent, and surgery, respectively. The advantage of surgery over the other approaches was statistically significant. Although these retrospective data do not provide a definitive answer as to whether there is any potential benefit of radiotherapy in medically inoperable early-stage NSCLC, only 4 of the 49 patients who were observed were alive at the time of review. Cancer was recorded as the cause of death in 26 of 41 observed patients for whom a cause of death was recorded. Currently, observation is not a standard option for patients who have no contraindications to treatment.

Definitive Conventional Radiotherapy

Several authors have reported results for patients treated with radiation alone for early-stage NSCLC. Selected results are summarized in Table 2 (14–22). Overall, results with conventional radiotherapy are not comparable to results from surgical series. Although techniques and doses have varied considerably between institutions, a proportion of patients have long-term disease control with standard fractionated radiotherapy. However, local control and distant metastases remain significant problems in these patients.

Sibley et al. (14) reported the Duke experience in treating early-stage NSCLC with radiotherapy alone. These authors reviewed 141 patients with stage I tumors that were medically inoperable but treated with radiotherapy without surgery or initial chemotherapy. The rates of 2-year and 5-year cause-specific survival (CSS) were 60% and 32%, with corresponding OS of 39% and 13%, respectively. On further analysis, increasing the radiotherapy dose seemed to predict for improved CSS, although this was not statistically significant. On analyzing the patterns of first failure for the 55 patients with failure, 42% failed locally only, 38% had a distant failure only, and regional-nodal failure alone accounted for 7%.

A meta-analysis published by Rowell and Williams (23) focused on the effectiveness of radical radiotherapy for stage I or II NSCLC. In the studies reviewed, rates of 5-year OS ranged from 0% to 42%, and rates of CSS (when reported) were 13% to 39%. Results varied by stage, with T1 tumors demonstrating 5-year OS rates of between

TABLE 2 Published results of conventional definitive radiotherapy for early-stage non–small cell lung cancer

Study	Therapy Details	*n*	Clinical Stage	Survival (Time)	Local Failure	Distant Metastasis
Sibley et al. (14)	50–80 Gy (median 64 Gy); 1.2 Gy twice daily to 3 Gy daily	141	Stage I	39% (2 y) 13% (5 y)	22%[a]	23%[a]
Hayakawa et al. (15)	60–81 Gy; 2 Gy daily	36	Stage I	42% (3 y) 23% (5 y)	28%[b]	36%
Jeremic et al. (16)	69.6 Gy; 1.2 twice daily	49	Stage I	T1: 76% (2 y), 37% (5 y) T2: 50% (2 y), 24% (5 y)	T1: 29%[b] T2: 62%[b]	25% (at 5 y)
Slotman et al. (17)	48 Gy; 4 Gy daily	31	Stage I	72% (2 y) 42% (3 y) 8% (5 y)	6%	16%
Morita et al. (18)	55–75 Gy; mostly 2 Gy daily	149	Stage I	34% (3 y) 22% (5 y)	44%	
Krol et al. (19)	60 Gy (3 Gy daily; 3-wk break at fraction 10) or 65 Gy (2.5 Gy daily)	108	Peripheral Stage I	49% (2 y) 31% (3 y) 15% (5 y)	67%	33%
Kaskowitz et al. (20)	39–79.2 Gy	53	Stage I	43% (2 y) 19% (3 y) 6% (5 y)	51% (3-yr PFS)	32%
Kupelian et al. (21)	Median 63 Gy	71	T1–4 N0	19% (3 y) 12% (5 y)	T1: 11%[c] T2: 39%[c] T3: 58%[c] T4: 45%[c]	
Rosenthal et al. (22)	18–65 Gy (median 60 Gy)	62	T1–2 N1	33% (2 y) 20% (3 y) 12% (5 y)	55%	31%[a]

PFS, progression-free survival.
[a]Includes first failures only; [b]5-year local failure; [c]3-year rate.

29% and 37%, compared with 4% to 24% for T2 lesions. Although the reported rates of local failure were quite broad (6%–70%), it remained a significant problem in most reports. This meta-analysis also emphasizes the problem associated with the later development of distant metastasis: 16% to 40% of patients with initial stage I disease failed distantly, with rates of distant disease of 25% to >50% among patients with stage IIA or IIB disease.

Overall, results for primary radiotherapy in early-stage NSCLC have been disappointing. Although a few patients enjoy durable long-term results, when radiotherapy is compared with surgery local control remains a significant issue in most patients.

Radiation Dose and Fractionation

Given the relatively poor prognosis of patients treated with definitive radiotherapy for NSCLC, several efforts have been made to improve the results for early-stage patients who cannot have surgery. Results for patients treated with higher doses and altered fractionation schemes have been reported.

Traditionally, fractionated radiotherapy for NSCLC has generally consisted of doses of 1.8 to 2.0 Gy per fraction given 5 days per week for a total dose of approximately 60 to 66 Gy. In the past, higher doses have been avoided due to concern for normal tissue toxicity. With the development of modern treatment planning systems and conformal radiotherapy, interest has turned to treating with higher doses in hopes of being able to improve tumor control.

A phase 2 dose escalation study using three-dimensional conformal radiation therapy (3DCRT) at the University of Michigan enrolled 104 patients with stage I to III NSCLC between 1992 and 1999 (24). Twenty-five patients also received neoadjuvant chemotherapy. Patients were escalated in 5 groups depending on the volume of normal lung irradiated. At the time of the analysis, 63 patients had completed the protocol and were assessable. With doses ranging from 63 to 102.9 Gy, there were 23 patients who failed in the planning target volume (PTV) at first failure. This included 9 of 16 assessable patients at a dose level of 69.3 Gy, 2 of 10 at a level of 75.6 Gy, 4 of 12 at a level of 84 Gy, and 1 of 8 at a level of 92.4 Gy. Only 2 patients experienced grade 3 pneumonitis. Another dose escalation study from Memorial Sloan-Kettering Cancer Center included 104 patients with stage I to III NSCLC treated with 3DCRT (25). The authors found a maximum tolerated dose (MTD) of 84 Gy, with the higher dose level of 90 Gy having excessive pulmonary toxicity. Their data suggest an improvement in OS with doses of 80 Gy or more. The Radiation Therapy Oncology Group (RTOG) conducted a dose escalation trial using 3DCRT for NSCLC (26). Fraction size was 2.15 Gy. They concluded that a dose of 83.8 Gy could be safely delivered in patients in whom the volume of lung receiving 20 Gy or more (V20) was <25%, and that a dose of 77.4 Gy could be safely used in patients with V20 values from 25% to 36%. They were unable to demonstrate a dose response for tumor control. Locoregional control remained a problem, with 2-year rates of 50% to 78%. The authors speculated that a lack of benefit for a higher dose may have been due to the prolonged treatment times, with treatment taking 8 weeks or more to complete.

In the previously mentioned meta-analysis of radiotherapy for early-stage NSCLC, radiation dose correlated with the ability of achieving complete response with rates of 60% in patients treated to 72 Gy compared with 32% if only 60 Gy was given (23).

Altered fractionation regimens have also been used in early medically inoperable NSCLC. Sause et al. published results for 161 patients with lung cancer treated mostly with 12 fractions of 4 Gy each. Of these patients, 16% had stage I tumors, and 22% had stage II. Of the 113 patients at risk, at 4 years, 10.6% were still alive at that time. For patients with NSCLC and negative supraclavicular nodes, 18.3% of patients were alive at 4 years (27). In another report, by Slotman et al., 31 patients with T1–2 disease were treated using hypofractionation to a dose of 48 Gy delivered in 12 fractions (17). The 3-year OS and CSS were 42% and 76%, respectively. Cheung et al. also used a dose of 48 Gy in 12 fractions for 33 patients with T1–2 N0 NSCLC. The 2-year OS was 46%, and recurrence-free survival was 40% (28). In a randomized trial testing continuous, hyperfractionated accelerated radiotherapy versus conventional dose radiotherapy, OS was improved with the altered fractionation technique (29). This trial included stages I to III NSCLC, and in the subgroup analysis there was no evidence that this benefit was limited to any particular stage.

Chemoradiotherapy

In advanced-stage NSCLC, chemoradiotherapy has an established role in the definitive management of disease. Given the relatively poor results of primary radiotherapy alone in early-stage NSCLC compared with surgery, chemoradiotherapy has also been tested for these patients. At the Peter MacCallum Cancer Centre, 39 patients were treated with chemoradiotherapy and 34 with radiotherapy alone for inoperable stage I NSCLC between 2000 and 2004 (30). Radiotherapy consisted of 60 Gy in 30 fractions in the chemoradiotherapy group and either that same regimen or 50 to 55 Gy in 20 fractions in the radiotherapy alone group. Chemotherapy was delivered concurrent with radiation and consisted of either single-agent carboplatin or a cisplatinum-based regimen. The patients treated with chemoradiotherapy experienced a local progression-free survival at 2 years of 66%, compared with 55% with radiotherapy alone, with corresponding 2-year rates of distant progression-free survival of 60% and 63%. This experience highlights that local and distant disease control remain problematic even with the addition of chemotherapy to radiotherapy.

Stereotactic Body Radiotherapy

SBRT is becoming more common in the treatment of patients with early-stage NSCLC who are not surgical candidates. As mentioned, published experiences using limited radiotherapy fields with conventional fractionation have reported only marginal rates of local control. With elimination of large elective nodal fields, attention has been placed on focal treatments with higher doses per fraction. SBRT has been used to treat clinically staged T1–2 or select T3 patients without nodal disease. Selected published results are presented in Table 3 (31–40). Overall, local control following SBRT for early-stage lung cancer has demonstrated rates of 80% to 95% at 2 to 3 years.

Uematsu et al. (41) treated 131 patients with stage I disease with stereotactic radiotherapy. In most cases, doses of 50 to 60 Gy in 5 to 10 fractions were prescribed. With a median follow-up of 90 months in living patients, the 5-year and 10-year CSSs were 78% and 74%, respectively. Local progression was found in 5 patients on follow-up imaging.

A large series published by Onishi et al. (38) summarizes the results of 257 patients treated with total doses of 30 to 84 Gy at the isocenter in 1 to 14 fractions at 14 institutions in Japan. Dose per fraction varied from 4.4 to 35 Gy. The authors calculated the biologically effective dose (BED) using the linear quadratic (LQ) model with an $\alpha:\beta$ ratio of 10. For surgically operable patients, OS was 70.8% for patients treated with a BED ≥100 Gy but was only 30.2% if a BED dose of <100 Gy was used. The authors also reported a statistically significant difference in local and distant failures favoring higher doses when patients who received BEDs of ≥100 Gy were compared with patients who received <100 Gy.

Prospective data from a phase 1 trial have been reported from Indiana University (42). Forty-seven patients with medically inoperable stage I NSCLC were treated on this dose escalation protocol. Patients received three fractions of radiation delivered to the target, with a starting total dose of 24 Gy. For patients with T1 tumors, no MTD was achieved despite reaching a dose level of 60 Gy. The patients with T2 tumors did meet an MTD of 66 Gy in tumors 5 to 7 cm. For smaller T2 lesions no MTD was achieved despite testing to 66 Gy. Local failures were observed in 4 of 19 T1 tumors and 6 of 28 T2 tumors. Control seemed to be related to the radiation dose. Of the 10 local failures, 9 patients had a fractional dose of ≤16 Gy. Only one failure occurred at higher doses.

Indiana University also completed a phase 2 trial of their three-fraction technique. Seventy patients were treated on this protocol (37). Clinically staged T1 tumors received 60 Gy, whereas T2 tumors were treated with 66 Gy. They observed excellent local control at 2 years (95%). Toxicity results, however,

TABLE 3 Published results with stereotactic body radiotherapy for early-stage non–small cell lung cancer

Study	Fraction Size	Total Dose	*n*	Follow-UP (Years)	Clinical Stage	2-Year Survival (%)	2-Year LC (%)
Uematsu et al. (31)	5–12 Gy	50–60 Gy @ 80% IDL	50	3	T1–2 N0	77[a]	94
Onimaru et al. (32)	6–7.5 Gy	48–60 Gy @ isocenter	17	2	T1–2 N0	42	85
Wulf et al. (33)	10–26 Gy	26–37.5 Gy	20	2	I–II	32	92
Xia et al. (34)	5 Gy	50 Gy @ 50% IDL	43	3	I (n = 25) II (n = 18)	91 64	96 93
Hoyer et al. (35)	15 Gy	45 Gy @ isocenter	40	2.4	Early stage	48	85
Nagata et al. (36)	12 Gy	48 Gy @ isocenter	45	3	T1 N0 (n = 32) T2 N0 (n = 13)	84 72	95 100
Timmerman et al. (37)	20–22 Gy	60–66 Gy @ PTV periphery	70	1.5	T1 N0 (n = 35) T2 N0 (n = 35)	55	95
Onishi et al. (38)	4.4–35 Gy	30–84 Gy @ isocenter	257	3	T1 N0 (n = 164) T2 N0 (n = 93)	82 83	 85
Lee et al. (39)	10 Gy	30–40 Gy @ PTV periphery	9	1.5	T1–2 N0	100	90
Baumann et al. (40)	10–20 Gy	30–48 Gy @ 65% IDL	141	2.75	T1 (n = 56) T2 (n = 85)	68	100 85

IDL, isodose line; LC, local control; PTV, planning tumor volume.
[a]Two-year survival was 88% in those medically operable.

caused concern about using high doses in centrally located tumors. Grade 3 to 5 toxicity was observed in a total of 14 patients. Tumor location was subdivided into central and peripheral location. Central tumor location was within 2 cm of the proximal bronchial tree. The 2-year freedom from severe toxicity was 83% in peripheral tumors, whereas it was only 54% in central tumors.

Researchers from Stanford have performed a phase 1 dose escalation study for single-fraction radiosurgery (43). Patients with either early-stage NSCLC or solitary lung metastases were eligible. At doses of >20 Gy freedom from local progression at 1 year was 91%, compared with only 54% for doses <20 Gy.

Experience from Japan using somewhat lower total doses of radiation has been reported. In a phase 1/2 trial of 45 patients treated at Kyoto University, Nagata et al. (36) reported success using a dose of 48 Gy delivered in four fractions. The 5-year local relapse-free rate was 95% for T1 lung cancers and 100% for T2. The 5-year disease-free survival was 72% and 71% for T1 and T2 tumors, respectively. A Japanese Clinical Oncology Group (JCOG) trial (0403) is currently testing this dose fractionation in a multi-institutional setting.

Some have raised concern that the surgical correlate of SBRT would be a wedge resection. This is alarming given the evidence of superior local control of anatomic resections in early-stage NSCLC, as demonstrated in a randomized controlled trial (7). Timmerman et al. (44) have presented a rationale for why SBRT is not similar to a wedge resection, which would explain the high rate of tumor control with SBRT reported in the literature. As those authors have pointed out, although the prescription dose is applied to a target, the dose falloff that inevitably occurs with SBRT will cover areas of potential microscopic spread that are not apparent on imaging.

The published results for SBRT for early-stage NSCLC have been very encouraging in terms of local control and toxicity. As data mature, results of longer follow-up will become available with better characterization of late toxicity. At the current time, SBRT remains a viable option for patients with T1–2 N0 tumors or T3 N0 tumors (by the criterion of chest wall invasion) that are ≤5 cm who cannot undergo surgery. Although not considered standard for medically operable patients, SBRT is actively being compared with surgery in two separate phase 3 trials.

Radiobiologic Considerations in SBRT

Conventionally fractionated (doses of around 2 Gy per day) radiation therapy has traditionally been used because of several theoretical advantages. First, normal tissue has a greater capability of repairing sublethal damage than cancer cells. Such a regimen given over weeks also allows for cancer cells to redistribute to G2 and M phases of the cell cycle, which are regarded as being more radiosensitive. Fractionated radiotherapy may also allow for reoxygenation of partially hypoxic tumors, thus potentially increasing the effectiveness of the radiation delivered. However, in dose escalation with standard fractionation the protracted radiation course may allow cancer cells more time to repair and repopulate.

Probably the most widely accepted and used model for radiation dose response has been the LQ model. This has been described elsewhere (45) and is commonly used to compare doses among different radiation fractionations. However, many question the utility of this model in the setting of high doses per fraction. As pointed out by Park et al. (46), the LQ model predicts for a continuous response curve even at higher doses per fraction, despite clinical data suggesting a more linear relationship between dose and the log of the proportion of surviving cells. Thus, according to the LQ model, radiation effects in this range would be overestimated. These same authors have suggested a different model to help account for this, the universal survival curve. In this model there is a transition zone designated Dt. At doses less than Dt the LQ model predominates and is used to predict radiation effects. However, at higher doses the multitarget model is implemented. Further work in the area of describing radiobiologic principles at high doses per fraction will aid in accurate and reproducible prediction models for use in clinical and research settings.

■ TOXICITY

Conventional Radiotherapy

Radiation injury to normal lung tissue is a dose-limiting toxicity for patients receiving treatment to the thorax. This lung injury includes both radiation pneumonitis and late pulmonary fibrosis. Acute radiation pneumonitis classically presents 1 to 6 months after exposure. Patients suspected of radiation pneumonitis should receive a full workup for other causes of lung injury. Treatment of symptomatic radiation pneumonitis often involves the administration of steroids. Presenting symptoms can include dyspnea, cough, or low-grade fever, and radiographic changes can be seen. Lung fibrosis is thought to be due to chronic injury and is typically a late manifestation (>1 year).

Much investigation has gone into predicting risk of lung toxicity with different doses of radiation. In addition to the amount of radiation, patient factors such as pulmonary function should be considered. Some authors have reported a relationship between the volume of lung receiving a certain dose or the mean lung dose (MLD) and the risk of lung injury or toxicity. Washington University performed a prospective study in 99 patients treated with radiation doses of 50 to 70 Gy in 1.8 to 2.0 Gy per fraction (47). Grade ≥2 pneumonitis occurred in 14%, 17%, and 20% of patients at 6, 12, and 24 months, respectively. Important predictors for lung injury included the V20, MLD, and effective lung dose. Lower lobe location also increased the risk as compared with upper lobe location. On multivariate analysis, V20 appeared to be the best predictor of pneumonitis. With V20s of <22%, 22% to 31%, 32% to 40%, and >40% the incidence of pneumonitis ≥grade 2 at 2 years was 0%, 7%, 13%, and 36%, respectively. Grade 3 to 5 toxicity was not seen until the V20 was >32%. If the MLD was <20 Gy the incidence of pneumonitis ≥grade 2 was 8%, but it increased to 24% if the MLD was >20 Gy. Subsequently, the RTOG completed a phase 1–2 dose escalation study (RTOG 93-11) (26). The dose delivered was largely dependent on the V20. For patients with a V20 <25% the incidence of lung toxicity at 18 months was 7%, 16%, 0%, and 13% for patients treated with doses of 70.9, 77.4, 83.8, and 90.3 Gy, respectively. Patients with V20 of 25% to 30% had an incidence of 15% for doses of 70.9 or 77.4 Gy. On multivariate analysis MLD and V20 remained prognostic of late lung toxicity.

Radiation-induced lung injury was recently reviewed in an article by Ghafoori et al. (48). They noted that most studies do document a decline in PFTs after radiotherapy. Changes in forced expiratory volume in 1 second (FEV_1) can occur 3 to 6 months out, but some patients will improve with time. D_{LCO} may change more than the FEV_1 and does not appear to demonstrate the same recovery. Changes after radiation are consistent with a restrictive process as the FEV_1 to forced vital capacity ratio remains normal. They found evidence in the literature correlating lung injury to multiple dosimetric parameters including MLD and the volume of lung receiving a certain dose of radiation.

Concurrently administered chemotherapy has been associated with a higher risk of radiation pneumonitis. Tsujino et al. (49) retrospectively reviewed 65 patients who received concurrent chemotherapy. In this report, grade ≥2 pneumonitis increased with an increase in V20. In patients with V20 of ≤20%, 21% to 25%, 26% to 30%, and ≥31% the corresponding rates were 8.7%, 18.3%, 51%, and 85%, respectively. These rates of toxicity are higher than would have been estimated on the basis of radiation alone.

Other side effects are also considered when giving thoracic radiation. Depending on the irradiated volume or the use of chemotherapy, esophagitis can be a risk and may require analgesics or intravenous fluid supplementation. Fatigue can be common in patients receiving radiotherapy. One of the most feared complications of radiation is radiation injury to the spinal cord. This has generally been considered to have a ≤5% late complication rate at a dose level of 45 to 50 Gy. In addition, toxicities such as brachial plexopathy and radiation effect on the bone marrow, skin, or heart are potential complications depending on the location, dose, and use of chemotherapy.

Lung SBRT

Several prospective trials have documented toxicity data for a three-fraction regimen of SBRT. Timmerman et al. published the preliminary results of a phase 1 trial of SBRT for NSCLC done at Indiana University (50). The dose ranged from 24 to 60 Gy in three fractions. Fatigue was reported in all 37 patients. One patient was diagnosed with an asymptomatic pericardial effusion after radiation. Six patients (16%) were treated with medical therapy that included steroid therapy for pulmonary symptoms. Data from this trial are pertinent in that they describe changes in PFTs obtained prospectively. Ten patients (27%) had at least a 10% acute worsening of one or more test parameters. Most of these patients (70%) returned to their pretreatment baseline with time. Other documented side effects included pain and discomfort from abdominal compression devices, and dermatitis 2 to 3 weeks after therapy (grade 3 in one patient). One patient experienced grade 3 hypoxemia, and another developed symptomatic radiation pneumonitis requiring hospitalization. All therapy-related side effects were recognized within 6 weeks. No late effects were noted at the time of publication.

McGarry et al. (42) published updated results of this trial with 47 patients enrolled and noted no definitive relationship between dose and toxicity. In the updated report they found three patients with grade 2 pneumonitis, bronchitis, or pneumonia. One patient had a grade 2 pericardial effusion, and another had a grade 3 pericardial effusion. A patient with a total dose of 72 Gy experienced grade 3 tracheal necrosis. Other grade 3 events included four patients with pneumonitis or hypoxia and one patient with dermatitis.

Concern about toxicity at high doses of SBRT in centrally located tumors was generated by phase 2 data published by Timmerman et al. (37). Grade 3 to 5 toxicity was noted in 14 of 70 patients treated with SBRT for early-stage lung cancer. Patients with T1 tumors received 60 Gy in three fractions, and T2 tumors were treated with a slightly higher dose of 66 Gy in the same number of treatments. Both univariate analysis and multivariate analysis indicated that tumor location was a strong predictor of high-grade toxicity. The 2-year freedom from severe toxicity was 83% in peripheral tumors, whereas it was only 54% in central tumors. Eight patients had grade 3 events, including a decline in PFTs, pneumonia, pleural effusion, apnea, or skin reactions. Unfortunately, six patients had grade 5 events (death) that were scored as related to treatment. Four died of bacterial pneumonia, one had a pericardial effusion, and one patient with a tumor recurrence died with hemoptysis. Four of the six deaths were among patients with perihilar/central tumors.

Results of toxicity from RTOG 0236 have been published in abstract form. This was a multi-institutional, prospective trial of SBRT in medically inoperable stage T1–3 NSCLC with peripheral location (51). Prescription dose was 60 Gy in three fractions. Of the patients in this trial, 2% experienced grade 4 and 13% had grade 3 pulmonary or upper respiratory toxicity at a median follow-up of 8.7 months. In addition, there was one patient with grade 3 dermatitis and one with grade 3 syncope that were noted to be related to treatment. No treatment-related deaths were observed.

Whyte et al. (52) have published results of a prospective phase 1 trial of single-fraction SBRT at a dose of 15 Gy using the Cyberknife system at two institutions. At a median follow-up of 7 months no grade 3 or 4 complications were observed related to radiotherapy. Four patients experienced complications related to fiducial placement, three with pneumothoraces and one with an emphysema exacerbation.

In a Stanford phase 1 dose escalation study for single-fraction radiosurgery all late toxicity was seen at a dose of >20 Gy and was mostly seen in patients with central tumors or patients who had received previous irradiation to a volume of at least 50 cc (43). There were three late grade 5 toxicities (one patient with a tracheoesophageal fistula, one with pneumonitis and a pleural effusion, and one with a pulmonary embolism and pneumonitis). All three received chemotherapy at some point, and two had received prior radiotherapy to the thorax. Other late toxicity included pneumonitis, atrial fibrillation, and a pleural effusion.

Recent work has attempted to characterize lung injury after SBRT. Guckenberger et al. (53) evaluated lung injury in 70 patients who underwent stereotactic radiotherapy or radiosurgery in the lungs. Symptomatic pneumonitis was found in 10% of patients. Median time to onset of symptoms was 5 months. “Spotted-streaky” consolidation was present radiographically in 32%, 34%, and 41% of patients at 3, 6, and 9 months, respectively. After 12 months this pattern went away in most patients. A dense consolidation pattern appeared at 6 months, with retraction at 9 months. Fibrotic remodeling went on for years after treatment. Similar to conventional radiotherapy, there may be a relationship between risk of radiation pneumonitis after SBRT and the MLD (54).

Toxicity risks with lung SBRT are related to the location of the tumor. Chest wall toxicity, including pain and rib fractures, has been reported following SBRT for peripheral lesions (55). The volume of chest wall receiving ≥30 Gy has been shown to correlate with severe toxicity in patients treated with three to five fractions (56). The median time to onset of chest wall toxicity was reported as 7.3 months. Pettersson et al. (57) analyzed 13 rib fractures in 7 of 33 patients treated with 45 Gy in three fractions. They described a relationship between the risk of fracture and the dose to 2 cm^3 of rib. The risk was near 0%, 5%, and 50% for patients when that dose was <7 Gy per fraction, 9.1 Gy per fraction, and 16.6 Gy per fraction, respectively. Treatment of apical tumors can be associated with injury to the brachial plexus. Forquer et al. (58) found that for patients treated with three to four fractions, the 2-year risk of brachial plexopathy was 46% and 8%, respectively, for patients with maximum BED of >100 or <100 Gy (calculated with an α:β ratio of 3) to the brachial plexus, respectively. Median onset of plexopathy in this report was 7 months from SBRT.

The risk of acute skin toxicity was highlighted in a report of 50 patients treated at Memorial Sloan-Kettering Cancer Center (59). Patients received either 60 Gy in three fractions or 44 to 48 Gy in four fractions using three to seven coplanar beams. Skin toxicity grade 1 was found in 38% of patients. Higher-grade toxicity was less common, with 8% experiencing grade 2 toxicity, 4% experiencing grade 3, and 2% with grade 4. Risk factors for grade ≥2 acute skin toxicity included location within 5 cm of the skin of the posterior chest wall, the use of only three beams, and a maximum back skin dose that was ≥50% of the prescribed dose. These effects developed within 3 to 6 weeks of treatment. The authors postulated that the immobilization devices used may have had a dose buildup effect, thus explaining the high rate of skin toxicity and the association of toxicity with the skin dose on the back in this series of patients.

Overall, acute toxicity for SBRT is felt to be reasonably low. One review of SBRT toxicity included 15 lung studies with 683 patients (60). Although various techniques and doses were employed, estimates of acute toxicity for patients undergoing SBRT were summarized. Overall, up to 8% of all patients had grade 1 or 2 toxicity. Many of those patients had grade 1 events that lasted for a short time after treatment such as anorexia, fever, chills, and general malaise. Other common low-grade toxicities included grade 1 cough, pain, and skin erythema and grade 2 pneumonitis, pain, esophagitis, and dermatitis. Two patients had minor bone fractures. Although many patients had radiographic changes after SBRT, symptomatic manifestations were not common. The reported rates of grade 3 to 5 toxicity were 0% to 8% acutely and 0% to 7% for chronic effects. Commonly reported high-grade events included pneumonitis, hypoxia, and dermatitis. Two deaths were found in the literature in this review, for a treatment-related mortality of 0.3%. One death was related to a radiation-induced esophageal ulcer at a dose to the isocenter of 48 Gy in eight fractions (32). The other death was a fatal bleeding from the pulmonary artery 9 months after SBRT in a patient who had been previously irradiated (61).

■ TECHNIQUES

Conventional Radiotherapy Techniques

A typical setup approach for conventional radiotherapy involves the use of an immobilization device such as a VacLoc bag or an Alpha cradle with the patient in the supine position. The arms-up, or arms-above-the-head, position may allow different beam arrangements, depending on the tumor location. Patients should be instructed to maintain a calm, regular pattern of breathing for the simulation procedure as well as actual treatments. Four-dimensional CT (4DCT) at the time of simulation can collect data on tumor motion for use during the planning of radiotherapy volumes.

In the past, radiation to elective nodal sites was delivered in an attempt to eradicate subclinical disease. Several reports have questioned the need for treating uninvolved areas. Slotman et al. reported on 31 patients with T1–2 N0 NSCLC treated with a dose of 48 Gy in 12 fractions (17). The radiation fields did not electively include the hilum or mediastinum. Only two patients (6%) had a regional recurrence. Others have reported similar low rates of regional failures after limited-field radiotherapy for inoperable NSCLC (19,62,63). Elimination of elective nodal treatment is now commonly accepted.

Target volumes in radiotherapy include gross tumor volume (GTV), clinical tumor volume (CTV), internal target volume (ITV), and PTV. GTV is the actual gross tumor, which should be delineated using information from imaging. The CTV includes areas of potential microscopic disease spread. For NSCLC this should include the surrounding normal-appearing rim of tissue. According to a study by Giraud et al. (64), a CTV expanded from the GTV by 6 mm for SCCs and 8 mm for adenocarcinomas is needed in order to include 95% of microscopic extension. The ITV is the CTV with an internal margin (IM) added to account for physiologic motion. Information from 4DCT is often obtained to define the IM. Finally, the PTV is created beyond the CTV and IM with an expansion to account for setup error. The PTV margin depends on the type of immobilization, use of image guidance, and other institution-specific parameters.

Multifield conformal external beam radiotherapy is used to deliver dose to the PTV while observing the tolerance of normal tissues. Beam energies are typically in the range of 6 to 10 MV. During the previous two-dimensional treatment planning era, dose was given with an anterior and a posterior beam until the spinal cord tolerance was met, and then an oblique angle was use to deliver dose exclusive of the spinal cord. In the modern three-dimensional planning era the choice of beam angles and weighting can be more individualized prospectively on the basis of the location of the tumor and distance to critical structures. Selected normal tissue dose constraints from the National Comprehensive Cancer Network (NCCN) guidelines are shown in Table 4. Under some circumstances intensity-modulated radiation therapy (IMRT) may help in sparing organs at risk from potential radiation injury.

SBRT Techniques

SBRT Setup, Localization, and Delivery

The simulation and treatment of SBRT involves similar general principles to those used for conventional radiotherapy. In the setup, localization, and delivery of lung SBRT several key elements require consideration:

1. Three-dimensional target verification. After a plan is developed from the patient simulation procedure, verification of target structures is performed with each fraction. A number of image-guided technologies are available to facilitate this process.
2. Measures to account for respiratory motion. As the lung moves with respiration, respiratory motion becomes an important factor. There are several techniques to address respiratory motion.
3. Immobilization. Many institutions use a stereotactic frame for immobilization during SBRT. Unlike the setting of intracranial stereotactic radiotherapy and radiosurgery, SBRT in the lung involves a much less static target. Fixed frames are generally not used. Frameless stereotaxy can be done with technology capable of localizing fiducial markers in space.
4. Treatment delivery. Several systems exist to deliver the high doses of radiosurgery. These systems often incorporate technologies for any of the above elements of SBRT.

Technology for SBRT and image-guided radiotherapy (IGRT) is developing rapidly. A more complete review of technology, planning, and image guidance is provided in several recent texts (65–67). A summary of these principles is provided below as they pertain to lung SBRT.

With delivery of high doses per fraction comes the need for precise setup. Compared with intracranial stereotactic radiosurgery, where immobilization is often fixed, less invasive methods have been applied in the setting of SBRT for thoracic tumors. Often this is accomplished with whole-body vacuum molds that may have other components such as an abdominal pressure pillow, reference indicators to aid

TABLE 4 NCCN recommended normal tissue dose constraints

Radiation Therapy Alone		Radiation Therapy With Chemotherapy	
Spinal cord	50 Gy	Spinal cord	45 Gy
Lung	20 Gy < 40%	Lung	20 Gy < 35%
Heart	40 Gy < 100%	Heart	40 Gy < 50%
	50 Gy < 50%		
Esophagus	60 Gy < 50%	Esophagus	55 Gy < 50%
Liver	30 Gy < 40%		
Kidney	20 Gy < 50% of both Kidneys or < 25% of one side if the other kidney is not functional		

in localization, and vacuum seals that cover the top of patients. Currently there are several such frames used in clinical practice. The Elekta stereotactic body frame consists of a vacuum mattress along with a reference system that aids in localization of internal targets and a template that can be applied for controlling movement of the diaphragm. Another available device is the Medical Intelligence BodyFIX system. This has a full-body vacuum pillow below the patient and a vacuum seal on the top of the patient. With advanced imaging, many centers now no longer use the external fiducial systems that were previously common for localization.

When thoracic malignancies are being treated, respiratory motion must be taken into consideration. A common method to perform this task is 4DCT, which incorporates the three standard geometric dimensions with a fourth dimension, time. Typically, technology for monitoring the timing of target motion throughout the respiratory cycle is employed. As described by Khan, data can be acquired either prospectively or retrospectively (65). Acquiring data prospectively involves taking the scanning CT data from only one phase of the respiratory cycle, whereas in retrospective gating the data are obtained throughout the respiratory cycle and subsequently registered with respiratory motion.

Other recent strategies have involved systems for respiratory gating in which respiration is monitored during treatment. The system will turn the beam on only during a specific portion of the respiratory cycle. Several centers are now equipped with respiratory gating. Others have used breath-holding techniques in which the treatment is given only when the patient holds his or her breath. For patients with excessive respiratory motion, methods such as abdominal compression can be used. A compression device is placed on the torso and adequate pressure is applied to minimized diaphragm movement.

Several methods of image guidance for SBRT are used in clinical practice. Most modern treatment systems are equipped with both megavoltage and kilovoltage imagers. Fluoroscopic-based IGRT is capable of detecting fiducials, which can be placed at or near target structures for localization. Some facilities use in-room high-resolution CT scanners for pretreatment verification. Data from either the megavoltage imager or kilovoltage imager can be reconstructed to produce megavoltage or kilovoltage cone beam CT images, respectively.

Linear accelerators are now widespread and have been used for delivering high-dose SBRT at many centers. Often, standard linear accelerators are used with immobilization devices and IGRT to accomplish this task. Several systems are commercially available, each with various supporting technologies to accomplish similar goals.

Brainlab AG has developed the Exactrac/Novalis Body system for delivery of highly accurate image-guided stereotactic radiotherapy and radiosurgery. This isocentric system performs infrared (IR) tracking and kilovoltage radiographic imaging. The IR-based optical positioning component consists of two IR cameras on the ceiling for detection of IR markers. Bony landmarks or implanted fiducials can be localized by stereoscopic x-ray tubes mounted in the floor with opposing detectors attached to the ceiling. The information from the x-ray detectors and the IR tracking system can be combined to monitor the position of the target. Required adjustments can be applied by means of a robotic couch with capabilities in three rotational and three translational dimensions. The system can align the target in real time and has capabilities to facilitate respiratory gating. A Novalis treatment machine also exists with a 6-MV linear accelerator incorporating a mini-microleaf collimator. This machine can be used for conformal beam capabilities, dynamic field shaping, and IMRT. For a more detailed discussion of this system the reader is referred to a review by Slotman et al. (67).

The Cyberknife system, produced by Accuray, consists of a 6-MV linear accelerator mounted on a robotic arm. It has two orthogonal x-ray tubes mounted on the ceiling, with opposing silicon detectors. An X-band linear accelerator with a cylindrical collimator is used, with the advantage of being lightweight and small. The robotic arm with six degrees of rotation can produce a variety of nonisocentric beams. With inverse planning to select and give weight to each beam, highly conformal plans can be achieved. Images can be obtained to verify patient setup or to track target or fiducial motion. A built-in IR tracking system allows for tracking of motion during treatment, and the system can adjust for intratreatment target motion.

Helical tomotherapy has a gantry that rotates similarly to a CT, with a built-in 6-MV linear accelerator. Translational movement of the couch produces a spiral motion, and the system also has a multileaf collimator. Currently a commercially available tomotherapy unit is produced by TomoTherapy that also has capabilities for acquiring CT images using megavoltage x-rays. Thus, tomotherapy brings together IMRT and megavoltage-CT IGRT into one treatment delivery system.

SBRT Target Volumes, Planning, and Dosimetry

Quality dosimetry is important in SBRT given the need for a rapid dose falloff from the high doses used. Dose prescription and planning techniques have varied among centers. The main technique used in the United States has been to prescribe to a PTV. In the University of Indiana trials the CTV was the GTV (37,50). The PTV was created from the GTV by a 5-mm expansion axially and 10-mm expansion in the craniocaudal dimension. Beam arrangement used multiple noncoplanar, nonopposing beams with apertures formed directly to the PTV with no margin. Weighting of the beams was roughly equal and the dose was prescribed such that 95% of the PTV volume was covered by the 80% isodose line. The RTOG developed a similar, alternative method for the 0236 protocol. The protocol specifies a dose of 60 Gy in three fractions separated by a period of 40 hours to 8 days. In general the protocol requires a minimum field dimension of 3.5 cm. GTV is contoured on the pulmonary windows of the CT and equals the CTV. The PTV is created by expanding this volume by 5 mm axially and 10 mm in the craniocaudal dimension. Seven to 10 beams of equal weighting are placed around a common isocenter. Although noncoplanar, nonopposing beams are preferred, they are not required. No margin is applied from the PTV to the edges of the beam. The dose is prescribed such that 95% of the PTV receives the prescription dose, and 99% of the volume receives 90% of the prescription dose. Thus a dose higher than prescription will be delivered to the center of the PTV with this method. Representative treatment approaches for peripheral and central tumors using SBRT are provided in Figures 2 and 3. Selected normal tissue dose constraints used in RTOG 0236 are shown in Table 5.

In contrast, the more common approach in Japan has been to prescribe to the isocenter to apply a more uniform dose across the target. Nagata et al. (36,68) describe the technique at Kyoto University. They focus 6 to 10 noncoplanar 6-MV beams around an isocenter. An ITV is constructed by including an IM and a CTV. PTV expansion from the ITV is created by extending 5 mm in the axial dimension and 8 to 10 mm in the craniocaudal dimension. The target dose homogeneity is within 20% in the ITV. A dose of 48 Gy in four fractions is prescribed to the isocenter.

Some interest has been generated in the use of protons for lung SBRT. Macdonald et al. (69) compared the technique used in RTOG 0236 with proton beam plans for the same patients. One-field, two-field, or three-field proton plans were constructed for treatment comparison. PTV coverage was similar between the two modalities. The protons did have the advantage of less lung tissue receiving lower-dose radiation. Skin surface dose and rib dose were higher but may have been a function of having fewer beams, not of the use of protons.

Radiation dose as commonly prescribed in many protocols was calculated using algorithms that assume tissue density to be that of water. Such an assumption is inaccurate in the thorax, where lung tissue density differs significantly from that of water. A more accurate prediction of dose would take into account the heterogeneity of normal tissue densities. The RTOG recalculated the dose given to patients in their trial with heterogeneity corrections and found the dose to be 54 Gy (51). At our institution, where dose planning is currently done with heterogeneity corrections, a dose of 54 Gy in three fractions is given for peripheral tumors.

■ SUMMARY AND TREATMENT ALGORITHM

A treatment diagram is illustrated in Table 6. The standard treatment for early-stage NSCLC is surgery. For patients who either refuse surgery or are medically inoperable, radiation is generally recommended. The NCCN recommends definitive doses of up to 77.4 Gy (2 to 2.15 Gy per fraction) without chemotherapy or 74 Gy (2 Gy per fraction) with chemotherapy. The addition of chemotherapy should be considered on the basis of patient tolerability. Local control remains a problem at these doses, even with chemotherapy. SBRT represents a promising and relatively new choice for patients with early-stage NSCLC. Patients with peripheral T1–2 or T3 (by the criterion of chest wall invasion) tumors ≤5 cm

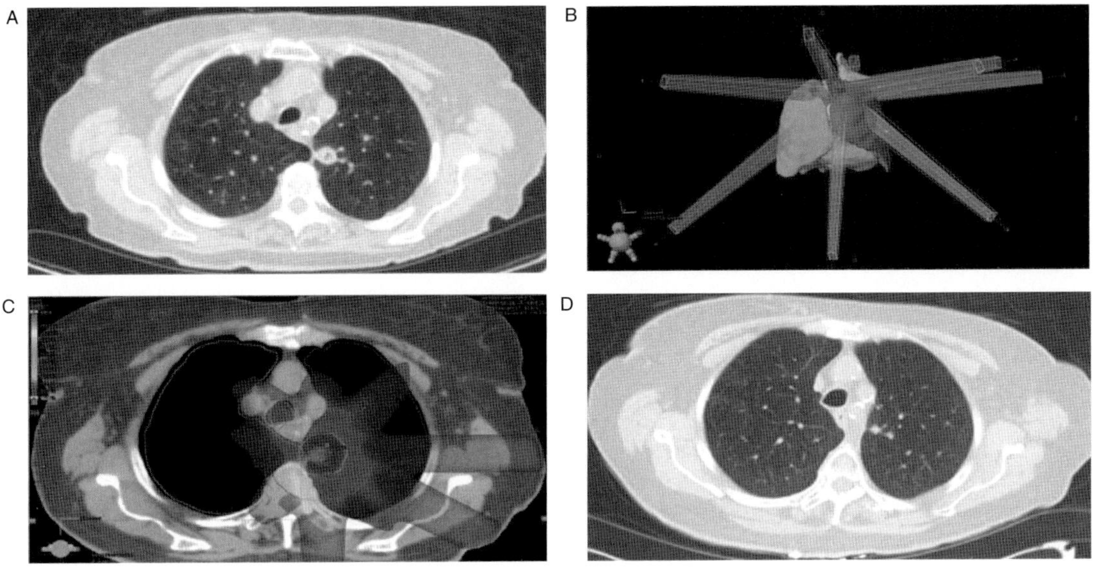

FIGURE 2 Representative images from the use of stereotactic body radiotherapy to definitively treat a centrally located primary non–small cell lung cancer, including (A) the pretherapy tumor on axial computed tomography (CT) image, (B) representative beam arrangement from treatment plan, (C) representative dose distribution based on a prescription dose of 48 Gy in four fractions, and (D) 15-month follow-up axial CT image.

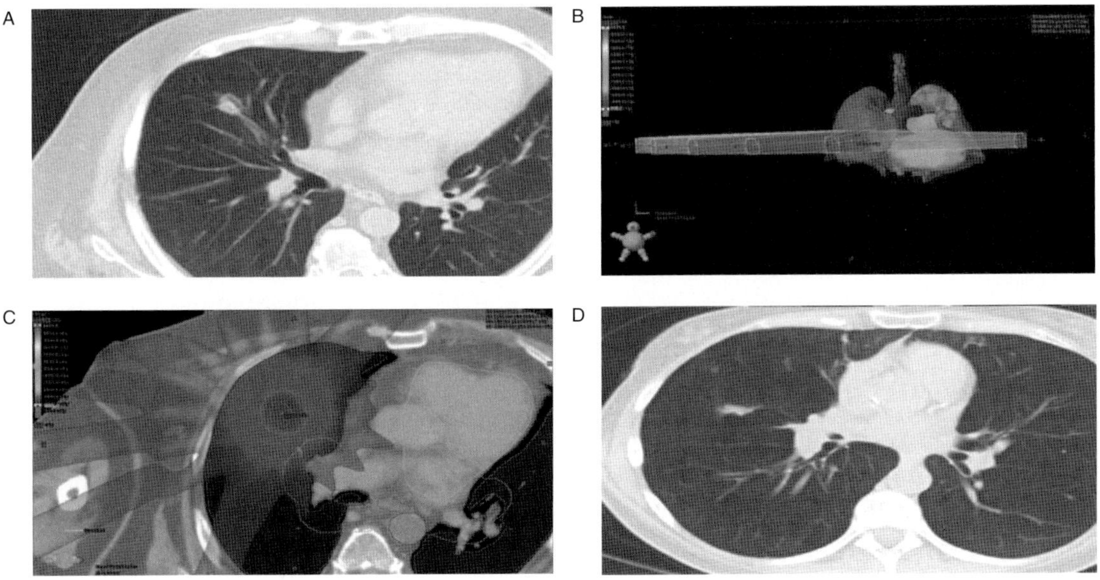

FIGURE 3 Representative images from the use of stereotactic body radiotherapy to definitively treat a peripherally located primary non–small cell lung cancer, including (A) the pretherapy tumor on axial computed tomography (CT) image, (B) representative beam arrangement from treatment plan, (C) representative dose distribution based on a prescription dose of 54 Gy in three fractions, and (D) 15-month follow-up axial CT image.

TABLE 5 Selected tissue constraints for 3-fraction stereotactic body radiotherapy

Spinal cord (any point)	18 Gy (6 Gy per fraction)
Esophagus (any point)	27 Gy (9 Gy per fraction)
Ipsilateral brachial plexus (any point)	24 Gy (8 Gy per fraction)
Heart (any point)	30 Gy (10 Gy per fraction)
Trachea and ipsilateral bronchus (any point)	30 Gy (10 Gy per fraction)

TABLE 6 Algorithm for potential treatment options for a patient with early-stage non–small cell lung cancer. (Adapted from NCCN guidelines, 2009.)

Treatment Algorithm for Early Stage NSCLC
T1-2 N0-1 Medically Operable[a]
• Surgery
T1-2 N0-1 Medically Inoperable
• Curative radiotherapy with or without chemotherapy is recommended when patients have adequate life expectancy and performance status
– without chemotherapy the radiation dose is up to 77.4 Gy in 2 to 2.15 Gy fractions (V20 should be ≤ 35%)
– with chemotherapy the radiation dose is up to 74 Gy in 2 Gy fractions
• SBRT can be considered for node-negative peripheral lesions ≤ 5 cm

[a]NCCN recommendeds that the distinction of medically operable or inoperable be made by a thoracic surgeon.

without evidence of nodal or distant metastasis are candidates for treatment with SBRT when surgery is not pursued.

■ FUTURE DIRECTIONS

The Problem of Distant Metastases After SBRT

Even after surgical therapy for stage I NSCLC, many patients may harbor micrometastatic disease. As recently described by Bradley et al. (70), metastatic disease represents a significant problem for early-stage NSCLC treated with SBRT. This report included 70 patients with T1–3 lesions with a median follow-up of 19 months. Although the 3-year actuarial local control was 83%, a total of 20 patients had a distant failure. Distant recurrence alone was the most common failure pattern and was found in 14 patients.

Several trials have evaluated the role of adjuvant chemotherapy after surgery for NSCLC. A randomized trial from Japan on patients with stage I NSCLC treated with adjuvant combination uracil and tegafur after surgery showed an improvement in OS for the 979 patients randomized (P = .04) (71). On subset analysis the patients with stage IB tumors benefited in terms of OS (hazard ratio .48; 95% confidence interval 0.29 to 0.81). Such a benefit could not be demonstrated for stage IA. This chemotherapy regimen is not in use in the United States or Europe. The CALGB performed a trial (CALGB 9633) aimed at assessing the role of adjuvant chemotherapy for stage IB NSCLC (72). They randomized 344 patients after surgery with lobectomy or pneumonectomy to either receive adjuvant chemotherapy or observation. The regimen used consisted of paclitaxel and carboplatin. Although an early analysis indicated promising results for chemotherapy, the final report did not demonstrate a significant survival benefit from adding chemotherapy. On an unplanned subgroup analysis a survival benefit was suggested for patients with larger tumors (>4 cm). Several other trials with broader inclusion criteria that have analyzed patients with stage IB NSCLC on subset analysis have failed to find a statistically significant benefit (73–75). A recent pooled analysis of five trials had similar findings of no benefit in stage IB disease (76). Currently, chemotherapy as adjuvant therapy after surgery for stage IB (<4 cm) NSCLC cannot be considered standard.

In contrast to the literature on the role of chemotherapy after surgery, the role of adjuvant systemic therapy for patients treated with SBRT for NSCLC has not been tested in a randomized fashion. Certainly, metastatic relapse of disease remains problematic. A challenge for the future will be designing and implementing effective systemic therapy to improve outcomes for these patients.

Other Trials

The RTOG has recently initiated several protocols for SBRT in the setting of early-stage NSCLC. As highlighted above, doses of around 60 Gy in three fractions have generated concerns about excessive toxicity for centrally located tumors. RTOG 0813 is a phase 1/2 dose escalation trial for tumors in this location. The starting dose is set at 50 Gy in 10-Gy fractions. The primary endpoint is to find the MTD for these patients. The RTOG is combining efforts with the North Central Cancer Treatment Group (NCCTG) in planning a randomized phase 2 study comparing a dose of 34 Gy in a single fraction with 48 Gy in four fractions for medically inoperable patients with peripheral T1–2 tumors.

Given the success of treating patients with medically inoperable early-stage NSCLC, the RTOG has designed a protocol to test SBRT in patients who are candidates for surgery. This trial includes patients with T1–3 tumors ≤5 cm in size and will treat with a dose of 60 Gy in three fractions. T3 tumors are eligible only if they have chest wall invasion. No randomized trials have compared SBRT with surgery for medically operable patients, but two trials are actively testing the comparison; one, a corporate-sponsored trial, is active in the United States, and the other is actively enrolling in the Netherlands.

REFERENCES

1. Jemal A, Siegel R, Ward E, et al. Cancer statistics, 2009. *CA Cancer J Clin.* 2009;59(4):225–249.
2. Alberg AJ, Samet JM. Epidemiology of lung cancer. *Chest.* 2003;123(1)(suppl):21S–49S.
3. Travis WD, Brambilla E, Müller-Hermelink HK, Harris CC, eds; World Health Organization; International Agency for Research on Cancer. *Pathology and Genetics of Tumours of the Lung, Pleura, Thymus, and Heart.* Lyon: IARC Press; 2004.
4. Brambilla E, Travis WD, Colby TV, et al. The new World Health Organization classification of lung tumours. *Eur Respir J.* 2001;18(6):1059–1068.
5. Greene FL; American Joint Committee on Cancer; American Cancer Society. *AJCC Cancer Staging Manual.* New York: Springer; 2002.
6. Okada M, Nishio W, Sakamoto T, et al. Effect of tumor size on prognosis in patients with non-small cell lung cancer: the role of segmentectomy as a type of lesser resection. *J Thorac Cardiovasc Surg.* 2005;129(1): 87–93.
7. Ginsberg RJ, Rubinstein LV. Randomized trial of lobectomy versus limited resection for T1 N0 non-small cell lung cancer. Lung Cancer Study Group. *Ann Thorac Surg.* 1995;60(3):615–622; discussion 622–623.
8. Gajra A, Newman N, Gamble GP, et al. Impact of tumor size on survival in stage IA non-small cell lung cancer: a case for subdividing stage IA disease. *Lung Cancer.* 2003;42(1):51–57.
9. Port JL, Kent MS, Korst RJ, et al. Tumor size predicts survival within stage IA non-small cell lung cancer. *Chest.* 2003;124(5):1828–1833.
10. Miller DL, Rowland CM, Deschamps C, et al. Surgical treatment of non–small cell lung cancer 1 cm or less in diameter. *Ann Thorac Surg.* 2002;73(5):1545–1550.
11. Fernando HC, Santos RS, Benfield JR, et al. Lobar and sublobar resection with and without brachytherapy for small stage IA non–small cell lung cancer. *J Thorac Cardiovasc Surg.* 2005;129(2):261–267.
12. Keenan RJ, Landreneau RJ, Maley RH Jr, et al. Segmental resection spares pulmonary function in patients with stage I lung cancer. *Ann Thorac Surg.* 2004;78(1):228–233; discussion 233.
13. McGarry RC, Song G, des Rosiers P, et al. Observation-only management of early stage, medically inoperable lung cancer: poor outcome. *Chest.* 2002;121(4): 1155–1158.
14. Sibley GS, Jamieson TA, Marks LB, et al. Radiotherapy alone for medically inoperable stage I non-small-cell lung cancer: the Duke experience. *Int J Radiat Oncol Biol Phys.* 1998 Jan 1;40(1):149–154.
15. Hayakawa K, Mitsuhashi N, Saito Y, et al. Limited field irradiation for medically inoperable patients with peripheral stage I non–small cell lung cancer. *Lung Cancer.* 1999;26(3):137–142.
16. Jeremic B, Shibamoto Y, Acimovic L, et al. Hyperfractionated radiotherapy alone for clinical stage I nonsmall cell lung cancer. *Int J Radiat Oncol Biol Phys.* 1997; 38(3):521.
17. Slotman BJ, Antonisse IE, Njo KH. Limited field irradiation in early stage (T1–2 N0) non–small cell lung cancer. *Radiother Oncol.* 1996;41(1):41–44.
18. Morita K, Fuwa N, Suzuki Y, et al. Radical radiotherapy for medically inoperable non–small cell lung cancer in clinical stage I: a retrospective analysis of 149 patients. *Radiother Oncol.* 1997;42(1):31–36.
19. Krol ADG, Aussems P, Noordijk EM, et al. Local irradiation alone for peripheral stage I lung cancer: could we omit the elective regional nodal irradiation? *Int J Radiat Oncol Biol Phys.* 1996;34(2):297.

20. Kaskowitz L, Graham MV, Emami B, et al. Radiation therapy alone for stage I non–small cell lung cancer. *Int J Radiat Oncol Biol Phys*. 1993;27(3):517–523.
21. Kupelian PA, Komaki R, Allen P. Prognostic factors in the treatment of node-negative nonsmall cell lung carcinoma with radiotherapy alone. *Int J Radiat Oncol Biol Phys*. 1996;36(3):607.
22. Rosenthal SA, Curran WJ Jr, Herbert SH, et al. Clinical stage II non–small cell lung cancer treated with radiation therapy alone. The significance of clinically staged ipsilateral hilar adenopathy (N1 disease). *Cancer*. 1992; 70(10):2410–2417.
23. Rowell NP, Williams CJ. Radical radiotherapy for stage I/II non–small cell lung cancer in patients not sufficiently fit for or declining surgery (medically inoperable): a systematic review. *Thorax*. 2001;56(8): 628–638.
24. Hayman JA, Martel MK, Ten Haken RK, et al. Dose escalation in non-small-cell lung cancer using three-dimensional conformal radiation therapy: update of a phase I trial. *J Clin Oncol*. 2001;19(1):127–136.
25. Rosenzweig KE, Fox JL, Yorke E, et al. Results of a phase I dose-escalation study using three-dimensional conformal radiotherapy in the treatment of inoperable nonsmall cell lung carcinoma. *Cancer*. 2005;103(10):2118–2127.
26. Bradley J, Graham MV, Winter K, et al. Toxicity and outcome results of RTOG 9311: a phase I-II dose-escalation study using three-dimensional conformal radiotherapy in patients with inoperable non-small-cell lung carcinoma. *Int J Radiat Oncol Biol Phys*. 2005;61(2):318–328.
27. Sause WT, Sweeney RA, Plenk HP, et al. Radiotherapy of bronchogenic carcinoma. Analysis of a treatment schedule designed for use with hyperbaric oxygen. *Radiology*. 1981;140(1):209–212.
28. Cheung PCF, Yeung LTF, Basrur V, et al. Accelerated hypofractionation for early-stage non-small-cell lung cancer. *Int J Radiat Oncol Biol Phys*. 2002;54(4):1014.
29. Saunders M, Dische S, Barrett A, et al. Continuous, hyperfractionated, accelerated radiotherapy (CHART) versus conventional radiotherapy in non-small cell lung cancer: mature data from the randomised multicentre trial. CHART Steering Committee. *Radiother Oncol*. 1999;52(2):137–148.
30. Campeau MP, Herschtal A, Wheeler G, et al. Local control and survival following concomitant chemoradiotherapy in inoperable stage I non-small-cell lung cancer. *Int J Radiat Oncol Biol Phys*. 2009;74(5):1371–1375.
31. Uematsu M, Shioda A, Suda A, et al. Computed tomography-guided frameless stereotactic radiotherapy for stage I non–small cell lung cancer: a 5-year experience. *Int J Radiat Oncol Biol Phys*. 2001;51(3):666–670.
32. Onimaru R, Shirato H, Shimizu S, et al. Tolerance of organs at risk in small-volume, hypofractionated, image-guided radiotherapy for primary and metastatic lung cancers. *Int J Radiat Oncol Biol Phys*. 2003;56(1): 126–135.
33. Wulf J, Haedinger U, Oppitz U, et al. Stereotactic radiotherapy for primary lung cancer and pulmonary metastases: a noninvasive treatment approach in medically inoperable patients. *Int J Radiat Oncol Biol Phys*. 2004;60(1):186–196.
34. Xia T, Li H, Sun Q, et al. Promising clinical outcome of stereotactic body radiation therapy for patients with inoperable stage I/II non-small-cell lung cancer. *Int J Radiat Oncol Biol Phys*. 2006;66(1):117–125.
35. Hoyer MRH, Hansen ATOL, Petersen JNH, et al. Prospective study on stereotactic radiotherapy of limited-stage non-small-cell lung cancer. *Int J Radiat Oncol Biol Phys*. 2006;66(4):S128.
36. Nagata Y, Takayama K, Matsuo Y, et al. Clinical outcomes of a phase I/II study of 48 Gy of stereotactic body radiotherapy in 4 fractions for primary lung cancer using a stereotactic body frame. *Int J Radiat Oncol Biol Phys*. 2005;63(5):1427–1431.
37. Timmerman R, McGarry R, Yiannoutsos C, et al. Excessive toxicity when treating central tumors in a phase II study of stereotactic body radiation therapy for medically inoperable early-stage lung cancer. *J Clin Oncol*. 2006;24(30):4833–4839.
38. Onishi H, Shirato H, Nagata Y, et al. Hypofractionated stereotactic radiotherapy (HypoFXSRT) for stage I non-small cell lung cancer: updated results of 257 patients in a Japanese multi-institutional study. *J Thorac Oncol*. 2007;2(7)(suppl 3):S94–S100.
39. Lee SW, Choi EK, Park HJ, et al. Stereotactic body frame based fractionated radiosurgery on consecutive days for primary or metastatic tumors in the lung. *Lung Cancer*. 2003;40(3):309–315.
40. Baumann P, Nyman J, Lax I, et al. Factors important for efficacy of stereotactic body radiotherapy of medically inoperable stage I lung cancer. A retrospective analysis of patients treated in the Nordic countries. *Acta Oncol*. 2006;45(7):787–795.
41. Uematsu M, Fukui T, Tahara K, et al. Long-term results of computed tomography guided hypofractionated stereotactic radiotherapy for stage I non-small cell lung cancers. *Int J Radiat Oncol Biol Phys*. 2008;72(1):S37.
42. McGarry RC, Papiez L, Williams M, et al. Stereotactic body radiation therapy of early-stage non-small-cell lung carcinoma: phase I study. *Int J Radiat Oncol Biol Phys*. 2005;63(4):1010–1015.
43. Le QT, Loo BW, Ho A, et al. Results of a phase I dose-escalation study using single-fraction stereotactic radiotherapy for lung tumors. *J Thorac Oncol*. 2006;1(8): 802–809.
44. Timmerman RD, Park C, Kavanagh BD. The North American experience with stereotactic body radiation therapy in non–small cell lung cancer. *J Thorac Oncol*. 2007;2(7)(suppl 3):S101–S112.
45. Douglas BG, Fowler JF. The effect of multiple small doses of x rays on skin reactions in the mouse and a basic interpretation. *Radiat Res*. 1976;66(2):401–426.
46. Park C, Papiez L, Zhang S, et al. Universal survival curve and single fraction equivalent dose: useful tools in understanding potency of ablative radiotherapy. *Int J Radiat Oncol Biol Phys*. 2008;70(3):847–852.
47. Graham MV, Purdy JA, Emami B, et al. Clinical dose-volume histogram analysis for pneumonitis after 3D

treatment for non–small cell lung cancer (NSCLC). *Int J Radiat Oncol Biol Phys.* 1999;45(2):323–329.
48. Ghafoori P, Marks LB, Vujaskovic Z, et al. Radiation-induced lung injury. Assessment, management, and prevention. *Oncology* (Williston Park). 2008;22(1):37–47.
49. Tsujino K, Hirota S, Endo M, et al. Predictive value of dose-volume histogram parameters for predicting radiation pneumonitis after concurrent chemoradiation for lung cancer. *Int J Radiat Oncol Biol Phys.* 2003;55(1): 110–115.
50. Timmerman R, Papiez L, McGarry R, et al. Extracranial stereotactic radioablation: results of a phase I study in medically inoperable stage I non–small cell lung cancer. *Chest.* 2003;124(5):1946–1955.
51. Timmerman RD, Paulus R, Galvin J, et al. Toxicity analysis of RTOG 0236 using stereotactic body radiation therapy to treat medically inoperable early stage lung cancer patients. *Int J Radiat Oncol Biol Phys.* 2007;69(3)(suppl 1):S86.
52. Whyte RI, Crownover R, Murphy MJ, et al. Stereotactic radiosurgery for lung tumors: preliminary report of a phase I trial. *Ann Thorac Surg.* 2003;75(4):1097–1101.
53. Guckenberger M, Heilman K, Wulf J, et al. Pulmonary injury and tumor response after stereotactic body radiotherapy (SBRT): results of a serial follow-up CT study. *Radiother Oncol.* 2007;85(3):435–442.
54. Borst GR, Ishikawa M, Nijkamp J, et al. Radiation pneumonitis in patients treated for malignant pulmonary lesions with hypofractionated radiation therapy. *Radiother Oncol.* 2009;91(3):307–313.
55. Voroney JPJ, Hope A, Dahele MR, et al. Pain and rib fracture after stereotactic radiotherapy for peripheral non–small cell lung cancer. *Int J Radiat Oncol Biol Phys.* 2008;72(1):S35.
56. Dunlap NE, Biedermann GB, Yang W, et al. Chest wall volume receiving more than 30 Gy predicts risk of severe pain and/or rib fracture following lung SBRT [abstract 77]. *Int J Radiat Oncol Biol Phys.* 2008;72(1):S36.
57. Pettersson N, Nyman J, Johansson K-A. Radiation-induced rib fractures after hypofractionated stereotactic body radiation therapy of non–small cell lung cancer: a dose- and volume-response analysis. *Radiother Oncol.* 2009;91(3):360–368.
58. Forquer JA, Fakiris AJ, Timmerman RD, et al. Brachial plexopathy (BP) from stereotactic body radiotherapy (SBRT) in early-stage NSCLC: dose-limiting toxicity in apical tumor sites [abstract 78]. *Int J Radiat Oncol Biol Phys.* 2008;72(1):S36.
59. Hoppe BS, Laser B, Kowalski AV, et al. Acute skin toxicity following stereotactic body radiation therapy for stage I non-small-cell lung cancer: who's at risk? *Int J Radiat Oncol Biol Phys.* 2008;72(5):1283–1286.
60. Carey Sampson M, Katz A, Constine LS. Stereotactic body radiation therapy for extracranial oligometastases: does the sword have a double edge? *Semin Radiat Oncol.* 2006;16(2):67–76.
61. Wulf J, Hädinger U, Oppitz U, et al. Stereotactic radiotherapy of targets in the lung and liver. *Strahlenther Onkol.* 2001;177(12):645–655.
62. Bradley JD, Wahab S, Lockett MA, et al. Elective nodal failures are uncommon in medically inoperable patients with stage I non-small-cell lung carcinoma treated with limited radiotherapy fields. *Int J Radiat Oncol Biol Phys.* 2003;56(2):342–347.
63. Rosenzweig KE, Sura S, Jackson A, et al. Involved-field radiation therapy for inoperable non-small-cell lung cancer. *J Clin Oncol.* 2007;25(35):5557.
64. Giraud P, Antoine M, Larrouy A, et al. Evaluation of microscopic tumor extension in non-small-cell lung cancer for three-dimensional conformal radiotherapy planning. *Int J Radiat Oncol Biol Phys.* 2000;48(4):1015–1024.
65. Khan FM. *The Physics of Radiation Therapy.* 4th ed. Baltimore, MD: Lippincott Williams & Wilkins; 2009.
66. Kavanagh BD, Timmerman RD. *Stereotactic Body Radiation Therapy.* Philadelphia, PA: Lippincott Williams & Wilkins; 2005.
67. Slotman BJ, Solberg T, Verellen D. *Extracranial Stereotactic Radiotherapy and Radiosurgery.* Boca Raton, FL: Taylor & Francis; 2006.
68. Nagata Y, Matsuo Y, Takayama K, et al. Current status of stereotactic body radiotherapy for lung cancer. *Int J Clin Oncol.* 2007;12(1):3–7.
69. Macdonald O, Garces YI, Miller J, et al. Dose characteristics of proton beam radiotherapy and stereotactic body radiotherapy in primary non–small cell lung carcinoma (NSCLC): a comparative analysis. *Int J Radiat Oncol Biol Phys.* 2008;72(1)(suppl 1):S618.
70. Bradley JD, El Naqa I, Trovo M, et al. SBRT for early-stage NSCLC: the predominant failure pattern is distant. *Int J Radiat Oncol Biol Phys.* 2008;72(1)(suppl 1):S37–S38.
71. Kato H, Ichinose Y, Ohta M, et al. A randomized trial of adjuvant chemotherapy with uracil-tegafur for adenocarcinoma of the lung. *N Engl J Med.* 2004;350(17):1713–1721.
72. Strauss GM, Herndon JE II, Maddaus MA, et al. Adjuvant paclitaxel plus carboplatin compared with observation in stage IB non-small-cell lung cancer: CALGB 9633 with the Cancer and Leukemia Group B, Radiation Therapy Oncology Group, and North Central Cancer Treatment Group Study Groups. *J Clin Oncol.* 2008;26(31):5043–5051.
73. Arriagada R, Bergman B, Dunant A, et al. Cisplatin-based adjuvant chemotherapy in patients with completely resected non-small-cell lung cancer. *N Engl J Med.* 2004;350(4):351–360.
74. Winton T, Livingston R, Johnson D, et al. Vinorelbine plus cisplatin vs. observation in resected non-small-cell lung cancer. *N Engl J Med.* 2005;352(25):2589–2597.
75. Douillard JY, Rosell R, De Lena M, et al. Adjuvant vinorelbine plus cisplatin versus observation in patients with completely resected stage IB-IIIA non-small-cell lung cancer (Adjuvant Navelbine International Trialist Association [ANITA]): a randomised controlled trial. *Lancet Oncol.* 2006;7(9):719–727.
76. Pignon J-P, Tribodet H, Scagliotti GV, et al. Lung adjuvant cisplatin evaluation: a pooled analysis by the LACE collaborative group. *J Clin Oncol.* 2008;26(21):3552.

demos MEDICAL

RADIATION MEDICINE ROUNDS

Radiotherapy for the Locally Advanced Non–Small Cell Lung Cancer

Kenneth R. Olivier* and Yolanda I. Garces
Mayo Clinic, Rochester, MN

ABSTRACT

Pathology and Natural History: Non–small cell lung cancer (NSCLC) is an important topic for radiation oncologists. Patients with advanced NSCLC have node positive lung cancer and no evidence of metastatic spread of their disease. The majority of NSCLC is caused by tobacco smoking, a preventable habit, and secondarily by Radon gas, a preventable environmental exposure.

Evaluation and Staging: Symptoms present at diagnosis suggest the extent of the disease and can be prognostic for survival. Imaging studies to evaluate the extent of disease include computed tomography (CT) and positron emission tomography (PET). The sensitivity and specificity of these tests are important to remember when considering the method of biopsy and when making treatment recommendations. No imaging study is replacement for tissue biopsies, and there are several reasonable approaches to obtaining biopsy. These should be tailored to the location of the primary and to the additional information they might reveal.

Therapy: Therapy for advanced NSCLC has had a variety of iterations over the past 50 years. Radiotherapy (RT) was proven to be beneficial when compared with observation, even when using the earliest technology of RT. Chemotherapy adds to the benefit of RT: the benefit is evident when given sequentially (chemotherapy first), but the benefit is even greater when given concurrently. RT given concurrently with chemotherapy is the standard of care. The patterns of failure don't give clear evidence as to the nature of the benefit, and work is ongoing in this respect. RT dose-response data suggests that higher doses may favorably influence patient survival. The Radiation Therapy Oncology Group (RTOG) is leading a multicooperative group phase III trial which will hopefully clarify whether higher RT dose improves patient survival.

Algorithm: RT planning of advanced NSCLC has unique challenges. Motion of targets creates the need for unique volumes and methods of motion assessment. Newer technology such as intensity modulated RT (IMRT), image guided RT, and proton therapy may improve patient care. Ultimately, the therapeutic index is improved when the greatest RT dose is administered in the least amount of time while sparing the adjacent normal tissue.

INTRODUCTION

Non–small cell lung cancer (NSCLC) remains an important topic for radiation oncologists around the world. For the purposes of this chapter, the definition of advanced NSCLC is patients presenting with stage IIA to IIIB disease using the International Association for the Study of Lung Cancer (IASLC) (see Table 1) (1), and are not considered surgically resectable. Using this definition, advanced NSCLC is the most common presentation of patients (1). Despite many of the advances made over the past several decades,

*Corresponding author, Department of Radiation Oncology, Mayo Clinic, 200 1st St. SW, Rochester, MN 55905
E-mail address: olivier.kenneth@mayo.edu

Radiation Medicine Rounds 1 (2010) 21–38.

DOI: 10.5003/2151–4208.1.1.21

TABLE 1A TNM staging for lung cancer

Descriptors	Definitions	Subgroups*
T	**Primary tumor**	
T0	No primary tumor	
T1	Tumor ≤ 3 cm,† surrounded by lung or visceral pleura, not more proximal than the lobar bronchus	
T1a	Tumor ≤ 2 cm†	T1a
T1b	Tumor > 2 but ≤3 cm †	T1b
T2	Tumor > 3 but ≤ 7 cm† or tumor with any of the following‡: Invades visceral pleura, involves main bronchus ≥ 2 cm distal to the carina, atelectasis/obstructive pneumonia extending to hilum but not involving the entire lung	
T2a	Tumor > 3 but ≤ 5 cm†	T2a
T2b	Tumor > 5 but ≤ 7 cm†	T2b
T3	Tumor > 7 cm;	$T3_{>7}$
	or directly invading chest wall, diaphragm, phrenic nerve, mediastinal pleura, or parietal pericardium;	$T3_{Inv}$
	or tumor in the main bronchus < 2 cm distal to the carina§:	$T3_{Centr}$
	or atelectasis/obstructive pneumonitis of entire lung;	$T3_{Centr}$
	or separate tumor nodules in the same lobe	$T3_{Satell}$
T4	Tumor of any size with invasion of heart, great vessels, trachea, recurrent laryngeal nerve, esophagus, vertebral body, or carina;	$T4_{Inv}$
	or separate tumor nodules in a different ipsilateral lobe	$T4_{Ipsi\ Nod}$
N	**Regional lymph nodes**	
N0	No regional node metastasis	
N1	Metastasis in ipsilateral peribronchial and/or perihilar lymph nodes and intrapulmonary nodes, including involvement by direct extension	
N2	Metastasis in ipsilateral mediastinal and/or subcarinal lymph nodes	
N3	Metastasis in contralateral mediastinal, contralateral hilar, ipsilateral or contralateral scalene, or supraclavicular lymph nodes	
M	**Distant metastasis**	
M0	No distant metastasis	
M1a	Separate tumor nodules in a contralateral lobe; or tumor with pleural nodules or malignant pleural dissemination ‖	$M1^{a}_{Contr\ Nod}$ $M1^{a}_{pi\ Dissem}$
M1b	Distant metastasis	M1b
Special situations		
TX, NX, MX	T, N, or M status not able to be assessed	
T1s	Focus of *in situ* cancer	T1s
T1§	Superficial spreading tumor of any size but confined to the wall of the trachea or mainstem bronchus	$T1_{ss}$

*These subgroup labels are not defined in the IASLC publications2–5 but are added here to facilitate a clear discussion.
†In the greatest dimension.
‡T2 tumors with these features are classified as T2a if ≤ 5 cm.
§The uncommon superficial spreading tumor in central airways is classified as T1.
‖Pleural effusions are excluded that are cytologically negative, nonbloody, transudative, and clinically judged not to be due to cancer.

TABLE 1B Incidence of TNM at presentation

	Descriptors, % of all			
Stage Groups	**T**	**N**	**M**	**Patients, %***
Ia	T1a,b	N0	M0	15
Ib	T2a	N0	M0	13
IIa	T1a,b	N1	M0	2
	T2a	N1	M0	4
	T2b	N0	M0	4
IIb	T2b	N1	M0	2
	T3	N0	M0	14
IIIa	T1–3	N2	M0	20
	T3	N1	M0	6
	T4	N0,1	M0	2
IIIb	T4	N2	M0	1
	T1–4	N3	M0	3
IV	T_{Any}	N_{Any}	M1a,b	14

*Percentage of patients in IASLC database according to best stage (rounded to nearest integer).

Source: From Ref. 5.

the overall prognosis for patients with advanced NSCLC remains poor. This is a source of both concern and motivation for the oncologic community, as advances in this disease would greatly affect a large number of patients.

Etiology

In 2009, the American Cancer society predicts 219,000 people will be diagnosed and 160,000 people die in the United States of lung cancer (2). While the incidence for both men and women is less than prostate and breast cancers respectively, lung cancer has the dubious distinction of having the highest cancer-related mortality. The yearly mortality of lung cancer in the United States is greater than breast and prostate cancer combined (see Figure 1). More impressive is the fact that the majority of these diagnoses and deaths are avoidable. The primary risk factor for the development of lung cancer is smoking tobacco, accounting for greater than 80% of cases. The World Health Organization (WHO) estimates that 50% of regular smokers will die of smoking-related illness (3). While this highly addictive recreational drug is linked to other cancers, its contribution to lung cancer is the most impressive (see Figure 1). As you can see from the figure, the mortality rate has been dropping since 1990, and much of this reduction has been attributed to successful campaigns for reducing tobacco use in the United States. Although it is encouraging to see that the incidence and mortality of lung cancer in the United States is dropping, the incidence of tobacco use is increasing in many developing countries, such as China and India, which already account for 40% of all tobacco consumption worldwide (3). As such, NSCLC, together with the other health problems caused by tobacco, will remain an important global issue for the foreseeable future. The second most common cause of NSCLC is exposure to radon. This odorless radioactive gas is a byproduct of decay of radium and is linked to 15% to 20% of the lung cancers presenting in the United States. Jonathan Samet has written an excellent summary on the topic, if the reader wishes a more thorough discussion of radon and NSCLC (4). Despite the obvious importance of tobacco and radon, inheritance and genetic susceptibility do play a role in the development of lung cancer. This appears to be especially true in patients developing cancer before the age of 60 years, patients with adenocarcinomas, and patients with more than two first-degree relatives with lung cancer. The reported relative risk of having two first-degree relatives is 2.2). The genes responsible for this genetic susceptibility appear to be on chromosome 6q23–25. Subramanian and Govindian (6) have published an excellent review of the literature on lung cancer in never smokers that nicely details the topic. It would serve as an excellent starting point for readers interested in more information.

Presentation

The presenting complaints of patients with NSCLC can vary broadly. In a series of 678 lung cancer patients (7), 32% present with symptoms consistent with metastatic disease, 27% presented with nonspecific symptoms such as weight loss and fatigue, 27% presented with symptoms attributable to the primary thoracic tumor (cough, hemoptysis), and only 6% were asymptomatic at the time of diagnosis. The symptoms attributable to the primary cancer are frequently cough and dyspnea. Other presenting complaints may be more associated with specific presentations such as arm pain, with weakness in patients with an NCLC in the superior sulcus.

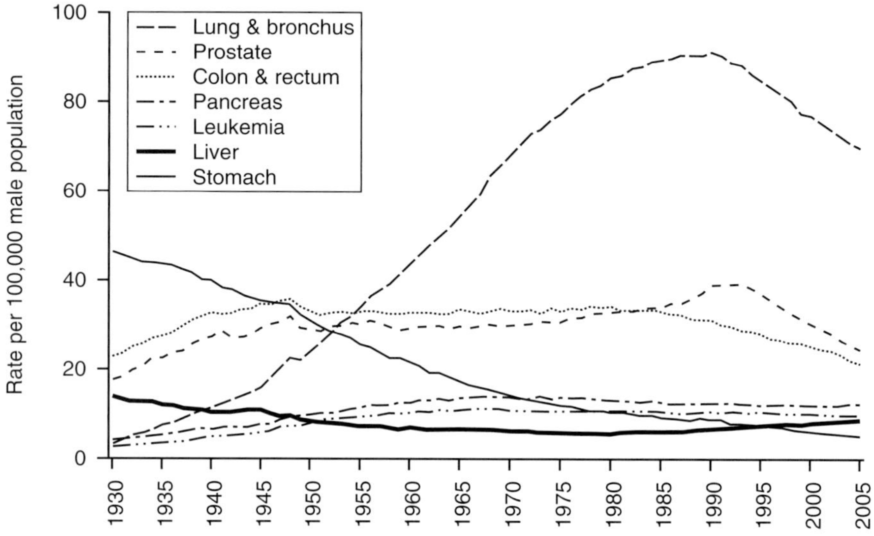

*Per 100,000, age adjusted to the 2000 US standard population

FIGURE 1A Age-adjusted death rates. *Males by site, United States, 1930–2005.

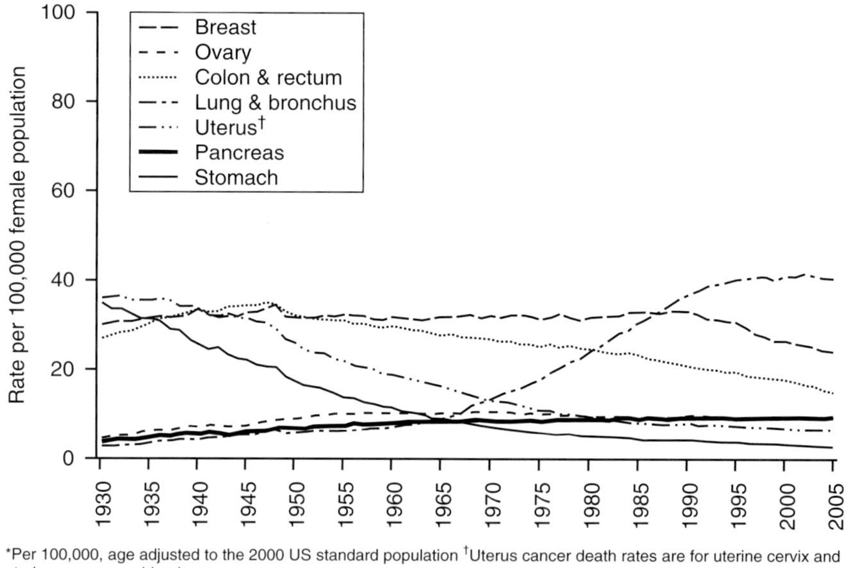

*Per 100,000, age adjusted to the 2000 US standard population †Uterus cancer death rates are for uterine cervix and uterine corpus combined

FIGURE 1B Age-adjusted cancer death rates. *Females by site, United States, 1930–2005.

All of these symptoms are relatively nonspecific, however, and may be indicative of such common illnesses as bronchitis or pneumonia. The Veterans Administration (VA) compared presenting complaints and disease characteristics in 5,000 patients treated on early VA lung trials (8). The most important prognostic factors were performance status, extent of disease, and weight loss. This cemented the importance

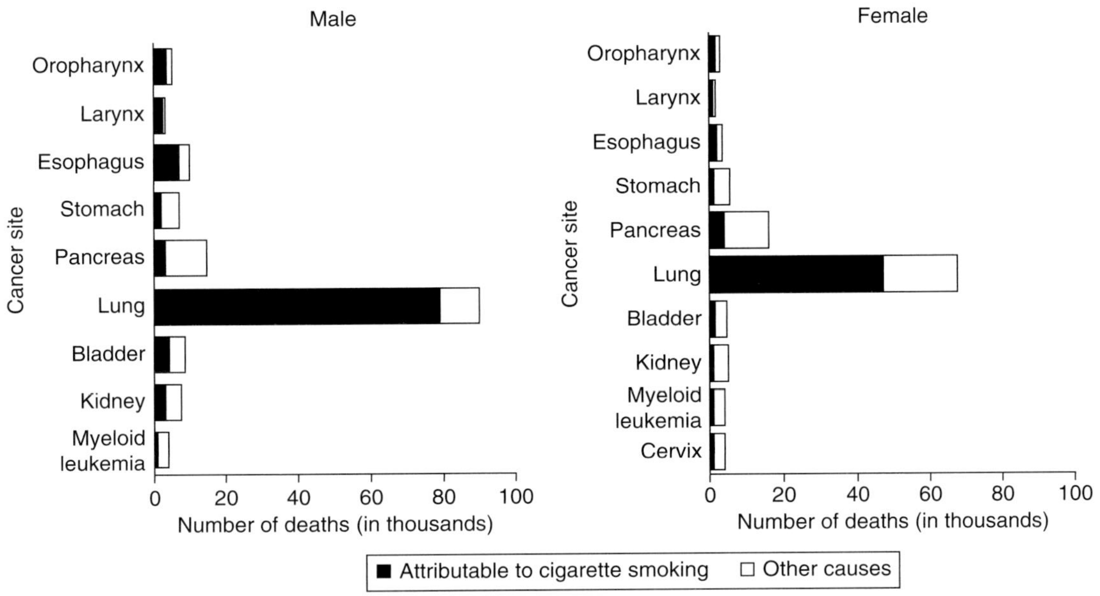

FIGURE 1C Annual number of cancer deaths attributable to smoking by sex and site, United States, 2000–2004. From Ref. 2.

of performance status and weight loss in the initial assessment of patients with advanced NSCLC.

Workup

The workup of patients typically begins with a chest x-ray done by the primary doctor while evaluating the patient for the above complaints. Typically, this will reveal the presence of a mass and possibly of widened mediastinum suggestive of mediastinal adenopathy. The sensitivity of CXR is approximately 54% with a specificity of 99% in patients deemed "suspicious" based on CXR (9). Comparison with prior chest x-rays is important, when possible, to assess for interval changes.

The chest x-ray should be followed with a computed tomography (CT) of the chest. These are typically done with contrast, extend through the liver, and are evaluated on both lung windows and mediastinal windows. Several characteristics suggest lung cancer on CT. The primary mass typically has a spiculated rim (alternatively called corona radiata), size >2 cm, absence of calcifications, and increase in size over multiple imaging studies (10). Lymph nodes are commonly deemed "positive" on CT if they are >1.0 cm in size. The ability for CT to accurately stage the mediastinum is mediocre, however. The pooled sensitivity and specificity of CT for lymph node assessment is 51% and 85%, respectively (11). This is particularly salient as radiation oncologists rely on CT definitions for our target volumes.

When the CT is suggestive of a primary lung cancer, the next appropriate imaging study is a positron emission tomography (PET) scan. The PET scan doesn't replace the necessity of biopsies, but can be informative as to the true stage of the patient. A seminal study by Pieterman et al. (12) compared the performance of PET to that of CT for the staging of lung cancer. In comparing the two diagnostic modalities in 106 patients, Pieterman et al. found PET superior to CT in every parameter. The sensitivity and specificity of PET for mediastinal adenopathy was 91% and 86%, respectively, compared with 75% and 66% for CT scans. The positive predictive value was 74% and the negative predictive value was 95%. PET scanning identified previously unsuspected metastases in 10% of the studied patients. Most often today, the PET and CT are performed together with both providing complementary information.

The American College of Surgeons Oncology Group (ACOSOG) (13) conducted a prospective trial to assess the utility of PET in patients diagnosed with stage I–III NSCLC (ACOSOG Z0050). Patients who had enrolled received a CT scan of the chest, and bone scan routinely. Any abnormality seen on those two radiographic exams was followed up with MRI or biopsy for confirmation. If patients were deemed resectable based on that workup, they were enrolled and they received a PET scan. PET was significantly better at detecting N1, N2/N3 disease (48% and 52%) in the study population as compared with CT (13% and 32%, respectively, $P = .0041$). Despite the rigorous workup, 6% of patients were upstaged by the PET scan (confirmed by biopsy), but 6% of patients diagnosed with metastases by PET were subsequently found to be benign histology, underscoring the need to follow-up on positive PET findings.

An MRI of the brain is of questionable value in patients with NSCLC and with no evidence of cranial metastases on the basis history and physical examination. Only 10% of patients with no CNS symptoms will have brain metastases at diagnosis (11), but an early diagnosis of this pattern of spread again spares the patient unneeded therapy and can direct an early intervention to the developing brain metastases and is a commonly required examination for clinical trial entrance. Some authors have recommended routine MRI only for adenocarcinoma and large cell carcinoma where the incidence of asymptomatic brain metastases may approach 20% (14). Most trials do include either CT or MRI of the brain during staging.

Laboratory examinations are helpful in determining a patient's fitness for CT. Typically, a complete blood count (CBC) assessment of renal function with BUN and creatinine, and liver function tests provide the required picture. Hematologic toxicity is common during combined modality therapy and, therefore, weekly CBCs are imperative to ensure the patient's safety and toxicity of the treatment.

■ DIAGNOSIS

Sputum

Sputum testing, historically, was often a first step in attempting to establish a diagnosis. Although not as commonly used today, it is noninvasive and requires no separate procedure. Sputum testing typically requires three separate specimens, and the yield is improved in patients with central tumors and/or hemoptysis. Overall, the sensitivity of detecting cancer with sputum is 66% on average with 99% specificity. As stated above, it is more useful in patients with central tumors as compared with peripheral tumors (sensitivity 74% vs. 49%) (15).

Bronchoscopy

In current medical practice, bronchoscopy is often the first step in obtaining a diagnosis of NSCLC. It is useful for both sampling the primary cancer as well as assessing the nodal involvement. Typically, bronchoscopy has three components when assessing the primary cancer: washings, brushings, and biopsy. The sensitivity of these components are 48%, 59%, and 74%, respectively (16). Endobronchial biopsy sensitivity is influenced by location of the primary cancer. Central lesions are more reliably biopsied successfully than are peripheral lesions. In the case of larger (>2cm) peripheral lesions, the sensitivity is 66%, and for smaller peripheral lesions, the sensitivity is 33% (16).

The assessment of mediastinal lymph nodes with bronchoscopy is commonly performed. This is done via a Wang needle biopsy and is most useful for subcarinal lymph nodes (station 7), and hilar lymph nodes (station 9), but can assess paratracheal lymph nodes in skilled hands.

Transthoracic Needle Biopsy (TTNA)

TTNA can be performed via either fluoroscopy or CT guidance. Both are associated with high sensitivity, with CT having a lightly higher sensitivity and is more frequently practiced (92% for CT, 88% for fluoroscopy) (15). The sensitivity suffers from lesion size, as smaller lesions are less reliably biopsied as compared with larger lesions. This difference may be as large as 94% for lesions >1.5 cm and 78% for lesions ≤1.5 cm (17). The false positive rate of TTNA ranges from 10% to 20%. This is more salient for unresectable patients with T1 cancers, where other methods of diagnosis may not be feasible.

Pathology

Non–small cell is somewhat of a garbage bin of histologies. In essence, it contains all the histologies of primary parenchymal lung cancers that aren't small cell lung cancer (SCLC). While this does highlight the unique pathology, natural history, and treatment regimens of SCLC, it does little to help distinguish the different natural histories of NSCLC. Using WHO's 2004 definitions (18), NSCLC histologies include the following:

- Squamous Cell Carcinoma
  - Variants: papillary, clear cell, small cell and basaloid
- Adenocarcinoma
  - Variants: mixed, acinar, papillary, bronchio-alveolar, solid with mucin
- Large Cell
  - Variants: large cell neuroendocrine, mixed cell neuroendocrine, basaloid, lymphoepithelioma-like, clear cell, large cell with rhabdoid features.
- Adenosquamous carcinoma
- Sarcomatoid carcinoma
  - Variants: pleomorphic, spindle cell, giant cell, carcinosarcoma, and pulmonary blastoma.

Adenocarcinomas are currently the most common type of NSCLC, followed by squamous cell carcinomas (SCC). This reverses the previous predominance of SCC (18). An additional consideration when discussing the pathology of NSCLC is how to determine the tissue of origin when there is a history of other malignancies. Determining whether the new mass is a recurrence or a new primary greatly impacts the direction of care for the patient. Immunohistochemistry can be helpful in this regard (19). Approximately 85% of adenocarcinomas of the lung stain with Thyroglobulin Transcription Factor 1 (TTF-1). Cytokeratin 7 and 20 (CK-7, CK-20) are also used to help in the diagnosis, as most adenocarcinomas of the lung are CK-7 positive and CK-20 negative. An excellent review written by Beasley on this topic is recommended for further reading (19).

THERAPY

Radiotherapy Versus Observation

Radiotherapy (RT) for lung cancer has evolved over the preceding decades, both in terms of dose and volume. For patients with advanced NCLC, the changes in therapy have been dramatic, but without the same transformative effect on survival. With poor survival in all patients with advanced NSCLC, a reasonable question to ask is whether any therapy is useful. The question of RT alone versus observation has been addressed in a couple of phase 3 randomized trials and provides not only useful information about the utility of RT, but also answers the common patient question of "how long will I live if I don't do anything." The original study was conducted by the VA and enrolled 554 patients with locally advanced, but nonmetastatic lung CA (20). The investigators compared 40 to 50 Gy of RT to observation and noted a benefit in survival at 1 year for RT patients (18%) versus untreated patients (14%). The median survival was 20 weeks for RT versus 14 weeks for observation (P = .05). The surprisingly short survival for patients treated with RT can primarily be attributed to the age of the trial. The vast majority of patients were treated with orthovoltage RT (90%), making it not surprising that survival advantage seen is very modest.

A more modern version of the trial was recently conducted in France (21). Between the years 1992 and 1996, this trial enrolled 240 patients with unresectable stage III NSCLC and randomized them to three arms: 50 Gy delivered in 2 Gy per fractions (79 patients), 40 Gy split course (20 Gy in 4 Gy per fractions followed by a 4-week break then another 20 Gy in 4 Gy per fractions, 81 patients), and observation (80 patients). Patients assigned to observation were given RT for palliation (20 Gy in 5 Gy fractions), if symptoms developed later. The median survival for this trial by arm was 12 months versus 9 months versus 6 months, respectively (50 Gy vs. 40 Gy split course vs. observation). There was a statistically significant difference in survival for all the groups. RT provided a doubling of the median survival in patients treated with conventional doses, and untreated advanced NCLC patients typically survived for 6 months after diagnosis, if not initially treated.

RT Versus Sequential Chemotherapy and RT

Although RT prolonged survival when compared with observation, the prognosis remained so dismal that adding additional therapies was a logical next step. Chemotherapy delivered prior to the RT has been evaluated in several trials. The first of these was the Cancer and Leukemia Group B (CALGB) 8433 trial published by Dillman et al. (22,23) comparing induction chemotherapy with cisplatin (100 mg/m^2

given on days 1 and 29) and vinblastine (5 mg/m^2 given on days 1, 8, 15, 22, 29) followed by RT (day 50) to RT alone (day 1). The dose of RT was 60 Gy in 2 Gy per fractions (40 Gy to pre-chemotherapy volumes, with 20 Gy boost to residual mass after induction chemotherapy). The rate of response between the two regimens was statistically identical (56% for CMT, 43% for RT alone), but the median survival was improved with induction chemotherapy at 13.7 months versus 9.6 months for RT alone. Toxicity was mild in both treatment groups. The rate of serious infections was higher in patients receiving chemotherapy (7% vs. 3%), as was the rate of nausea and vomiting (5% vs. 0%). The rate of severe esophagitis or pneumonitis was 1% in both arms. Induction chemotherapy did not interfere with the delivery of the RT, as 88% of patients completed the RT with induction chemotherapy and 87% completed the regimen with RT alone. The rate of major deviation with the RT delivery was high in both arms (21% in the chemo group, 23% in the RT group). Of the patients with major deviations, six survived to 2 years, with all but one having been on the induction chemotherapy arm. Limited data was collected on patterns of failure for this study, but suggested no significant difference between the two treatment arms.

An intergroup trial was designed to confirm the results of the CALGB study and to test the utility of hyperfractionated RT (24). This trial had three randomized arms: induction chemotherapy followed by 60 Gy of RT, RT of 60 Gy without chemotherapy, and 69.6 Gy of RT given at 1.2 Gy twice daily. The chemotherapy consisted of cisplatin and vineblastine at the same dose delivered in CALBG trial. The toxicity of the therapies was deemed acceptable. There were six patients with grade 4 radiation toxicities, of which four were esophagitis in patients treated up to 69.6 Gy. Overall survival was improved in the patients receiving induction chemotherapy ($P = .04$). Median survival on the three arms was 13.2 months (induction chemotherapy), 12 months (69.6 Gy HFX), and 11.4 months (60 Gy alone). A notable footnote to this trial was the effect of therapy for the subset of patients with SCC. In those patients the 5-year survival was 9% with HFX RT alone, compared with 2% on the other two arms.

Le Chevalier et al. (25) also examined the role of induction chemotherapy prior to radiation. In a randomized phase 3 trial, patients received either radiation alone or chemotherapy followed by radiation and additional three cycles. The radiation was 65 Gy in 26 fractions of 2.5 Gy. RT volumes included a comprehensive field of the tumor, bilateral hila, mediastinum, and bilateral supraclavicular fossae to 40 Gy. A boost of 15 Gy was then given to the tumor, mediastinum, and bilateral hilla. A second boost of 10 Gy was given to the tumor, mediastinum, and ipsilateral hilum. Induction chemotherapy was vindesine (1.5 mg/m^2 on days 1, 2), lomustine (50 mg/m^2 on day 2, and 25 mg/m^2 on day 3), cisplatin (100 mg/m^2 on day 2), and cyclophosphamide (200 mg/m^2 on days 2–4) for three cycles prior to RT. This same regimen was given following the radiation. The toxicity of the treatment was primarily hematologic for the patients receiving chemotherapy. The differences in toxicity from the RT were essentially the same in the two arms, with the predominant toxicity being esophagitis. The first report of this trial showed no significant difference in survival between the arms despite a strong trend for improved survival with the chemotherapy (median survival 12 months for CMT, 10 months for RT alone). A second analysis at 5 years from enrollment revealed the survival difference had attained statistical significance at $P < .02$ (26). This was attributed to a strongly significant difference in the rate of distant metastases between the two arms favoring the chemotherapy containing arm ($P < .001$).

RT Combined With Chemotherapy

The current standard of care for patients with advanced NSCLC is RT administered concurrent with chemotherapy. The primary trial informing this regimen is the results of Radiation Therapy Oncology Group (RTOG) 94-10 (27,28). An important caveat of this trial is that it remains unpublished and therefore the final results, and many important issues of the trial, are unknown. What is known is that this trial was a phase 3 randomized trial with three separate arms: The concurrent arm (CON-QD): 60 Gy in 2 Gy per fractions given concurrently with cisplatin (100 mg/m^2 given on days 1 and 29, same as the CALGB 8433 and intergroup study listed above) and vinblastine (5 mg/m^2 given weekly for 5 weeks). The sequential arm (SEQ) was the same chemotherapy regimen as CON given for two cycles with RT starting on day 50. The third arm consisted of hyperfractionated RT 69.6 Gy in 1.2 Gy per fractions given twice daily (similar to the intergroup trial) concurrent with cisplatin (50 mg/m2 given on days 1, 8, 29, and 36) with etoposide (50 mg BID for 10 weeks) (CON-BID). There is some limited data on toxicity available through presented abstracts. The rate of grade 3 or higher nonhematologic toxicity was 63% for CON-BID, 50% for CON-QD, and 31% in SEQ. There was no reported difference in late toxicity between the arms. The survival results favor CON-QD versus CON-BID or SEQ, with median survival of 17 months, 15.2 months, and 14.6 months, respectively. The patterns of failure data suggest an improvement in local control for CON-BID (29). This was true only for patients with SCCs. Nonsquamous histologies had a similar pattern of failure across the three arms.

The other phase 3 randomized trial looking at sequential therapy versus concurrent was conducted in Japan. Furuse et al. (30) used vindesine (3 mg/m^2 on days 1 and 8), cisplatin (80 mg/m^2 on day 1), and mitomycin C (8 mg/m^2 on day 1). This was given concurrently with 56 Gy in 2 Gy per fractions, or sequentially after two cycles of chemotherapy. The concurrent RT was done with a planned 10-day break after 14 treatments (commonly called "split course"). The sequentially treated patients had no planned breaks. The trial enrolled 315 eligible patients. Myleosupression was the only toxicity that was significantly higher on the CON arm compared to the SEQ arm (P = .001). Interestingly, the rate of esophagitis was the same between the two arms, and this is likely attributable to the use of split course RT in the CON arm. Survival favored the CON, with a median survival of 16.5 months versus 13.3 months with SEQ therapy (P = .04). The patterns of failure for the trial show equivalent local control between the two arms. The rate of distant metastatic disease was the same between the two arms, with a higher rate of brain metastases in the CON arm relative to the SEQ arm (19% vs. 9%, P = .018).

Both randomized trials found survival benefits when chemotherapy is used concurrently with the RT. An important question is what is the origin of the benefit? Most thoracic radiation oncologists believe that the benefit from concurrent chemotherapy is the sensitization of the tumor to the radiation rather than an effect on distant disease. This is clearly true in head and neck cancers (31,32); however, the data to support this in lung cancer is less convincing. Patterns of failure are more ambiguous in lung cancer than for head and neck cancers. The investigators at the RTOG have published two articles comparing toxicities and patterns of first failure for several conducted trials. The first compared standard RT, hyperfractionated RT (HFX), and sequential chemotherapy followed by RT (SEQ) (33). Patients treated with SEQ had significantly less distant metastases (excluding brain metastases) as compared with RT or HFX (P = .045). There was no difference in local failures between the groups, and the toxicity was comparable. The second study examined RTOG studies looking at SEQ versus CON and divided the patients into SEQ, induction chemotherapy followed by concurrent chemotherapy with RT (IND-CON), and chemotherapy concurrent with hyperfractionated RT (CON-BID) (34). In this analysis of five different trials there was no difference in patterns of failure among the groups. Nonhematologic toxicity was significantly higher in both the concurrent arms as compared with the sequential arm (P < .0001 and P = .0005, respectively). So where does that leave us? We have two phase 3 trials showing a significant survival advantage to CON over SEQ, but the patterns of failure are ambiguous as to why the benefit is present. Meanwhile, the benefit we see is not as dramatic as we might hope. Table 2 compares the above listed trials. The consistency of

TABLE 2 Comparison of median survival on selected clinical trials

Treatment	Median Surivial
Observation:	
Roswit et al. (1968) [20]	3.5 mon
Reinfus et al. (1999) [21]	6 mon
RT alone:	
Roswit et al. (1968) [20]	5 mon
Reinfus et al. (1999) [21]	12 mon
Dillman et al. (1990) [22]	9.6 mon
Sause et al. (1995) [24]	11.4 mon
Le Chevalier et al. (1991) [25]	10 mon
Induction chemotherapy followed by RT:	
Dillman et al. (1990) [22]	13.7 mon
Sause et al. (1995) [24]	13.2 mon
Le Chevalier et al. (1991) [25]	12 mon
RTOG 94-10 (2000) [27]	14.6 mon
Furuse et al. (1999) [30]	13.3 mon
Concurrent chemotherapy with RT:	
RTOG 94-10 (2000) [27]	17 mon
Furuse et al. (1999) [30]	16.5 mon

the data is impressive, especially when you consider the data covers 40 years of therapy for lung cancer. If the benefit of concurrent chemotherapy is solely a result of local control then the need for it may change as technology changes and we become better able to deliver tumor ablative doses (see the Stereotactic Body Radiotherapy [SBRT] section in Chapter 1). If that was true chemotherapy could be moved to sequential once again, where it has a proven benefit for lung cancer patients who have had surgery (35,36). Maybe as local control improves to levels seen in surgery, as it has with SBRT in early stage disease, the way we integrate chemotherapy may change.

Dose

Having established the utility of RT for NCLC, the necessity of chemotherapy, and having introduced the ambiguity of why and how it all works together, a reasonable question is what dose is the correct dose when treating definitively. Much of our current understanding of dose comes from the RTOG study 73-01 (37,38). Patients with stage III and medically inoperable stages I and II NSCLC were randomly assigned to receive either 40 Gy split course (20 Gy in 5 Gy fractions followed by 2 week break, then 20 Gy in 5 Gy fractions), or 40 Gy, 50 Gy, or 60 Gy given daily in 2 Gy per fractions. The trial enrolled 383 patients from 1973 to 1978. The design diagrams for the fields are shown in Figure 2 and are instructive as to the changes RT has undergone since the time of this trial. There was an improvement in local control with 60 Gy as compared with the other regimens (35% local failure vs. 49%, 53%, and 58% for 50 Gy, 40 Gy, and 40 Gy split course, respectively). The initial report showed a survival advantage at 3 years for the 60 Gy regimen, but that improvement was lost with additional follow-up. The overall survival for all the regimens was 6% at 5 years. The dose of 60 Gy given in 2 Gy per fractions was deemed to be the superior regimen and that dose continues to be the most commonly used in the United States. While this tells us which of the four dose tested was superior in terms of local control, it doesn't tell us which is the best dose to optimize survival. Given the poor local control using a local modality (RT), it is a reasonable conclusion that increasing the RT dose may improve local control, and such an improvement may lead to longer survival.

The RTOG conducted a dose escalation trial for 3D conformal RT (3D CRT) using RT alone (39). Chemotherapy prior to the radiation was allowed, but no chemotherapy was given concurrent with the RT. This well-designed trial escalated dose base on amount of lung receiving 20 Gy (V20). For the patients with V20 <25%, the maximum tolerated dose (MTD) was 88.2 Gy, for patients with V20 of 25% to 36%, the MTD was 77.4 Gy. Local failure (cancer progressed in treated field) was still present in 38% of patients.

With the advent of concurrent chemotherapy and RT the question of dose is again salient. There are two well-done phase 2 dose escalation trials available for guidance. The North Central Cancer Treatment Group (NCCTG) conducted a dose escalation trial using concurrent carboplatin (AUC=2) and paclitaxel (50 mg/m^2) given weekly with escalating doses of RT given in 2 Gy per fractions. This trial treated involved sites only (no ENI) and began at 70 Gy. The maximum tolerated dose was found to be 74 Gy (40) with the dose limiting toxicity (DLT) being grade 3 pneumonitis (1/6 patients treated to 74 Gy). Limited patterns of failure were presented (median followup was 28 mon), but local failure was seen in only 15% of patients.

Investigators at the RTOG conducted a similar phase 1 dose escalation trial for patients with advanced NSCLC (41). The chemotherapy regimen used was identical to the NCCTG study. The RTOG reported that the MTD was 74 Gy at 2 Gy fraction, identical to the NCCTG results. The data on patterns of failure and survival are not available from this trial. It is reassuring that the results of these two trials concluded on an identical MTD. In addition, Stinchcombe et al. (42) reported a phase 1/2 trial which included 62 patients with stage III disease. All patients receive induction and concurrent carboplatin and paclitaxel, and the majority of these patients received 74 Gy/37 daily fractions. The median survival time was quite favorable at 25 months. The results of these trials made up portions of the rationale behind a phase 3 clinical trial (RTOG 0617/NCCTG N0628/CALGB 30609/ECOG R0617), which is comparing 60 Gy to 74 Gy when combined with chemotherapy.

Prophylactic Cranial Irradiation (PCI)

Patients with lung cancer commonly develop brain metastases. After curative lung cancer treatment, up to 30% of patients can develop brain metastases, often

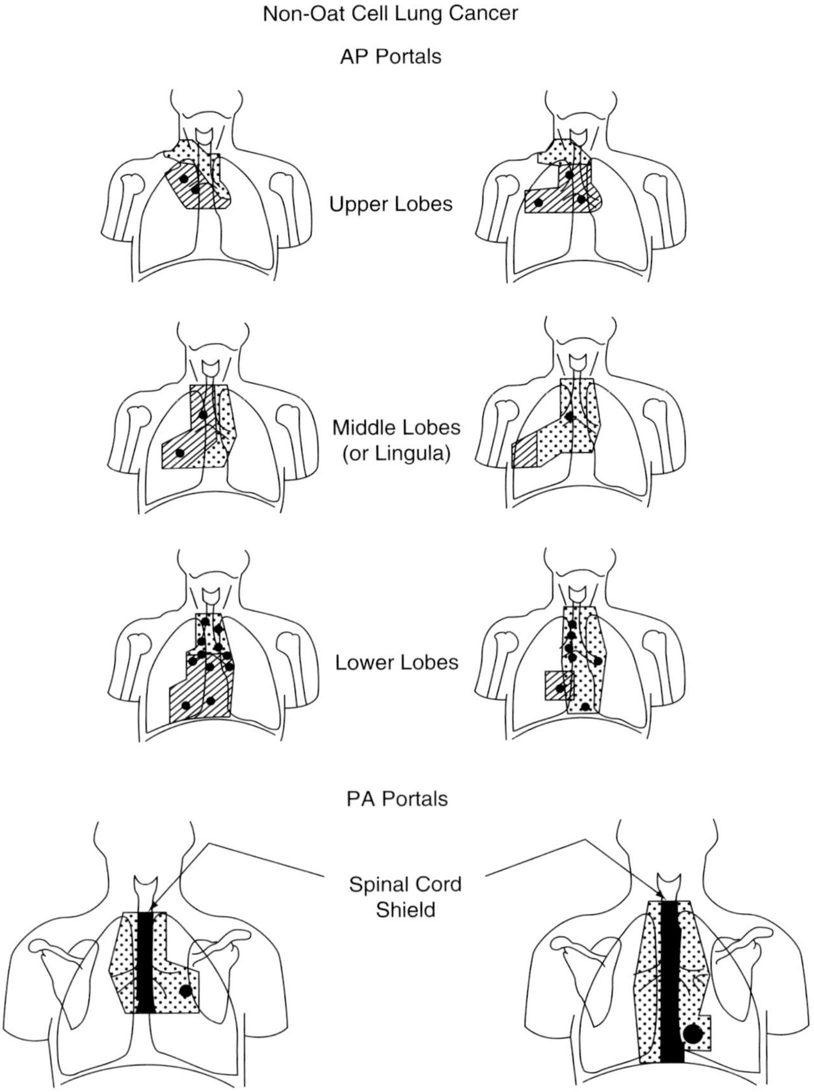

FIGURE 2 Examples of portals used to treat primary lung tumor and regional lymph nodes From Ref. 1.

as their only site of metastatic disease. Furthermore, approximately 50% of patients who develop brain metastases do so within 16 weeks of completing treatment for primary advanced lung cancer (43). Although NSCLC and SCLC have this same propensity for the brain, PCI is viewed very differently for patients with NSCLC and SCLC.

First, PCI cannot be recommended for patients with NSCLC. A Cochrane review on four studies found that among 791 patients, PCI was able to reduce brain failure rates from 11% to 23% without PCI and to 1% to 6% with PCI. No impact was seen on overall survival among three out of the four trials (44). Studies were developed to address this problem by offering PCI to patients with advanced NSCLC. One of these studies was closed early due to accrual issues, despite the collaboration of many other cooperative groups (Radiation Therapy Oncology Group L-0214; ClinicalTrials.gov identifier: NCT00048997). Patients with stage IIIA or IIIB NSCLC without disease progression after locoregional treatment with surgery and/or radiation therapy with or without chemotherapy were eligible for this trial. Participants were randomized to PCI or observation and stratified by stage (IIIA or IIIB), histology (nonsquamous or squamous), and therapy (surgery or no surgery). PCI was delivered to a total dose of 30Gy at 2Gy per fraction, once daily. The primary endpoint was survival (OS). Secondary endpoints included disease-free survival (DFS), incidence of brain metastases, neuropsychological and QOL impact of PCI. The total accrual was 356 patients of the planned 1,058. Of these 340 patients were evaluable. One year OS (75.6% and 76.9% for PCI and observation, $P = .86$) and 1 year DFS (56.4% and 51.2% for PCI and observation, $P = .11$) were not statistically significantly different. However, the incidence of brain metastases at 1 year was statistically significantly different with brain relapse of 7.7% for PCI versus 18% for observation ($P = .004$). Patients in the observation arm were 2.52 times more likely to develop brain metastases than those in the PCI arm (odds ratio = 2.52, [95% CI = 1.32–4.80]). There were no significant differences at 1 year between the two arms amongst any QOL components (45). Therefore, PCI is unlikely to become part of our routine practice for patients with locally advanced NSCLC; although, some authors suggest that it can be given to high-risk patients on an individual basis (46).

TREATMENT PLANNING OF THORACIC RT

Simulation

Radiation oncology is a rapidly evolving field, quickly adapting to the advances in treatment planning and delivery that has resulted primarily from advancing computing power and advanced imaging. The "state of the art" yesterday may not be the current state of the art. The process of simulation has seen evolution as dramatic as seen in treatment planning and delivery systems. This is exemplified by the field designs seen in RTOG 73-01 (Figure 2). Simulation for that trial consisted of simple chest x-rays taken with the patient supine. Target definition was made with a wax pencil and was usually completed before the patient left the department after the simulation. Now the common standard is CT-based simulation for all of radiation oncology, and wax pencils are now only used by old professors to show residents what it was like "back in my day." For thoracic RT, the optimal simulation includes four-dimensional CTs (4D CT) when available. The use of traditional thin slice CTs results in volume errors, as the tumor moves in and out of the CT slice during respiration. This creates errors in GTV assessment (47) due to this "interplay" of tumor motion and the progression of the CT, for example the tumor may be at deep inspiration during one slice, and mid expiration during the next slice. The byproduct of that error is that the GTV may appear to increase and decrease in diameter in the chest. A 4D CT is a standard CT (which gives three dimensions) plus a fourth variable/dimension of time. The variable of time is added by the use of a respiratory trace. This is done by measuring the motion of a light sensor, or by using bellows to monitor a breathing cycle. The breathing cycle (from peak to peak) is then broken into 10 phases, representing the different percentages of the respiratory cycle. The CT is able to correlate patient position to respiratory position (i.e., patient is at couch position—10 cm while at respiratory position of 10% of the respiratory cycle) and then "bins" 10 CT such that a complete CT is generated for each respiratory position (i.e., a full CT at 10% of the respiratory cycle). The result of all this hard work on the part of the planning session is that a cine loop of the CTs is obtainable showing the motion of the tumor through a respiratory cycle. Each of the CTs can be used for contouring, allowing the radiation oncologists to track tumor position over the respiratory cycle. More on target delineation is listed below.

Target Volumes

ICRU report 62 (48) provides a thorough discussion of treatment volumes defined for radiation oncology dose delivery. In Figure 3 we clarify some of the definitions of the ICRU report 62, and add a more practical definition which we commonly use in clinical practice. Some discussion about these individual volumes as they relate to the treatment of advanced NSCLC is worth reviewing.

GTV

GTV is the gross tumor volume and is a radiographic volume, that is the tumor you see on radiographic exams (CT, MRI, x-ray, etc.). Although MRI can be used for tumor assessment in lung cancer, the

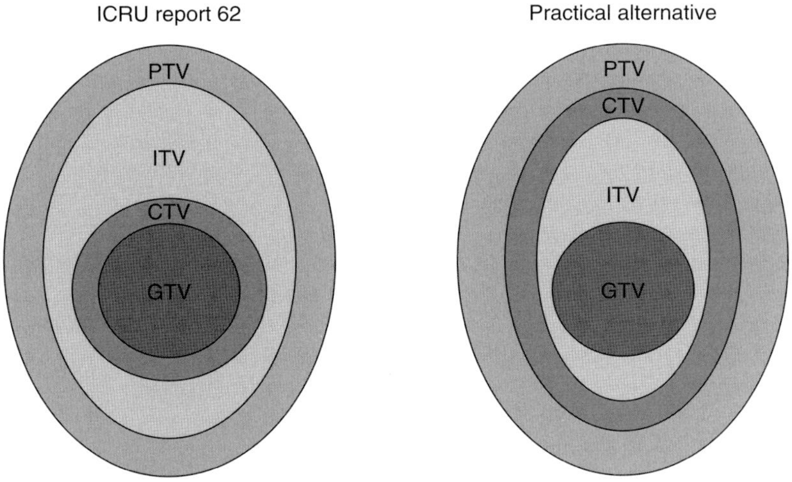

FIGURE 3 Comparison of target volume definitions.

majority of practicing radiation oncologists use CT imaging to define the GTV. Generally speaking, the GTV does not consider time or motion as a function of its volume (distinguishing it from the ITV described below). It is frequently appropriate to make separate GTVs for the primary tumor itself and for the nodal disease. These separate GTVs can then be independently expanded for the CTVs and ITVs as described below.

CTV

CTV is the clinical target volume. This volume includes the GTV but has additional expansion to cover other tissue deemed to be at high risk of microscopic disease. Whereas GTV and typically ITV are radiographic margins, CTV is an intellectual margin. The CTV may include a margin around the primary tumor to cover microscopic spread as well as nodal stations deemed to be at high risk of harboring microscopic disease. In regards to the CTV to include around primary tumors, there are two excellent articles looking at appropriate CTVs for primary lung cancers (49,50). Both are recommended to the interested reader. The authors used radiographic volumes and compared it to the pathologic volumes to estimate the microscopic extension of tumor cells surrounding the primary tumor. It is encouraging how closely these two authors agree with regard to appropriate volumes to cover 95% of tumors. Grills et al. (49) found the microscopic extension was best correlated with histologic grade, with low grade tumors requiring larger margins to cover creaping bronchioaveolar carcinoma (BAC), whereas nuclear grade 2 and 3 tumors required 7 and 2 mm, respectively, to cover the true CTV. The authors Giruard et al. (49) found a difference in microscopic extension based on squamous versus adenocarcinomas. In their review, margins of 6 mm were required for squamous histologies, and 8 mm were required for adenocarcinomas. For a practical summation, we typically use 7 mm to accommodate both data sets. A couple of important caveats are appropriate to remember here as well. First, these volumes are for microscopic extension in open lung. Hence, the 7 mm expansion around an ITV would be pulled in to 2–3 mm if the CTV came in contact with solid thoracic structures such as the chest wall or mediastinum. As such this volume should be reviewed on each CT slice to ensure that unnecessary volumes are not being treated. That accommodation is frequently useful when trying to spare normal tissues such as the esophagus, spinal cord, brachial plexus, and other dose-limiting structures. Second, these data apply to primary lung tumors and not to mediastinal nodes. The microscopic extension around lymph nodes is typically 3 mm (51). Altering the CTV in accordance with the previous caveats will typically allow more sparing of normal tissues within the mediastinum such as the heart and esophagus.

A second important discussion regarding appropriate CTVs is the discussion of elective nodal irradiation (ENI). As stated above CTVs are intellectual volumes, and hence are prone to strong differences of opinion about the appropriateness of the different CTV definitions in NSCLC. ENI is the treatment of thoracic lymph node stations that are not radiographically involved with tumor at the time of simulation. Translated into the context of this chapter, ENI involves expanding the CTV to include lymph node stations that are not involved by cancer by CT or PET definitions. Historically, this meant treating the entire mediastinum similar to the fields shown in Figure 2 (73-01 fields). Currently it may mean treating the entire mediastinum, or may mean treating 1 to 2 lymph node stations beyond the GTV/ITV (52). Those in favor of treating elective nodal volumes point to surgical literature showing microscopic involvement of high-risk mediastinal lymph node station that appear normal on imaging, but are positive at time of mediastinal dissection. This rate is easily translatable from the negative predictive value of PET for assessment of the mediastinum (see above). Hence, excluding them from a CTV excludes tumor from planned RT volumes. On the surface exclusion of those volumes sounds like "a hear no evil, see no evil, speak no evil" approach to treatment planning. There is more to this story, however.

The opponents of ENI point to several lines of research when advocating for an involved field approach to NSCLC. First, patterns of failure studies have found isolated nodal failure rare. RTOG (53) reviewed the treatment fields of 1,705 patients treated on RTOG protocols and assessed the quality of mediastinal coverage. They found no correlation between nodal coverage and mediastinal failure or 2-year overall survival. Subsequently several institutions moved to treating only involved fields in an attempt toincrease dose and limit toxicity. Summed experience from these investigators (54,55) showed an isolated nodal failure rate of only 0% to 6%. This is contrasted to local failure rate of 27% to 62%. This is retrospective data, however, and subject to the quality of the follow-up data. University of Michigan conducted a prospective dose escalation trial using involved field RT (56). Results of this prospective trial with carefully defined follow-up showed no isolated regional failures, and no regional-distant failure in the 106 patients treated. Local failure, in contrast, was present in 54% of the patients despite dose escalation to more than 100 Gy. The RTOG conducted a similar dose escalation trial and omitted ENI from the treatment (39). In 179 patients, regional failure in elective nodal sites was <10%, whereas local failure was 38%. So, even when treating to the high doses used on phase I dose escalation trials, the failure rate inside the PTV is 3–5× higher than in elective nodal volumes. This low-failure rate may be explained by these sites receiving incidental RT while treating the non-ENI PTVs (57).

Second, the use of ENI increases treatment volumes and limits the possibilities of dose escalation. Grills et al. (58) compared full ENI plans to 3D conformal RT plans and intensity modulated RT (IMRT) plans. They found treating involved field (IF) RT only allowed them to escalate the dose by 80% when treating with 3D CRT and 130% when treating with IMRT, while keeping the risk of toxicity the same across the groups. A controversial trial related to this was recently published by Yuan et al. (59) and merits review. These investigators randomized 200 patients with stage III NSCLC to either 60–64 Gy treating ENI fields or 68–74 Gy of IF fields. Both arms were combined with platinum-based chemotherapy. The results showed improved 5-year local control (51% vs. 36%, $P = .032$), lower rate of pneumonitis (17% vs. 29%, $P = .044$), and an improved 2-year OS (25.6% vs. 39.4%, $P = .048$). The critics of this trial have correctly stated that the trial addresses the benefits of dose, rather than the benefits of field design. As such it doesn't establish that IF is superior to ENI, but rather that 68–74 Gy is superior to 60–64 Gy. However, it does point to the fact that dose was escalated by 10 Gy with with IF RT, which resulted in significant improvements in local control, survival, and toxicity.

Our conclusion of the data on ENI is that purposeful treatment of elective nodal sites is unnecessary. In patients treated intentionally with IF RT, significant doses of RT are delivered to the adjacent nodal sites and this may be enough to control microscopic disease. Local failure within the IF PTV is relatively high and this overshadows the small risk of isolated nodal failure in outside of the treatment target. As we improve RT techniques and begin to achieve local control rates similar to what we see in early stage NSCLC with SBRT, patterns of failure may change, and we may find a renewed need to consider ENI.

ITV

ITV is the internal target volume. For this definition, in terms of practical application in the use of RT, we disagree with the definition provided by ICRU report 62, which describes the ITV as a CTV expanded to cover motion. Hence, when planning a lung case following the ICRU report 62 strictly, the ITV volume is greater than the CTV volume. Patient-specific ITVs for NSCLC are typically derived using a 4D CT simulation. The ITV is then defined by examining the movement of the GTV over a typical respiratory cycle. The ITV then is a radiographic parameter defined by another radiographic parameter rather than a radiographic parameter, the addition of a CTV, and then migration to another radiographic parameter. The process of doing a 4D CT simulation takes long enough without adding unnecessary complication. For practical purposes, an ITV is the expansion of the GTV to account for motion through the respiratory cycle. In clinical practice, we recommend that the CTV be added to the ITV. The reason for the confusion was that the original authors of the ICRU report 62 anticipated that ITV would be defined by population-based statistical reports of tumor motion, rather than patient-specific motion. Indeed, they felt ITV would primarily be of interest to physicists studying organ motion and advised clinicians to consider only GTV, CTV, and PTV (60).

PTV

The PTV is margin around the CTV that accounts for the errors associated with therapy. These errors come in two types: Random errors associated with individuals' daily setup due to uncertainties in patient's tumor position and systematic errors associated with the errors inherent in the machine and daily setup. The PTVs are therefore specific both to the individual and to the institution. They are individual in that tumor position, presence of a cough, etc. influence daily error and hence the PTV volume chosen. They are institutional in that the way the treatment is delivered and verified influence the error and hence the PTV volume chosen. PTVs are typically prescribed as a uniform expansion of a CTV. As such, decreasing the required PTV volume can affect a treatment volume by a substantial amount. Methods to decrease the PTV have dramatically improved in recent years. The ways to reduce PTV can be broadly divided into two different categories: Patient-specific methods and delivery-specific methods.

Patient-specific methods primarily center on restricting or limiting the motion of the tumor. These include monitored breathing, breath hold, and gated therapy. Delivery-specific methods would include improved immobilization, abdominal compression, and image guidance with on-board imaging via KV x-ray or cone beam CT.

■ TREATMENT PLANNING

The fields shown for RTOG 73-01 would typically be described as two-dimensional (2D) treatment planning. There are no GTV-CTV-PTV considerations and no attempt to spare critical structures. For the most part, the days of 2D planning is past and modern RT for NSCLC incorporates three-dimensional (3D) planning. The previous section of this chapter details many of the considerations when generating 3D plans. These are used in conjunction with concerns about normal tissue toxicity (please see Chapter 13) to create the parameters of an acceptable plan. But what about other planning methods? Most radiation oncologists will have the tools to deliver intensity modulated RT (IMRT) in their facility. Is IMRT an acceptable alternative? What are the benefits and potential disadvantages in using IMRT in NSCLC?

The primary concerns with the use of IMRT in NSCLC involve "interplay" and increase in the integral dose to normal lung. Remember we briefly discussed interplay in the section above as it related to the simulation CT and the primary tumor. The concept here is essentially the same, with some different actors. The term "interplay" refers to the relationship between beamlets in an IMRT field and their motion relative to the motion of the target. If you imagine a cell in a tumor moving through the respiratory cycles, and then imagine the variety of beamlets in that are delivered in an IMRT field, you can imagine that a cell may move together with a beamlet, receiving more dose than was intended, or may move opposite the beamlet, receiving less dose or perhaps no dose during the delivery of the beamlet. It is primarily the possibility of underdosing as a result of interplay that concerns physicists and physicians alike. Whereas interplay affected the geometric shape of the GTV for simulation, the interplay in IMRT potentially affects dose delivered to the GTV.

For the most part this concern appears to be unfounded when calculating dose over a 30+ fraction regimen if an ITV is generated (61). Using the above example, individual cancer cells may be underdosed in one fraction, but overdosed in a subsequent fraction, averaging the error. In addition, IMRT appears to have benefits in terms of sparing normal tissues while escalating dose. In a comparison of 3D conformal plans with IMRT plans Grills et al. (58) saw a 15% improvement in lung V20 and a 40% improvement in esophagus V50 as compared with 3D conformal RT. This was at the expense of a slight increase in median lung dose. Other authors have seen a reduction in pneumonitis with the use of IMRT in conjunction with chemotherapy. Yom et al. (62) examined their experience using IMRT for 151 patients with NSCLC. When comparing the results with patients treated at the same institution with 3D conformal RT they saw a reduction in the risk of pneumonitis from 32% for 3D to only 8% with IMRT. In our clinical practice we begin planning patients with 3D conformal RT and switch to IMRT if we find the Lung V20 to exceed 30%. In those situations we have seen an improvement in V20 similar to what was seen by Grills et al. (58), and we believe the added expense is justifiable when compared to the increased risk of grade 3 pneumonitis.

PARTICLE THERAPY

Particle therapy, and particularly proton therapy, is becoming a hot topic for all of Radiation oncology. There is ample data on the feasibility of using protons for early stage NSCLC, but precious little data for advanced NSCLC. There are several dosimetry studies showing reduced dose to critical structures when using proton therapy (63,64), but we have yet to see a publication on patients treated with these techniques. Protons are uniquely dependent on density. The density of lung can vary dramatically depending on both phases of the respiratory cycle and the cardiac cycle (65). As such, looking at proton dosimetry simply on a static planning scan may not reveal all the dose ambiguities present during the delivery of the dose. We await the results of ongoing trials at MD Anderson and other particle centers.

REFERENCES

1. Detterbeck, FC, Boffa, DJ, Tanoue, LT. The new lung cancer staging system. *Chest.* 2009;136:260–271.
2. American Cancer Society. *Cancer Facts & Figures 2009.* Atlanta: American Cancer Society; 2009.
3. *WHO Report on the Global Tobacco Epidemic, 2008: The MPOWER package.* Geneva: World Health Organization; 2008.
4. Samet, JM. Radon and lung cancer. *J Natl Cancer Inst.* 1989;81:745–758.
5. Ann, GS, Michael, R, Ping, Y, Swanson, GM. Increased cancer risk among relatives of nonsmoking lung cancer cases. *Genet Epidemiol.* 1999;17:1–15.
6. Subramanian, J, Govindan, R. Lung cancer in never smokers: A Review. *J Clin Oncol.* 2007;25:561–570.
7. Carbone, PP, Frost, JK, Feinstein, AR, Higgins, GAJ, Selawry, OS. Lung cancer: perspectives and prospects. *Ann Intern Med.* 1970;73:1003–1024.
8. Stanley, KE. Prognostic factors for survival in patients with inoperable lung cancer. *J Natl Cancer Inst.* 1980;65:25–32.
9. Early lung cancer detection: summary and conclusions. *Am Rev Respir Dis.* 1984;130:565–570.
10. Ost, D, Fein, AM, Feinsilver, SH. The solitary pulmonary nodule. *N Engl J Med.* 2003;348:2535–2542.
11. Silvestri, GA, Gould, MK, Margolis, ML, et al. Noninvasive staging of non-small cell lung cancer. *Chest.* 2007;132:178S–201S.
12. Pieterman, RM, van Putten, JWG, Meuzelaar, JJ, et al. Preoperative staging of non-small-cell lung cancer with positron-emission tomography. *N Engl J Med.* 2000;343:254–261.
13. Reed, CE, Harpole, DH, Posther, KE, et al. Results of the American College of Surgeons Oncology Group Z0050 trial: the utility of positron emission tomography in staging potentially operable non-small cell lung cancer. *J Thorac Cardiovasc Surg.* 2003;126:1943–1951.
14. Hochstenbag, MMH, Twijnstra, A, Hofman, P, Wouters, EFM, ten Velde, GPM. MR-imaging of the brain of neurologic asymptomatic patients with large cell or adenocarcinoma of the lung. Does it influence prognosis and treatment? *Lung Cancer.* 2003;42:189–193.
15. Rivera, MP, Detterbeck, F, Mehta, AC. Diagnosis of lung cancer. *Chest.* 2003;123:129S–136S.
16. Schreiber, G, McCrory, DC. Performance characteristics of different modalities for diagnosis of suspected lung cancer. *Chest.* 2003;123:115S–128S.
17. Li, H, Boiselle, PM, Shepard, JO, Trotman-Dickenson, B, McLoud, TC. Diagnostic accuracy and safety of CT-guided percutaneous needle aspiration biopsy of the lung: comparison of small and large pulmonary nodules. *Am J Roentgenol.* 1996;167:105–109.
18. Beasley, MB, Brambilla, E, Travis, WD. The 2004 World Health Organization classification of lung tumors. *Semin Roentgenol.* 2005;40:90–97.
19. Beasley, MB. Immunohistochemistry of pulmonary and pleural neoplasia. *Arch Pathol Lab Med.* 2008;132:1062–1072.
20. Roswit, B, Patno, ME, Rapp, R, et al. The survival of patients with inoperable lung cancer: a large-scale randomized study of radiation therapy versus placebo. *Radiology.* 1968;90:688–697.
21. Reinfuss, M, Glinski, B, Kowalska, T, et al. [Radiotherapy for stage III, inoperable, asymptomatic small cell lung

cancer. Final results of a prospective randomized study (240 patients)]. *Cancer Radiother.* 1999;3:475–479.
22. Dillman, RO, Seagren, SL, Propert, KJ, et al. A randomized trial of induction chemotherapy plus high-dose radiation versus radiation alone in stage III non-small-cell lung cancer. *N Engl J Med.* 1990;323:940–945.
23. Dillman, RO, Seagren, SL, Propert, KJ, et al. A randomized trial of induction chemotherapy plus high-dose radiation versus radiation alone in stage III non-small-cell lung cancer. *N Engl J Med.* 1990;323:940–945.
24. Sause, W, Kolesar, P, Taylor, S, et al. Final results of phase III trial in regionally advanced unresectable non-small cell lung cancer. *Chest.* 2000;117:358–364.
25. Le Chevalier, T, Arriagada, R, Quoix, E, et al. Radiotherapy alone versus combined chemotherapy and radiotherapy in nonresectable non-small-cell lung cancer: first analysis of a randomized trial in 353 patients. *J Natl Cancer Inst.* 1991;83:417–423.
26. Chevalier, TL, Arriagada, R, Tarayre, M, et al. Signiicant effect of adjuvant chemotherapy on survival in locally advanced non-small-cell lung carcinoma. *J Natl Cancer Inst.* 1992;84:58.
27. Curran, W, Scott, C, Langer, C, et al. Phase III comparison of sequential vs concurrent chemoradiation for pts with unresected stage III non-small cell lung cancer (NSCLC): Report of Radiation Therapy Oncology Group (RTOG) 9410. *Lung Cancer.* 2000;29:93–93.
28. Komaki, R, Seiferheld, W, Ettinger, D, Lee, JS, Movsas, B, Sause, W. Randomized chemoradiation for patients with locally advanced inoperable non-small cell lung cancer (NSCLC): Long-term follow-up of RTOG 92–04. *Lung Cancer.* 2000;29:93–93.
29. Komaki, R, Seiferheld, W, Curran, W, et al. Sequential vs. concurrent chemotherapy and radiation therapy for inoperable non-small cell lung cancer (NSCLC): Analysis of failures in a phase III study (RTOG 9410). *Int J Radiat Oncol Biol Phys.* 2000;48:113–113.
30. Furuse, K, Fukuoka, M, Kawahara, M, et al. Phase III study of concurrent versus sequential thoracic radiotherapy in combination with mitomycin, vindesine, and cisplatin in unresectable stage III non-small-cell lung cancer. *J Clin Oncol.* 1999;17:2692–2699.
31. Denis, F, Garaud, P, Bardet, E, et al. Final results of the 94–01 French head and neck oncology and radiotherapy group randomized trial comparing radiotherapy alone with concomitant radiochemotherapy in advanced-stage oropharynx carcinoma. *J Clin Oncol.* 2004;22:69–76.
32. Brizel, DM, Albers, ME, Fisher, SR, et al. Hyperfractionated irradiation with or without concurrent chemotherapy for locally advanced head and neck cancer. *N Engl J Med.* 1998;338:1798–1804.
33. Komaki, R, Scott, CB, Sause, WT, et al. Induction cisplatin/vinblastine and irradiation vs. irradiation in unresectable squamous cell lung cancer: failure patterns by cell type in rtog 88–08/ECOG 4588. *Int J Radiat Oncol Biol Phys.* 1997;39:537–544.
34. Byhardt, RW, Scott, C, Sause, WT, et al. Response, toxicity, failure patterns, and survival in five radiation therapy oncology group (RTOG) trials of sequential and/or concurrent chemotherapy and radiotherapy for locally advanced non-small-cell carcinoma of the lung. *Int J Radiat Oncol Biol Phys.* 1998;42:469–478.
35. Winton, T, Livingston, R, Johnson, D, et al. Vinorelbine plus cisplatin vs. observation in resected non-small-cell lung cancer. *N Engl J Med.* 2005;352:2589–2597.
36. Strauss, GM, Herndon, J, Maddaus, MA, et al. Randomized clinical trial of adjuvant chemotherapy with paclitaxel and carboplatin following resection in stage IB non-small cell lung cancer (NSCLC): report of cancer and leukemia group B (CALGB) protocol 9633. *J Clin Oncol* (Meeting Abstracts). 2004;22:7019.
37. Perez, CA, Stanley, K, Rubin, P, et al. A prospective randomized study of various irradiation doses and fractionation schedules in the treatment of inoperable non-oat-cell carcinoma of the lung. Preliminary report by the radiation therapy oncology group. *Cancer.* 1980;45:2744–2753.
38. Perez, CA, Pajak, TF, Rubin, P, et al. Long-term observations of the patterns of failure in patients with unresectable non-oat cell carcinoma of the lung treated with definitive radiotherapy. Report by the radiation therapy oncology group. *Cancer.* 1987;59:1874–1881.
39. Bradley, J, Graham, MV, Winter, K, et al. Toxicity and outcome results of RTOG 9311: a phase I-II dose-escalation study using three-dimensional conformal radiotherapy in patients with inoperable non-small-cell lung carcinoma. *Int J Radiat Oncol Biol Phys.* 2005;61:318–328.
40. Schild, SE, McGinnis, WL, Graham, D, et al. Results of a phase I trial of concurrent chemotherapy and escalating doses of radiation for unresectable non-small-cell lung cancer. *Int J Radiat Oncol Biol Phys.* 2006;65:1106–1111.
41. Bradley, JD, Graham, M, Suzanne, S, et al. Phase I results of RTOG L-0117; a phase I/II dose intensification study using 3DCRT and concurrent chemotherapy for patients with Inoperable NSCLC. *J Clin Oncol* (Meeting Abstracts). 2005;23:7063–.
42. Stinchcombe, TE, Lee, CB, Moore, DT, et al. Long-term follow-up of a phase I/II trial of dose escalating three-dimensional conformal thoracic radiation therapy with induction and concurrent carboplatin and paclitaxel in unresectable stage IIIA/B non-small cell lung cancer. *J Thorac Oncol.* 2008;3:1279–1285.
43. Gaspar, LE, Chansky, K, Albain, KS, et al. Time from treatment to subsequent diagnosis of brain metastases in stage III non-small-cell lung cancer: a retrospective review by the Southwest Oncology Group. *J Clin Oncol.* 2005;23:2955–2961.
44. Lester, JF, MacBeth, FR, Coles, B. Prophylactic cranial irradiation for preventing brain metastases in patients undergoing radical treatment for non-small-cell lung cancer: a Cochrane Review. *Int J Radiat Oncol Biol Phys.* 2005;63:690–694.
45. Sun, A, Bae, K, Gore, E, et al. A phase III comparison of prophylactic cranial irradiation (PCI) versus observation in patients with locally advanced non-small cell lung cancer (LA-NSCLC). Initial analysis of primary and secondary endpoints: RTOG 0214. WCLC—13th World Conference on Lung Cancer, abstract C.6., August 2009 San Francisco 2009.

Cancer (UICC) stage I disease. Lung cancer is a disease of the elderly with a median age of 71 years at diagnosis (3).

The natural history of untreated SCLC included rapid tumor progression with a median survival of only 2 to 4 months (4). Until the late 1960s, physicians did not differentiate the management of small cell from non–small cell lung cancer (NSCLC), and clinical trials in the 1970s continued to include both major histologic types. It was recognized that most patients with SCLC had poor survival following resection and/or radiotherapy (RT) with little apparent survival benefit from either therapy. A major change in management occurred in the late 1960s and was linked to the recognition that SCLC was far more responsive to chemotherapy than NSCLC (5). Since that time, the standard of care for SCLC patients has included chemotherapy in addition to locoregional therapies.

■ PATHOLOGY AND PATHWAYS OF SPREAD

SCLC arises from neuroendocrine cells. The 2004 World Health Organization (WHO) Classification defined SCLC as, "a malignant epithelial tumor consisting of small cells with scant cytoplasm, ill-defined cell boarders, finely granular nuclear chromatin, and absent or inconspicuous nucleoli. The cells are round, oval, and spindle-shaped. Nuclear molding is prominent. Necrosis is extensive and the mitotic count is high. It occurs in two variants: small cell carcinoma and combined small cell carcinoma. The latter includes SCLC cells and any of the histologic types of NSCLC (6). The cells appear as small blue cells on hematoxylin and eosin staining and often appear as stacks of oats under that microscope leading to the name more often used in the older publications, "oat cell carcinoma." Electron microscopy shows dense-core neurosecretory granules. SCLC cells are immunoreactive for keratin, thyroid transcription factor 1, and epithelial membrane antigen.

■ BIOLOGIC CHARACTERISTICS/ MOLECULAR BIOLOGY

Cigarette smoke is a powerful mutagen that is strongly associated with the development of SCLC. Acquired hypermethylation of the promoter region of key genes has become a common mechanism that tumors use to inactivate tumor suppressor and other genes. A number of genetic mutations are frequently observed in SCLC tumors that frequently involve tumor suppressor genes (TSGs). The mutations lead to dysfunction of these suppressor molecules leading to the unrestricted tumor growth. The most common are deletions in the short arm of chromosome 3 in the 3p14–23 region (>80% of SCLC cases), inactivation of the *retinoblastoma (Rb)* gene on chromosome 13 (90%), and mutations of the *p53* tumor suppressor gene on the short arm of chromosome 17 (>80%) (Table 1) There has been substantial progress in understanding the relationship of these molecular abnormalities and the events leading normal bronchial epithelium to become invasive carcinoma. There has not yet been much progress made in preventing these events or reversing them, once they have taken place.

The chromosome 3 genetic deletions have been observed in both dysplastic and preneoplastic changes and have been demonstrated as the genetic mutation associated with the transformation of precancerous lesions into carcinoma. There has recently emerged evidence that the critical deletion in SCLC

TABLE 1 Molecular abnormalities in lung cancer

Molecular Abnormality	SCLC (%)	NSCLC (%)
Ras mutation	<1	30–40
Myc amplification	30	10
EGFR expression	NR	40–80
c-*erb*B-2 overexpression (HER-2)	10	30
c-kit/SCFR coexpression	70	15
Bcl-2 expression	95	35
p53 mutation	75–100	50
RB deletion (protein)	90	20
p16 inactivation	<1	70
COX-2 expression	NR	70
3p deletion	90	50
VEGF expression	>100-fold variation	
Matrix metalloproteinase (gelatinase)	50	65
Neuropeptides	90	NR

COX, cyclo-oxygenase; EGFR, epidermal growth factor receptors; NSCLC, non–small cell lung cancer; RB, retinoblastoma gene; SCFR, stem-cell factor receptor; SCLC, small cell lung cancer; VEGF, vascular endothelial growth factor. NR = not reported
Source: Adapted from Ref. 7.

and many other malignancies may be in a fragile portion of chromosome 3 known as the *Fragile histidine triad* gene (*FHIT* gene) deletion (8,9). Mutations in *FHIT* are found in many different cancers suggesting that defects in these genes may have a role in tumor development. However, the exact significance of *FHIT* mutations in cancer formation is unclear since aberrant *FHIT* genes have been found in both malignancies and normal noncancerous cells. Inactivation of the *Rb* gene most likely results in a loss of control of cell growth. It is believed that a functional *Rb* gene keeps the G1/S cell cycle boundary in check and that its inactivation will result in uncontrolled growth (10). The *p53* mutations specific to SCLC have also been observed in preneoplastic lesions and appear to most closely resemble *p53* mutations observed in other malignancies for which tobacco is a known carcinogen. It is likely that the mutations of *p53* in SCLC impair the ability of tumor cells to undergo apoptosis in response to various therapies (11). Another growth regulator, which is overexpressed in 95% of SCLC tumors, is BCL 2. It is believed that this overexpression prevents the tumor's apoptotic response to therapy (12). There are continuing research to develop therapies that target the tumor-specific biologic abnormalities.

In many non–small cell specimens, point mutations in the *ras* family of oncogenes have been observed (13). These mutations are rarely observed in SCLCs, but commonly, amplification or overexpression of the *myc* family of oncogenes is observed, most notably, c-*myc*, N-*myc*, and L-*myc*. It appears that abnormalities are more often observed in recurrent tumors, tumors with variant rather than classic SCLC, or tumors with a more aggressive and unfavorable prognosis. This has led to the concept that the overexpression of the *myc* oncogenes is a relatively late event in the pathogenesis of SCLC (14).

Another biologic feature that distinguishes small cell from NSCLC is the more common expression of neuroendocrine markers in SCLC. These neuroendocrine markers include enzymes (neuron-specific enolase and L-dopa decarboxylase), peptide hormones (gastrin-releasing peptide, arginine vasopressin), and surface markers such as neural cell adhesion molecule (NCAM). The two peptide hormones meet the criteria of autocrine growth factors, which require the production of a growth-promoting protein for which the producing cell has functional receptors. In the case of gastrin-releasing peptide, there is clear evidence that it is produced and secreted by many SCLC cells and then attaches to its cellular membrane receptors stimulating tumor growth (15). There are antibodies that have been developed against the abnormal proteins produced by tumors that are undergoing clinical testing (16). These antibodies could potentially block abnormal tumor biochemical functions such as the autocrine growth cycle.

■ CLINICAL MANIFESTATIONS/ PATIENT EVALUATION/STAGING

The presentation of patients with SCLC differs somewhat from those with NSCLC. These differences include fewer cases of SCLC diagnosed by imaging of asymptomatic patients, a shorter time from first thoracic symptoms to life-threatening symptoms, and the occasional presentation of SCLC with paraneoplastic symptoms. The signs and symptoms from either histology depend on the tumor location, bulk of the primary lesion, adenopathy, and/or metastatic disease. Because of the high frequency of nodal involvement with SCLC cases, patients frequently present with symptoms such as dyspnea, dysphagia, hoarseness, and superior vena cava syndrome. Patients also present with other thoracic symptoms, including cough, hemoptysis, chest pain, and weight loss.

SCLC is the most common solid tumor to have a number of associated paraneoplastic syndromes. Several of these are endocrinologic and neurologic. The most common endocrinologic abnormality is the syndrome of inappropriate secretion of antidiuretic hormone (SIADH). This condition results from the excessive secretion of ADH from tumor tissue, leading to severe hyponatremia with resultant hypo-osmolality. SIADH occurs in 11% to 46% of SCLC patients and typically resolves after response to anticancer therapy. Restriction of free water intake is critical to maintaining proper sodium concentrations before SIADH improves secondary to cancer therapy (17). Two less common endocrinologic syndromes are atrial natriuretic peptide (ANP) syndrome, which can produce hyponatremia, natriuresis, and hypotension, and ectopic adrenocorticotropic hormone (ACTH) production syndrome resulting in Cushing's syndrome. The former occurs in about 15% of SCLC cases and responds to therapy, whereas the latter occurs in 5% of cases and is associated with a poor prognosis (18).

The neurologic syndromes associated with SCLC include Lambert-Eaton syndrome, cerebellar degeneration syndrome, encephalomyelitis, sensory neuropathy, and cancer-associated retinopathy. Each of these is observed in well under 5% of all SCLC patients. Lambert-Eaton syndrome is an autoimmune disorder that affects calcium channels of the neuromuscular junction. Antibodies are directed against the calcium channels responsible for the presynaptic release of acetylcholine. These antibodies prevent the opening of calcium channels preventing the release of acetylcholine. Patients with Lambert-Eaton syndrome present with myasthenia gravis–like symptoms of proximal myopathy, autonomic dysfunction, and hyporeflexia. Like many paraneoplastic syndromes, this condition is generally improved with response to anticancer therapy, although there can also be symptomatic responses to anti-myasthenia therapies (19). The other neurologic syndromes are believed to be primarily autoimmune phenomena and most often respond poorly to cancer therapy (20,21). Table 2 summarizes these SCLC-associated syndromes.

SCLC can be diagnosed with histologic or cytologic sampling. In most cases, a diagnosis can be obtained via sputum expectoration, bronchoscopic sampling, or computed tomography (CT)–guided transthoracic needle aspiration. Rarely, mediastinoscopy or thoracotomy is required. Cytologic techniques have improved so much that bronchoscopic brush technique can usually distinguish small cell from NSCLC, as can the needle aspirate from a transthoracic needle. Once the diagnosis is established, there is no need for additional invasive mediastinal staging, as there sometimes is for NSCLC. This is due to the limited role of surgical resection in management.

The UICC/American Joint Commission on Cancer (AJCC) has been universally adopted for staging patients with NSCLC but is less frequently employed for SCLC. Instead, the 1973 Veterans Administration (VA) Lung Cancer Study Group's Staging System,which distinguishes between limited and extensive SCLC is more commonly used, despite its considerable imprecision (22). The initial definition of limited disease was an extent of intrathoracic disease encompassable within a "reasonable" radiation field. Such a vague definition allows for many interpretations, which have ranged from patients with ipsilateral pleural effusions and contralateral mediastinal, supraclavicular, and hilar adenopathy to only those without effusions and with ipsilateral adenopathy. Investigators in recent years have recognized the dangers of variable interpretations, and recent North American cooperative group trials require staging of SCLC patients with the standard TNM system prior to study entry. However, the categorization of SCLC patients into limited versus extensive stage disease has been extremely helpful for making rational treatment choices and designing trials.

Approximately, two-thirds of SCLC patients have extensive-stage or stage IV disease at presentation. This figure has increased from approximately 50% in the 1970s and 1980s, in part due to the greater sensitivity of screening techniques for metastatic disease. One of the principal goals of staging is to distinguish stages I–III from stage IV patients. This evaluation would typically include a

TABLE 2 Syndromes associated with SCLC

Syndrome	Major Problem	Frequency (%)	Improves with Therapy
SIADH	Hyponatremia, Hypo-osmolality	11 or more	
ANP Syndrome	Hyponatremia, Hypotension Natriuresis	15	yes
Ectopic ACTH production	Cushingoid Symptoms	5	rarely
Lambert-Eaton Syndrome	Myasthenia-like symptoms	<5	yes
Cb degeneration Syndrome	Cerebellar symptoms	<5	rarely
CA-Associated Retinopathy	Blindness	<5	rarely

ANP, atrial natriuretic peptide; CA, cancer; Cb, cerebellar; SIADH, syndrome of inappropriate antidiuretic hormone secretion.

Source: Schild, S, Curran, Chapter 40, Small Cell Lung Cancer. In: W. *Clinical Radiation Oncology* 2nd ed. Elsevier/Churchill Livingstone ©2007.

contrast-enhanced computed tomography (CT) scan of the thorax and upper abdomen (including the entire liver and both adrenal glands, bone scan, and either CT or magnetic resonance imaging (MRI) scan of the brain. In addition, serum studies would include a complete blood count with differential and complete chemistry screening panel. Bone marrow aspirates and biopsies have been advocated by some investigators but are not currently performed for limited SCLC in most current trials. If all of these investigations confirm that the patient has limited-stage SCLC, the patient should also undergo pulmonary function testing to confirm his or her ability to tolerate aggressive thoracic RT. Positron emission tomography (PET) scans are quite accurate for the staging of this SCLC. PET scan can aid in both the choice of appropriate therapy because of more accurate staging of disease and as an aid in the RT planning by better identifying the target (23). PET scanning does not replace either CT or MRI of the brain in staging. Because the background uptake of the tracer is quite high in the brain, metastases are difficult to distinguish from the brain itself. In addition, recent changes in Medicare guidelines regarding the indications for PET will allow much greater use of this very helpful imaging modality for SCLC. PET can now be used in Medicare patients for the initial staging of SCLC.

Investigators need to be cautioned regarding the influence of ever improving staging techniques on the interpretation of survival results. Many patients previously believed to have limited disease are currently "upstaged" to the extensive-disease category because of more sensitive staging studies. It is likely that their inclusion in the extensive-disease group and their exclusion from the limited disease category will improve survival rates of both groups. This effect is known as the "Will Rogers phenomenon," which was first described in oncology among patients with SCLC and is based on the quotation, "When the Okies left Oklahoma and moved to California, they raised the average IQ in both states." The implication being that the people who left Oklahoma were of lesser intellect than those left behind but more intelligent than the general population of California. One method of reducing the statistical distortions of the Will Rogers phenomenon (stage migration) is to compare survival outcome of entire populations rather than on a stage-by-stage basis. The best method of controlling for this potential bias is to perform properly stratified randomized trials.

There have been several efforts to identify prognostic factors other than staging as a means to better select patients for specific therapies. As with many malignancies, good performance status, young age, and female gender are associated with better prognosis, and these have been verified in large multivariate analyses (24–27). Among available laboratory tests, elevated lactate dehydrogenase (LDH) serum levels were most commonly associated with a poor prognosis, and hyponatremia and low albumin level were found in several studies to be independent adverse prognostic factors. The metastatic site found to be most unfavorable was the liver. Although such studies are valuable in understanding a disease, they are confounded by the extent and quality of imaging evaluation, available therapies, and selection of variables tested. Risk categories have been created by two different British groups, which include prognostic factors such as performance status and several laboratory tests such as LDH, alkaline phosphatase, and sodium level. The Mayo Clinic/North Central Cancer Treatment Group (NCCTG) recently evaluated 1598 patients with SCLC to determine prognostic factors. Multivariate analysis revealed that performance status, age, gender, greater number of metastatic sites, and baseline creatinine levels were all associated with survival of patients with extensive disease. Among patients with limited disease, only age and gender were associated with survival (27). One critical reason for determining prognostic factors is to use them for the proper patient stratification and selection when designing trials. This allows the investigators to decrease uncontrolled biases from clouding the results of well-designed trials.

■ PRIMARY THERAPY

Decisions regarding optimal therapy of patients with limited-stage SCLC must consider a patient's pulmonary and cardiac fitness, ability to tolerate specific chemotherapeutic agents, prior history of malignancies and their treatment, as well as patient age and performance status. Since the diagnosis of limited-stage disease by definition implies the potential ability to receive an aggressive course of thoracic RT, such treatment should be feasible. The issues discussed in the following sections have generally been studied in trials involving patients with ambulatory performance status (using mainly the Zubrod Performance Score of 0–1); no prior anticancer therapy; and acceptable organ (pulmonary, cardiac, renal, and hepatic) function. How these principles can be applied to patients not meeting those criteria should be determined on an individual basis.

Although performance status is an important prognostic factor among SCLC patients, a decline in performance status may be related to factors other than the malignancy. With the help of pulmonary physicians or other caregivers, a patient suffering from treatable conditions such as bronchitis, pneumonia, or an exacerbation of chronic obstructive lung disease can improve his or her performance status prior to the initiation of therapy. Such an improvement may in turn increase the likelihood of tolerating and benefiting from aggressive multimodality therapy. Recent weight loss among patients with a lung malignancy is usually considered a symptom of cancer-related cachexia and will only be reversible with a response to anticancer therapy. However, there can be more easily reversible causes of weight loss among these patients, including problems with dentition or dentures, oral candidiasis, thoracic pain requiring analgesia, or gastroesophageal reflux. Management of these problems is also likely to improve a patient's tolerance of therapy.

Use of Thoracic RT

After the demonstration in the late 1960s of activity of several chemotherapeutic agents and the poor prognosis of patients treated with surgery and/or radiation alone, multiagent chemotherapy became the primary therapy for all stages of SCLC (28,29). Unfortunately, recurrence inevitably followed the response to chemotherapy and these relapses were most frequent in areas of previous disease. This pattern of failure led investigators to reexamine the use of thoracic RT for limited-stage SCLC. Today, both RT and chemotherapy have central roles in the treatment of limited-stage SCLC (30,31). A series of randomized trials have been performed comparing chemotherapy alone with chemotherapy with thoracic RT (32–35). In 1992, two meta-analyses were published regarding the role of thoracic RT in addition to chemotherapy (2,35). They were based on randomized prospective studies that compared chemotherapy alone to chemotherapy plus thoracic RT. Pignon et.al. reported a 3-year survival rate of 14.3%, with combined modality therapy compared to 8.9% with chemotherapy alone (P = .001). This 5.4% absolute difference in 3-year survival rates was identical to the 5.4% difference in 2-year survival (P <.001) reported by Warde and Payne (2). While this 5.4% difference may seem rather small, it represented a 61% increase in the 3-year survival of 8.9% achieved with chemotherapy alone (35). In addition, the intrathoracic tumor control was improved by 25.3% in the RT arms (2).

Sequencing and Timing of Thoracic RT and Chemotherapy

Chemotherapy and thoracic RT can be and have been delivered concurrently, sequentially, or in an alternating manner. Potential advantages of concurrent delivery include the shorter overall treatment time, an increase in overall treatment intensity, and potential anticancer synergism between the various therapies. Disadvantages include the heightened risk of toxicity and the inability to assess the antitumor response rate of the chemotherapy alone. The Japanese Clinical Oncology Group (JCOG) performed a phase 3 trial in which limited-stage SCLC patients were randomized to sequential or concurrent therapy. All 231 patients received four cycles of etoposide and cisplatin (EP) every 3 weeks (sequential arm) or 4 weeks (concurrent arm) and were randomized to receive thoracic RT during the first cycle of chemotherapy in the concurrent arm or after the fourth cycle in the sequential arm. Thoracic RT consisted of 45 Gy (1.5 Gy twice daily) over 3 weeks. Concurrent therapy yielded better survival than sequential therapy (P = .097). The median survival time was 19.7 months in the sequential arm versus 27.2 months in the concurrent arm. The 5-year survival rate for patients treated sequentially was 18.3% compared to 23.7% for those treated concurrently. Hematologic toxicity was more severe in the concurrent arm. However, severe esophagitis was infrequent in both arms, occurring in 9% of the patients in the concurrent arm and 4% in the sequential arm. The authors (36) concluded that the findings strongly suggested that concurrent therapy was more effective for the treatment of limited-stage SCLC than sequential therapy. While the P value was not significant, the trend favors concurrent therapy, which is also consistent with the studies that examined this issue for NSCLC (37,38).

There have been multiple randomized trials that have addressed the issue of timing of thoracic RT during programs of concurrent chemotherapy and thoracic RT. In the trial conducted by the Cancer and Leukemia Group B (CALGB) from 1981 to 1984, 426 limited-stage SCLC patients were treated with cyclophosphamide (C), etoposide (E) or doxorubicin (A), and vincristine (V) and randomized to (Arm 1) no thoracic RT; (Arm 2) thoracic RT starting during cycle 1 of chemotherapy; or (Arm 3) thoracic RT starting during cycle 4 (32). The thoracic RT in both arms was 50 Gy administered over a period of 6 weeks. There was a survival advantage favoring arms 2 and 3 over the no-RT arm, with the best results achieved in arm 3. The 5-year survival rates were 3% for chemotherapy alone, 7% for early thoracic RT, and 13% for delayed thoracic RT. One criticism of this trial is that the doses of chemotherapy in arm 2 are intentionally reduced to lessen the risk of heightened toxicity during concurrent thoracic RT early in a chemotherapy program.

A National Cancer Institute of Canada (NCIC) trial compared thoracic RT (40 Gy/15 fractions in 3 weeks) applied during cycle 2 versus cycle 6 of an alternating chemotherapy regimen including CAV and cisplatin-etoposide (39). A survival advantage was noted for the patients randomized to cycle 2 thoracic RT, with median survival times of 16 versus 12 months and 4-year survival rates of 25% versus 15%.

James et al. (40) reported a trial of early versus late thoracic RT. A total of 325 limited stage (L-SCLC) patients were randomized to early thoracic RT with the 2nd course of chemotherapy versus late thoracic RT with the 6th course of chemotherapy. The chemotherapy was identical in each arm and included 6 cycles of cyclophosphamide, doxorubicin, and vincristine (CAV), alternating with cisplatin and etoposide on days 1 through 3. The thoracic RT dose was 40 Gy in 15 fractions in 3 weeks. Prophylactic cranial RT was given to responding patients. Median and 3-year survival were 13.5 months and 16% with early thoracic RT versus 15.1 months and 20% with late thoracic RT ($P = .18$).

Thus, conflicting results have been reported regarding the timing of thoracic RT. However, recent meta-analyses do help make sense of the contradictory data. One study analyzed randomized trials published after 1985 addressing the timing of thoracic RT relative to chemotherapy in limited-stage SCLC. Early thoracic RT was initiated <9 weeks after starting of chemotherapy and late thoracic RT >9 weeks. Seven trials (n = 1,524 patients) met the inclusion criteria and were included. The relative risk of survival for early thoracic RT compared to late thoracic RT for all studies was 1.17 (95% confidence interval (CI), 1.02–1.35, $P = .03$), indicating an increased 2-year survival for early versus late thoracic RT patients. This translated to a 5.2% (95% CI, 0.6%–9.7%, $P = .03$) improvement in the 2-year survival for early thoracic RT. This small but significant improvement in 2-year survival for early thoracic RT was similar in overall magnitude to the benefit of adding thoracic RT or prophylactic cranial irradiation to chemotherapy (41).

A subsequent meta-analysis also investigated timing factors for combined chemotherapy and RT, with respect to long-term survival of patients with limited-disease small cell lung cancer. Using meta-analysis methodology to compare results within phase 3 trials, the influence of the timing of chest radiation and the start of any treatment until the end of RT (SER) on local tumor control, survival, and esophagitis was analyzed. The SER was the most important predictor of outcome. There was a significantly higher 5-year survival rate in the shorter SER arms (relative risk [RR] = 0.62; 95% CI, 0.49 to 0.80; $P = .0003$), which was more than 20% when the SER was less than 30 days (upper bound of 95% CI, 90 days). A low SER was also associated with a higher incidence of severe esophagitis (RR = 0.55; 95% CI, 0.42 to 073; $P < .0001$). Each week of extension of the SER beyond that of the study arm with the shortest SER resulted in an overall absolute decrease in the 5-year survival rate of 1.83% +/– 0.18% (95% CI). Less time between the first day of chemotherapy and the last day of chest RT was associated with improved survival in limited-stage SCLC patients (42).

In summary, it would appear that the therapeutic window of opportunity for thoracic RT to optimally improve survival is early during the chemotherapy. There may be reasons to delay the initiation of concurrent thoracic RT in limited situations for patients with very large tumors, very limited pulmonary function, or postobstructive atelectasis. In all three instances, one may spare more normal lung by irradiating the tumors after a favorable response to a few cycles of chemotherapy.

Thoracic Radiation Therapy Dose

SCLC is considered a relatively radioresponsive malignancy because low doses of thoracic RT, previously used, produced encouraging responses.

Total thoracic RT doses for limited-stage SCLC have ranged from 25 to 30 Gy in 10 fractions in the 1970s to up to 70 Gy in 35 fractions in recent years. Doses in the lower end of this range may have been acceptable when chemotherapy was less effective and disseminated disease occurred earlier in the course of disease. Improvements in systemic therapy have increased the need for aggressive thoracic RT regimens that produce more durable responses. It was estimated by Choi and Carey (43) that the risk of intrathoracic tumor recurrence at total doses of 40 Gy or less was 80%, and this was confirmed in an NCIC limited-stage SCLC trial in which patients were randomized between 25 Gy in 10 fractions and 37.5 Gy in 15 fractions (44). The 2-year actuarial rates of local failure were 80% and 69%, respectively.

The most commonly administered doses of thoracic RT range from 45 to 70 Gy in 1.8 to 2.0 Gy daily fractions. Although a RT dose-response can be well demonstrated for tumor control below 40 Gy, it is difficult to conclusively establish an RT dose to tumor-control relationship in the range between 40 and 60 Gy in standard fractionation. Most randomized and nonrandomized trials estimate the local tumor control rates in this dose range as between 58% and 85% (45). A single-institution trial from Yale–New Haven Hospital reported a local tumor control rate of 96%, with a total RT dose in excess of 60 Gy (46). The CALGB conducted a phase 1 dose escalation of standard fractionation and found that a dose higher than 70 Gy was the maximal tolerated dose, with the given assumptions with respect to RT field definitions and chemotherapy employed (46). A subsequent study was performed and found 70 Gy tolerable and effective. Eligible patients received two cycles of induction paclitaxel and topotecan with granulocyte colony stimulating factor support, followed by three cycles of carboplatin and etoposide. Thoracic RT (70 Gy, 2 Gy/fx/7 weeks) was initiated with the first cycle of carboplatin and etoposide. Prophylactic cranial irradiation (PCI) was offered to patients achieving a complete response or good partial response. There was one treatment-related fatality. Nonhematologic grade 3/4 toxicities affecting more than 10% of patients, during or after thoracic RT, were dysphagia (16%/5%) and febrile neutropenia (12%/4%). The median overall survival was 22.4 months. They concluded that 70 Gy once-daily thoracic RT could be delivered safely in the cooperative group setting for patients with limited-stage SCLC. Initial efficacy data are encouraging. They presented the hypothesis that high-dose once-daily thoracic RT results in comparable or improved survival compared with twice-daily accelerated thoracic RT and warrants testing in a phase 3 trial (47).

Altered Fractionation

In addition to increasing the number of daily treatment, another means of intensifying therapy is the use of altered radiation fractionation. For limited-stage SCLC patients, most altered fractionation strategies have employed twice-daily fractionation with fraction sizes varying from 1.1 to 1.8 Gy and total doses ranging from 40 to 54 Gy. Most regimens have tested the principle of accelerated hyperfractionation, in which a twice-daily regimen allows the delivery of a standard total RT dose over a shortened period. Such a regimen should benefit patients with rapidly growing tumors such as SCLC with a small shoulder and a steep slope on its radiobiologic cell survival curve.

Several encouraging pilot studies led to the development of an Eastern Cooperative Group (ECOG)-led phase 3 trial testing the concept that accelerated hyperfractionation would improve tumor control for limited-stage SCLC patients. The experimental regimen was 45.0 Gy in 1.5 Gy twice daily fractions beginning on day 1 of a four-cycle regimen of etoposide and cisplatin (EP). The inter-fraction interval was 6 to 8 hours and the elapsed treatment time was 19 to 21 days. This regimen was piloted by Turrisi et al. (48), in 23 patients resulting in a median survival time of 25 months and a 5-year survival rate of 36%. A subsequent multi-institution phase 2 trial of the same regimen conducted by ECOG resulted in a 2-year survival rate of 36% (49). These results were considered sufficiently promising to launch the ECOG-led phase 3 trial (Intergroup Trial 0096) in 1988. A total of 419 patients were randomized between the thoracic RT regimens of 45.0 Gy in 1.8 Gy once-daily fractions versus 45.0 Gy in 30–1.5 Gy twice daily fractions. Of these, 8 treatments were often given with off cord oblique fields to limit the spinal cord to 36 Gy. In both arms the thoracic RT began on day 1 of a four-cycle course of cisplatin and etoposide. There was a significant survival advantage for the twice daily thoracic RT patients compared to the once daily thoracic RT patients, with 5-year survival rates of 26% versus 16%, respectively ($P = .04$). The median survival time was 19 months for the once-daily RT group and 23 months for the twice-daily RT group. The intrathoracic tumor failure rate was 36% for the twice-daily RT arm and 52% for the once-daily RT arm ($P = .06$). The principal difference in toxicity was a higher rate of grade 3 esophagitis in the twice-daily RT arm: 27% versus 11% ($P < .001$) (50). This study confirms the principle that an intensification of thoracic RT beyond the older standard of relatively low dose once daily RT can improve both local control and survival. This trial has altered the standard of care of limited-stage SCLC patients in the United States. Currently, this twice-daily dose-fractionation program is considered to be the standard by which all other programs are compared to.

The North Central Cancer Treatment Group (NCCTG) performed a trial (89-20-52) which has been misinterpreted as contradicting the findings of the Intergroup Trial 0096. The findings of these studies provide complimentary information regarding twice daily thoracic RT. This NCCTG trial included 310 patients with limited-stage SCLC initially treated with 3 cycles of EP (51). Subsequently, the 261 patients without significant progression were randomized to 2 cycles of EP plus either once daily thoracic RT (50.4Gy/28 fractions) or split-course twice daily RT (24 Gy/16 fractions followed by a 2.5 week break and then an additional 24 Gy/16 fractions). Patients then received a 6th cycle of EP followed by prophylactic cranial irradiation. The median and 5-year survival rates from randomization, were 20.6 months and 21% for patients who received once-daily RT compared to 20.6 months and 22% for those who received twice-daily RT($P = .68$). There were no significant differences in the rates of intrathoracic failure or distant failure between the treatment arms. There was no significant difference in the overall rates of grade 3 or greater (3+) or grade 4+ toxicity. Grade 3+esophagitis ($P = .05$) was more common in the BID arm as was grade 5 toxicity which occurred in 4/130 (3%) patients who received twice-daily RT compared to 0/131 (0%) who received once-daily RT ($P = .04$). The findings of these two randomized prospective studies comparing once-daily to twice-daily thoracic RT for limited-stage SCLC lead to the conclusion that continuous course twice-daily RT is better than once-daily RT, but split course twice-daily RT is not. This finding has precedence and is identical to the findings regarding twice-daily RT in head and neck cancer. The RTOG conducted a phase 3 randomized trial (RTOG 9003), in patients with locally advanced squamous cell carcinomas of the head and neck, which compared various RT regimens. Patients treated in the continuously administered twice-daily RT arms had better local-regional control than those treated with split course twice-daily or standard once-daily RT arms. This study also found that while continuously administered twice-daily RT was better than once-daily RT, split course twice-daily RT was not (52).

There has also been investigation of higher doses of twice-daily thoracic RT in an attempt to further improve outcome. NCCTG 95-20-53 was a phase 2 trial that included 6 cycles of cisplatin and etoposide (PE) (53). PCI (25 Gy/10 fractions) was delivered during cycle 3 to responding patients. Cycles 4 and 5 included concurrent chemotherapy and thoracic RT (30 Gy/20 twice-daily fractions followed by a 2-week break, and another 30 Gy/20 twice daily fractions). The 5-year survival rate of the 76 evaluable patients was 24% (median: 20 months). The 5-year survival rate of the 64 patients who received thoracic RT was 29% (median: 22 months). The 5-year cumulative incidence of in-field failure was 34%. This regimen included a high total dose of twice-daily thoracic RT, which resulted in a favorable 5-year survival rate. Local failure remains a problem that will require further investigation. Newer technology should allow the safe administration of greater doses of RT, which will improve patient outcome. Schild et al. (53) evaluated data from this trial (NCCTG 95-20-53) and others to demonstrate a relationship between RT dose fractionation and 5-year survival.

Thoracic RT decreases the tumor burden within the chest resulting in enhanced local control and survival. In spite of the addition of thoracic RT to chemotherapy, local failures occur in approximately one-third of patients treated with the currently accepted optimal therapy. Long-term survival occurs in about one-quarter of patients so treated. These results indicate the need for improved treatment strategies to combat this disease. In all situations in which RT affects a response, there exists a dose-response relationship much in the same way that drugs affect a physiologic outcome. Local control and subsequent survival are associated with both the timing of RT and dose-fractionation parameters.

When attempting to improve therapy, the goal should be obtain the longest possible patient survival with the least toxicity. Altering the fractionation pattern is one method used to improve the therapeutic index of RT. Some of the parameters used to develop a fractionation pattern include overall time, total dose, and fraction size. These factors can be adjusted for the proliferative nature of the tumor in question and the tolerance of the surrounding normal tissues. The biologically effective dose (BED)(formula shown below) can be used to compare the efficacy of various dose-fractionation regimens in providing tumor control (see Table 3). The first portion of the formula accounts for the efficacy provided by a particular fractionation program and the second part accounts for the decrease in efficacy related to the overall time RT is delivered compared to the potential doubling time of the tumor cells (53).

$$BED = (nd)(1+(d/(\alpha/\beta))-(0.693\ t\ /\alpha\ T_{pot})$$

n = the total number of fractions delivered
d = the dose per fraction (Gy)
α/β = 10 for acute effects and tumor control and 3 for chronic effects
α = 0.3 Gy
t = total days in which radiotherapy is delivered
T_{pot} = potential doubling time (5.6 days)

The potential doubling time (T_{pot}) for SCLC has been reported in the radiobiology literature to range from 2.6 to 8.6 days. Thus, a break in the RT decreases the BED and the efficacy of the regimen because a greater overall time of RT allows tumor repopulation to occur. The potential relationship between BED of thoracic RT and 5-year survival was evaluated for this trial and the randomized trials that included various thoracic RT programs. Studies selected included only phase 3 trials that administered platinum plus etoposide concurrently with thoracic RT reported between 1997 and 2004 (36,50,51,54,55). The Intergroup Trial 0096 compared once-daily to twice-daily RT and found that the twice-daily RT approach resulted in significantly better survival (50). NCCTG trial 89-20-52 compared once-daily to split-course twice-daily RT and found similar survival rates for both groups (51). The trials reported by Qiao et al. (55) and Takada et al. (36) compared sequential to concurrent administration of chemotherapy plus thoracic RT and concluded that concurrent therapy was superior. The trial of Jeremic et al. (54) compared the early versus late administration of twice-daily RT and concluded that the early administration of twice-daily RT was better. For the purposes of the following BED analysis, the early RT arm from Jeremic et al. was included as were the concurrent therapy arms from Qiao et al. (55) and Takada et al. (36). The RT regimens and 5-year survival rates derived from the 904 patients included in these trials are shown in Table 3 (36,50,51, 53–56). Then, the BED of the thoracic RT was plotted against the resulting 5-year survival reported in these studies (Figure 1). The Pearson Correlation Coefficient between BED and 5-year survival was 0.81 indicating a strong positive correlation.

Survival was used in this analysis rather than local control because of difficulties in objectively comparing local control rates reported in various studies. Some studies use chest radiographs and other

TABLE 3 Dose-fractionation, biologically effective doses (Gy10), and survival for patients with limited-stage small cell lung cancer

			RT Schedule				Corrected for Proliferation	
Source		**D (Gy)**	**d (Gy/fx)**	**No. of Fractions**	**t**	**No. of Patients**	**Gy10**	**5-Year Survival (%)**
Schild et al. 95-20-53	bid	60.0	1.5	40	40	64	52.50	29
Intergroup 0096	qd	45.0	1.8	25	33	206	39.49	16
Intergroup 0096	bid	45.0	1.5	30	19	211	43.91	26
NCCTG 89-20-52	qd	50.4	1.8	28	38	130	43.80	21
NCCTG 89-20-52	bid	48.0	1.5	32	38	131	39.53	22
Qiao et al.	qd	60.0	2.0	30	40	45	55.50	27
Jeremic et al.	bid	54.0	1.5	36	26	52	51.38	30
Takada et al.	bid	45.0	1.5	30	19	65	43.91	24

D, total dose of each regimen in Gy; d, dose per fraction; t, total no. of days of the RT regimen.

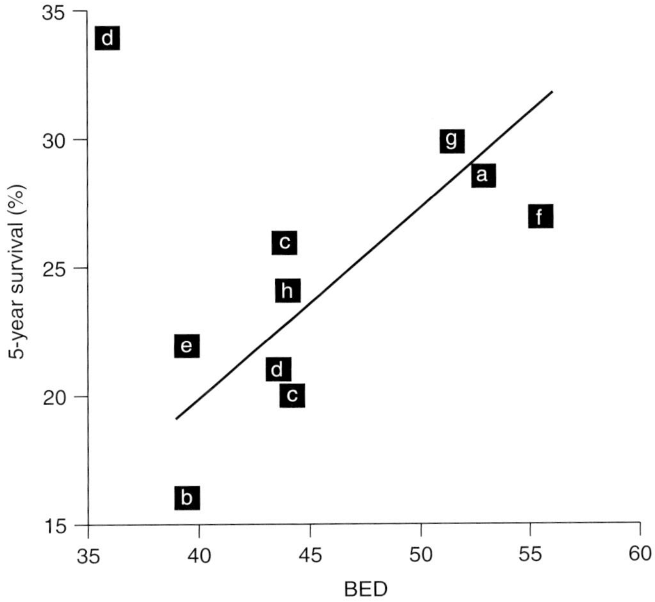

FIGURE 1 Five-year survival vs. biologically effective doses (BED) used in the thoracic radiotherapy programs found in Table 3. A spline fit function found that the equation of the line is 5-year survival in %= 10 + 0.76 x BED.

CTs to assess local control. PET or rebiopsy is likely to be more accurate in determining local control. However, survival is an objective endpoint that is difficult to misjudge.

One can go further in using a spline fit function to define a line that runs an average path between the various points each weighted by the number of patients on that trial. This line may very simplistically define the relationship between 5-year survival and BED. The equation of the line is 5-year survival in % = 10+0.76 × BED. The may be helpful to use in trying to estimate the probability of 5-year survival from a particular RT program used early and concurrently with cisplatin and etoposide.

There is at least one other study which found that dose-fractionation significantly influences survival (50). Komaki et al. (57) also reported that a greater BED was associated with survival in a multivariate analysis of the MD Anderson experience. CALGB and Radiation Therapy Oncology Group (RTOG) are leading a national trial (CALGB 30601/RTOG 0538) comparing the standard arm of 45 Gy/30 fractions twice daily to 70 Gy/35 once-daily fractions and 61.2 Gy in a mixed once- and twice-daily regimen.

Treatment Volumes and Normal Tissue Considerations

The ability of a limited-stage SCLC patient to tolerate increasingly aggressive RT regimens and higher total doses during concurrent chemotherapy is in part related to RT target volume selection (45). In the early 1980s, both CALGB and SWOG authors demonstrated poorer survival when patients were not treated with the recommended large fields employing elective nodal RT (58,59). Mira and Livingston (60) also demonstrated tumor failures just beyond the margins of the thoracic RT fields when the fields were designed following a response to chemotherapy. These reports lent further support for the need for generous thoracic RT fields. An example of such a field would be that the RT target volume for a patient with a tumor in the left upper lobe with ipsilateral hilar and mediastinal adenopathy might include only the tumor itself with a 2.0-cm margin, both hilar regions, the mediastinum from the thoracic inlet to at least the subcarinal region, and both supraclavicular regions. Such large fields were in part responsible for the acceptance of a moderate total RT dose as appropriate for SCLC, since the large volume irradiated precluded a substantial increase in dose.

In a report by the VA Surgical Oncology Group published in 1982, 5-year survival rates for patients with resected T1N0, T1 N1, and T2N0 small cell lesions were 60%, 31%, and 28%, respectively (75). All of these patients received the chemotherapy available in the 1970s postoperatively. A SWOG protocol enrolled 15 SCLC patients to undergo surgical resection followed by chemoradiation and found this group to have a better 2-year survival rate than a cohort of matched patients treated nonoperatively in other SWOG trials (45% vs. 14%) (76). Ichinose and colleagues (77) reported on 112 SCLC patients who underwent surgical resection and were then randomized between two chemotherapy regimens. Although the chemotherapy regimens produced comparable outcomes, the 3-year survival rates were encouraging for all enrolled patients: 65% for N0 disease, 52% for N1 disease, and 29% for N2 disease. Chandra et al. (78) also found a relatively favorable 5-year survival of 38% in patients with stages I and II SCLC who had resections performed. Each of these three reports suggests that for the rare SCLC patients with N0 or N1 disease, surgical resection followed by chemotherapy produces survival results that may be superior to nonoperative approaches. The role of postoperative thoracic RT in this setting remains uncertain. A pattern-of-failure study of patients with completely resected SCLC receiving postoperative chemotherapy alone would help clarify this issue.

At least four studies have evaluated the role of surgical resection of patients with L-SCLC following initial chemotherapy. In the three phase 2 trials conducted at Vanderbilt and the University of Toronto and on a multi-institutional basis, a post-chemotherapy pathologic N0 status or a pathologic complete response was associated with long-term survival (79–81). A randomized trial was conducted by the Lung Cancer Study Group (LCSG) in which L-SCLC patients achieving a partial or complete response to chemotherapy were randomized between resection and no resection (82). There was no survival difference between the arms, with a 2-year survival rate of 20% in both arms (P = .55). Based on this trial and on the proven survival benefit of concurrent thoracic RT, adjuvant surgery following chemotherapy is not recommended.

There is limited information regarding the role of surgical resection of intrathoracic recurrences. Shepherd and coworkers from the University of Toronto reported on 28 limited-stage SCLC patients who underwent salvage surgery following either a partial response to chemotherapy or subsequent progressive disease (83). Of these 28 patients 10 had NSCLC elements in their specimen. Their 5-year survival rate from the date of surgical salvage was 23%. There is only anecdotal information of surgical salvage of patients initially treated with both chemotherapy and thoracic RT. While there may be a role for resection in patients with stages I or II SCLC, it is unclear that surgical intervention would provide a benefit when compared with RT for similar volumes/stages of disease. While it appears that some patients may be salvaged after a partial response or local failure, surgical intervention at that point in care has not been widely used. This may be in part to the propensity of SCLC to spread to distant sites.

Prophylactic Cranial Irradiation

Prophylactic cranial irradiation (PCI) was initially introduced into practice in the 1960s for patients with acute lymphoblastic leukemia who had a high risk of failure in the central nervous system (CNS) (84). It was first tested for patients with SCLC in the 1970s following the recognition that brain metastases are frequent. The blood brain barrier prevents the penetration of most chemotherapeutic agents leaving the brain as a sanctuary site for relapse. The first trials demonstrated a substantial reduction in brain metastases, with one randomized trial of more than 200 patients conducted by ECOG revealing a decrease from 22% to 5% (85). Unfortunately, at the same time, a number of long-term survivors of SCLC were noted to have various neurologic abnormalities, including dementia, and many of these patients had received PCI (86,87). The lack of prospective evidence linking PCI to these changes as well as the uncertainty as to the optimal total PCI dose and fractionation and its optimal time of delivery contributed to a lack of enthusiasm for PCI.

Two large randomized trials evaluated both the therapeutic benefit and neurotoxicity of PCI for SCLC patients following response to initial therapy. In two French trials jointly coordinated to run parallel (PCI 85 and PCI 88), a total of 505 patients were randomized between PCI and no PCI following a complete response to chemotherapy (88). Most patients received 24.0 Gy in eight 3.0 Gy fractions. There was a highly significant reduction in overall and isolated brain relapse rates favoring the PCI-containing arms (40% vs. 59% and 39% vs. 57%, respectively; $P < .0001$) and a non-significant trend toward improved survival at 2 years (31% vs. 27%; $P = .10$). There was a slight increase in clinical asymptomatic imaging abnormalities but no significant CNS morbidity reported.

Gregor and associates reported on a 314-patient multi-center trial conducted in the United Kingdom (UK02) that randomized L-SCLC patients in remission after completion of chemotherapy between PCI and no PCI (89). Forty percent of the PCI patients received 30.0 Gy in 10 fractions, and other regimens ranged from 8 Gy in 1 fraction to 36.0 Gy in 18 fractions. At 2-year follow-up, a reduction in brain relapse was seen for the PCI arm from 52% to 29% ($P = .0002$). The advantage was greatest for the patients receiving the higher PCI doses, particularly 36.0 Gy in 18 fractions. There was also a non-significant trend in overall survival outcome favoring the PCI arm ($P = .14$). Detailed neuro-psychometric testing of both PCI patients and controls failed to demonstrate a substantial treatment-related deficit. There was, however, substantial impairment of function in up to 40% of patients prior to PCI, suggesting that factors other than PCI may contribute to neurologic dysfunction among SCLC patients. This may be due to the effects of this disease, therapy, and stress.

In addition to thoracic RT, PCI has been shown to positively influence survival in patients who achieve a complete response (CR). Auperin et al. (90) published a meta-analysis that included data from seven randomized prospective studies that compared PCI to no PCI after a CR was achieved. As in the thoracic RT meta-analyses, the 3-year survival rate was 5.4% better for those who received PCI at 20.7% compared with 15.3% for those who did not receive PCI ($P = .01$). While 5.4% appears small, it does reflect a 35% increase in 3-year survivors. A statistically significant PCI dose-response was noted for the risk of brain recurrence but not survival rates. Neurotoxicity was not evaluated in this analysis.

The European Organization for Research and Treatment of Cancer (EORTC) evaluated dose-fractionation patterns in an international phase 3 trial (91). Their randomized clinical trial compared the effect of standard versus higher PCI doses on the incidence of brain metastases. This trial included 720 patients with limited-stage SCLC in complete remission after chemotherapy and thoracic RT. They were randomly assigned to a standard ($n = 360$, 25 Gy in 10 daily fractions of 2.5 Gy) or higher PCI total dose ($n = 360$, 36 Gy) delivered using either conventional (18 daily fractions of 2 Gy) or accelerated hyperfractionated (24 fractions in 16 days with two daily sessions of 1.5 Gy separated by a minimum interval of 6 hours) RT. All of the treatment schedules excluded weekends. The primary endpoint was the incidence of brain metastases at 2 years. After a median follow-up of 39 months (range 0–89 months), 145 patients had brain metastases: 82 in the standard-dose group and 63 in the higher-dose group. There was no significant difference in the 2-year incidence of brain metastases between the standard PCI dose group and the higher-dose group, at 29% and 23%, respectively ($P = .18$). The 2-year overall survival was 42% in the standard-dose group and 37% in the higher-dose group ($P = .05$). The lower overall survival in the higher-dose group is probably due to increased cancer-related mortality: 189 patients in the standard group versus 218 in the higher-dose group died of progressive disease. The most common acute toxic events were fatigue (106 [30%] patients in the standard-dose group vs. 121 [34%] in the higher-dose group), headache (85 [24%] vs. 99 [28%]), and nausea or vomiting (80 [23%] vs. 101 [28%]). They concluded that while there was a significant reduction in the total incidence of brain metastases observed after higher-dose PCI, there was also a significant increase in mortality. Therefore, PCI at 25 Gy in 10 fractions should remain the standard of care in L-SCLC (91).

On the basis of the currently available data, it is recommended that SCLC patients achieving any degree of response to initial therapy should be offered PCI appears to significantly improve survival. The current standard dose-fractionation pattern is 25 Gy per 10 fractions.

■ TREATMENT ALGORITHM/ CONTROVERSIES/CLINICAL TRIALS

Limited-Stage Disease, Good Performance Status

Management of patients with SCLC is dependent on patient stage and medical fitness. For patients with good performance status and limited-stage disease (clinical stages I to IIIB, excluding those with a malignant pleural effusion), the recommended management would be concurrent thoracic RT with platinum-based chemotherapy. Specifically, the most widely accepted management in the United States includes four cycles of cisplatin and etoposide chemotherapy with twice-daily thoracic RT beginning early (41,42). The twice-daily RT would be delivered in 1.5 Gy fractions with an interfraction interval of at least 6 hours to a total dose of 45.0 Gy, with 8–10 of the 30 fractions sparing the spinal cord. This recommendation is based on the Intergroup Trial 0096 reported by Turrisi et al. (50). Encouraging patients to participate in a trial such as the current CALGB/RTOG trial (CALGB 30601/RTOG 0538) will help determine which of three thoracic RT regimens is best. For patients with huge tumors, postobstructive pneumonia, or atelectasis, there may be value in delaying initiation of thoracic RT until a later cycle of chemotherapy. This may be necessary in some cases to allow one to treat less normal lung if the initial tumor volume would require an excessively larger volume of normal lung to be treated. There are rare patients who have resection performed before RT. It is unknown whether adding thoracic RT improves the outcome of patients with completely resected SCLC. However, chemotherapy is generally administered after resection.

Limited-Stage Disease in Special Populations: The Elderly and Those With a Lower Performance Status

Treatment in fit elderly patients (>70 years of age) can be carried out in a manner similar to fit younger individuals. NCCTG 89-20-52 (described earlier) included 263 patients with L-SCLC and an ECOG performance status of <2 who were randomized to once-daily thoracic RT or split course twice-daily thoracic RT. The outcomes of the 209 (79%) younger patients (<70 years old) were compared with the 54 (21%) elderly patients (>70 years old). The overall incidence of grade >3 (3+) or grade >4 (4+) toxicity was not significantly greater in elderly patients. One specific toxicity, grade 4+ pneumonitis occurred in 0% of those <70 years compared to 6% of older patients (P = .008). Although hematologic toxicity was not significantly worse in those >70 years old, it was significantly worse in patients >65 years old compared with younger individuals (P = .03). Grade 5 toxicity occurred in 3 out of 54 (5.6%) patients >70 years old compared to 1 out of 209 (0.5%) younger individuals (P = .03). These deaths occurred due to pneumonitis in the three elderly patients and infection in the patient <70 years of age. The 2-year and 5-year survival rates were 48% and 22% in younger patients compared to 33% and 17% in older patients (P = .14). Survival was not significantly worse in older individuals. Fit elderly patients with L-SCLC can receive combined modality therapy, if carefully monitored, with a reasonable expectation of 5-year survival (92). Data on patients who are 80 years old or greater is scarce; therefore, some degree of caution in the very oldest patients is warranted.

Patients with lower performance status tolerate the aggressive twice-daily thoracic RT and platinum-based therapy more poorly than those with good performance status. However, there is still a likely benefit to concurrent chemoradiation for these patients, particularly if their reduced functional status is primarily due to their tumor burden. One reasonable option would be to deliver once-daily thoracic RT in 1.8 Gy fractions to 50 to 60 Gy, while sparing the spinal cord above 45 Gy. This could be delivered beginning with the first or second cycle of platinum-based chemotherapy. Judgment and flexibility are critical in attempting to fine-tune therapy to very old (>80 years) or poor performance status patients. It is also reasonable to administer sequential therapy for patients who could not tolerate the rigors of concurrent therapy.

Prophylactic Cranial Irradiation

Prophylactic cranial irradiation should be considered for all SCLC patients who have achieved any degree of response following initial management with chemotherapy or chemoradiation and without evidence of disease progression elsewhere. 25 Gy in 10 fractions is considered the most standard regimen (91).

Controversies/Clinical Trials

Issues addressed in current clinical trials include the benefit of twice-daily thoracic RT (45 Gy/30 twice daily fractions) versus higher BED thoracic RT regimens and the value of new systemic agents in the management of limited-stage SCLC. With the approval of PET for the initial staging of SCLC, there will be improvements in staging and the RT planning. Improvements in imaging allow one to better identify and target tumor while optimally sparing adjacent normal tissues.

A

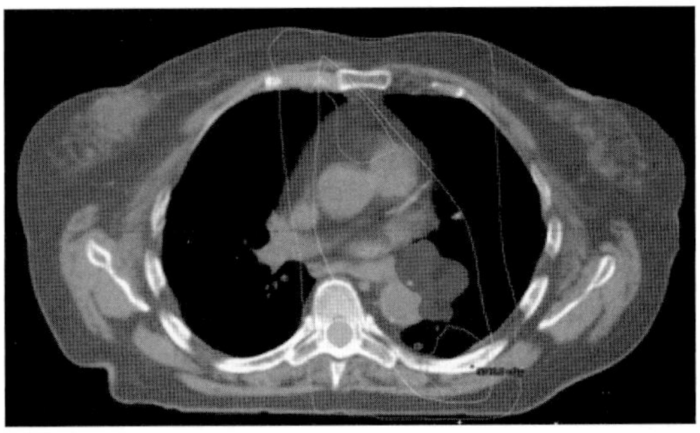

B

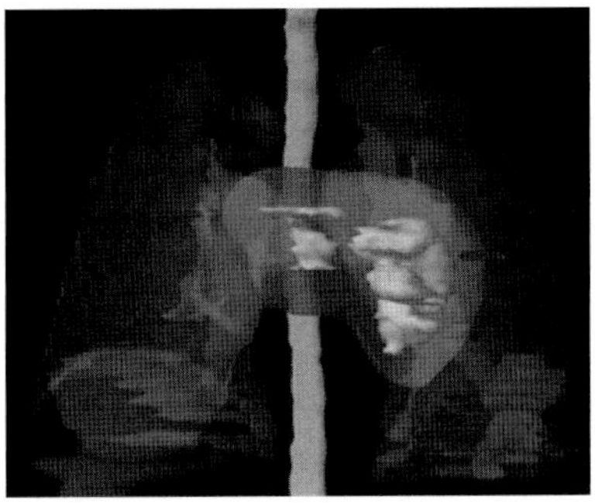

FIGURE 2 A. Dosimetric plan used for L-SCLC: AP: PA fields and opposed oblique fields (off the spinal cord). Doses shown are 48, 45, and 20 Gy. B. A dose cloud of 45 Gy is shown surrounding all gross disease detectable on PET/CT. Gross tumor received 45 Gy in 30 twice-daily fractions and the spinal cord received no more than 36 Gy.

REFERENCES

1. Jemal, A, Siegel, R, Ward, E, Hao, Y, Xu, J, Thun, MJ. Cancer statistics, 2009. *CA Cancer J Clin.* 2009;59(4):225–249.
2. Warde, P, Payne, D. Does thoracic irradiation improve survival and local control in limited-stage small-cell carcinoma of the lung? A meta-analysis. *J Clin Oncol.* 1992;10:890–895.
3. NCI. Cancer Statistics Review 1975–2002. Available at: http://seer.cancer.gov/csr/1975–2002/
4. http://www.cancer.gov/cancertopics/pdq/treatment/small-cell-lung/healthprofessional. Accessed January 9, 2009.
5. Green, RA, Humphrey, E, Close, H, Patno, ME. Alkylating agents in bronchogenic carcinoma. *Am J Med.* 1969;46:516–525.
6. Beasley, MB, Brambilla, E, Travis, WD. The 2004 World Health Organization classification of lung tumors. *Semin Roentgenol.* 2005;40:90–97.
7. Dy, GK, Adjei, AA. Novel targets for lung cancer therapy: part I. *J Clin Oncol.* 2002;20:2881–2894.
8. Hibi, K, Takahashi, T, Yamakawa, K, et al. Three distinct regions involved in 3p deletion in human lung cancer. *Oncogene.* 1992;7:445–449.
9. Sozzi, G, Veronese, ML, Negrini, M, et al. The *FHIT* gene *3p14.2* is abnormal in lung cancer. *Cell.* 1996;85:17–26.
10. Harbour, JW, Lai, SL, Whang-Peng, J, Gazdar, AF, Minna, JD, Kaye, FJ. Abnormalities in structure and expression of the human retinoblastoma gene in SCLC. *Science* (New York). 1988;241:353–357.
11. Gazdar, AF. Molecular markers for the diagnosis and prognosis of lung cancer. *Cancer.* 1992;69:1592–1599.
12. Ben-Ezra, JM, Kornstein, MJ, Grimes, MM, Krystal, G. Small cell carcinomas of the lung express the Bcl-2 protein. *Am J Pathol.* 1994;145:1036–1040.
13. Slebos, RJ, Kibbelaar, RE, Dalesio, O, et al. *K-ras* oncogene activation as a prognostic marker in adenocarcinoma of the lung. *N Engl J Med.* 1990;323:561–565.
14. Gazdar, AF. The molecular and cellular basis of human lung cancer. *Anticancer Res.* 1994;14:261–267.
15. Kelly, M, Linnoila, R, Avis, I. Antitumor activity of a monoclonal antibody directed against gastrin-releasing peptide in patients with small cell lung cancer. *Chest.* 1997;112:256–261.
16. Johnson, B, Kelly, M. Autocrine growth factors and neuroendocrine markers in the development of small cell lung cancer. *Oncology.* 1998;12:11–14.
17. List, AF, Hainsworth, JD, Davis, BW, Hande, KR, Greco, FA, Johnson, DH. The syndrome of inappropriate secretion of antidiuretic hormone (SIADH) in small-cell lung cancer. *J Clin Oncol.* 1986;4:1191–1198.
18. Dimopoulos, MA, Fernandez, JF, Samaan, NA, Holoye, PY, Vassilopoulou-Sellin, R. Paraneoplastic Cushing's syndrome as an adverse prognostic factor in patients who die early with small cell lung cancer. *Cancer.* 1992;69:66–71.
19. Patel, AM, Davila, DG, Peters, SG. Paraneoplastic syndromes associated with lung cancer. *Mayo Clin Proc.* 1993;68:278–287.
20. de la Monte, SM, Hutchins, GM, Moore, GW. Paraneoplastic syndromes and constitutional symptoms in prediction of metastatic behavior of small cell carcinoma of the lung. *Am J Med.* 1984;77:851–857.
21. Marchioli, CC, Graziano, SL. Paraneoplastic syndromes associated with small cell lung cancer. *Chest Surg Clin N Am.* 1997;7:65–80.
22. Stahel, R, Ginsberg, R, Havermann, K. Staging and prognostic factors in small cell lung cancer: A consensus. *Lung Cancer.* 1989;5:119–126.
23. Kamel, EM, Zwahlen, D, Wyss, MT, Stumpe, KD, von Schulthess, GK, Steinert, HC. Whole-body (18)F-FDG PET improves the management of patients with small cell lung cancer. *J Nucl Med.* 2003;44:1911–1917.
24. Albain, KS, Crowley, JJ, LeBlanc, M, Livingston, RB. Determinants of improved outcome in small-cell lung cancer: an analysis of the 2,580-patient Southwest Oncology Group data base. *J Clin Oncol.* 1990;8:1563–1574.
25. Souhami, RL, Bradbury, I, Geddes, DM, Spiro, SG, Harper, PG, Tobias, JS. Prognostic significance of laboratory parameters measured at diagnosis in small cell carcinoma of the lung. *Cancer Res.*1985;45:2878–2882.

26. Cerny, T, Blair, V, Anderson, H, Bramwell, V, Thatcher, N. Pretreatment prognostic factors and scoring system in 407 small-cell lung cancer patients. *Int J Cancer.* 1987;39:146–149.
27. Foster, NR, Mandrekar, SJ, Schild, SE, et al. Prognostic factors differ by tumor stage for small cell lung cancer: a pooled analysis of North Central Cancer Treatment Group trials. *Cancer.* 2009;115:2721–2731.
28. Edmondson, J, Lagakos, S, Selawry, O. Cyclophosphamide and CCNU in the treatment of inoperable small cell carcinoma and adenocarcinoma of the lung. *Cancer Treat Rep.* 1976;60:925–932.
29. Lowenbraun, S, Bartolucci, A, Smalley, RV, Lynn, M, Krauss, S, Durant, JR. The superiority of combination chemotherapy over single agent chemotherapy in small cell lung carcinoma. *Cancer.* 1979;44:406–413.
30. Souhami, RL, Geddes, DM, Spiro, SG, et al. RT in small cell cancer of the lung treated with combination chemotherapy: a controlled trial. *BMJ* (Clinical Research ed.) 1984;288:1643–1646.
31. Byhardt, RW, Cox, JD, PY, HO, Libnoch, JA. The role of consolidation irradiation in combined modality therapy of small cell carcinoma of the lung. *Int J Radiat Oncol Biol Phys.* 1982;8:1271–1276.
32. Perry, MC, Eaton, WL, Propert, KJ, et al. Chemotherapy with or without radiation therapy in limited small-cell carcinoma of the lung. *N Engl J Med.* 1987;316: 912–918.
33. Bunn, PA, Jr., Lichter, AS, Makuch, RW, et al. Chemotherapy alone or chemotherapy with chest radiation therapy in limited stage small cell lung cancer. A prospective, randomized trial. *Ann Intern Med.* 1987;106:655–662.
34. Perez, CA, Krauss, S, Bartolucci, AA, et al. Thoracic and elective brain irradiation with concomitant or delayed multiagent chemotherapy in the treatment of localized small cell carcinoma of the lung: a randomized prospective study by the Southeastern Cancer Study Group. *Cancer.* 1981;47:2407–2413.
35. Pignon, JP, Arriagada, R, Ihde, DC, et al. A meta-analysis of thoracic RT for small-cell lung cancer. *N Engl J Med.* 1992;327:1618–1624.
36. Takada, M, Fukuoka, M, Kawahara, M, et al. Phase 3 study of concurrent versus sequential thoracic RT in combination with cisplatin and etoposide for limited-stage small-cell lung cancer: results of the Japan Clinical Oncology Group Study 9104. *J Clin Oncol.* 2002;20:3054–3060.
37. Curran, WJ, Scott, CB, Langer, CJ, et al. Long-term benefit is observed in a phase 3 comparison of sequential vs concurrent chemo-radiation for patients with unresected stage III nsclc: RTOG 9410 (abstract #2499). 2003 annual meeting of ASCO, *Proc Am Soc Clin Oncol ASCO.* 2003;page 621.
38. Furuse, K, Fukuoka, M, Kawahara, M, et al. Phase 3 study of concurrent versus sequential thoracic RT in combination with mitomycin, vindesine, and cisplatin in unresectable stage III non-small-cell lung cancer. *J Clin Oncol.* 1999;17:2692–2699.
39. Murray, N, Coy, P, Pater, JL, et al. Importance of timing for thoracic irradiation in the combined modality treatment of limited-stage small-cell lung cancer. The National Cancer Institute of Canada Clinical Trials Group. *J Clin Oncol.* 1993;11:336–344.
40. James, L, Spiro, S, O'Donnell, K, Rudd, R. A randomised study of timing of thoracic irradiation in small cell lung cancer-study 8.Abstract: O-69 *Lung Cancer.* 2003;41:23.
41. Fried, DB, Morris, DE, Poole, C, et al. Systematic review evaluating the timing of thoracic radiation therapy in combined modality therapy for limited-stage small-cell lung cancer. *J Clin Oncol.* 2004;22:4837–4845.
42. De Ruysscher, D, Pijls-Johannesma, M, Bentzen, SM, et al. Time between the first day of chemotherapy and the last day of chest radiation is the most important predictor of survival in limited-disease small-cell lung cancer. *J Clin Oncol.* 2006;24:1057–1063.
43. Choi, NC, Carey, RW. Importance of radiation dose in achieving improved loco-regional tumor control in limited stage small-cell lung carcinoma: an update. *Int J Radiat Oncol Biol Phys.* 1989;17:307–310.
44. Coy, P, Hodson, I, Payne, DG, et al. The effect of dose of thoracic irradiation on recurrence in patients with limited stage small cell lung cancer. Initial results of a Canadian Multicenter Randomized Trial. *Int J Radiat Oncol Biol Phys.* 1988;14:219–226.
45. Lichter, AS, Turrisi, AT, 3rd. Small cell lung cancer: the influence of dose and treatment volume on outcome. *Semin Radiat Oncol.* 1995;5:44–49.
46. Choi, NC, Herndon, JE, 2nd, Rosenman, J, et al. Phase 1 study to determine the maximum-tolerated dose of radiation in standard daily and hyperfractionated-accelerated twice-daily radiation schedules with concurrent chemotherapy for limited-stage small-cell lung cancer. *J Clin Oncol.* 1998;16:3528–3536.
47. Bogart, JA, Herndon, JE, 2nd, Lyss, AP, et al. 70 Gy thoracic RT is feasible concurrent with chemotherapy for limited-stage small-cell lung cancer: analysis of cancer and leukemia group B study 39808. *Int J Radiat Oncol Biol Phys.* 2004;59:460–468.
48. Turrisi, AT, 3rd, Glover, DJ, Mason, BA. A preliminary report: concurrent twice-daily RT plus platinum-etoposide chemotherapy for limited small cell lung cancer. *Int J Radiat Oncol Biol Phys.* 1988;15:183–187.
49. Johnson, DH, Turrisi, AT, Chang, AY, et al. Alternating chemotherapy and twice-daily thoracic RT in limited-stage small-cell lung cancer: a pilot study of the Eastern Cooperative Oncology Group. *J Clin Oncol.* 1993;11:879–884.
50. Turrisi, AT, 3rd, Kim, K, Blum, R, et al. Twice-daily compared with once-daily thoracic RT in limited small-cell lung cancer treated concurrently with cisplatin and etoposide. *N Engl J Med.* 1999;340:265–271.
51. Schild, SE, Bonner, JA, Shanahan, TG, et al. Long-term results of a phase 3 trial comparing once-daily RT with twice-daily RT in limited-stage small-cell lung cancer. *Int J Radiat Oncol Biol Phys.* 2004;59:943–951.
52. Fu, KK, Pajak, TF, Trotti, A, et al. A Radiation Therapy Oncology Group (RTOG) phase 3 randomized study to compare hyperfractionation and two variants of accelerated fractionation to standard fractionation RT for head

and neck squamous cell carcinomas: first report of RTOG 9003. *Int J Radiat Oncol Biol Phys.* 2000;48:7–16.
53. Schild, SE, Bonner, JA, Hillman, S, et al. Results of a phase 2 study of high-dose thoracic radiation therapy with concurrent cisplatin and etoposide in limited-stage small-cell lung cancer (NCCTG 95-20-53). *J Clin Oncol.* 2007;25:3124–3129.
54. Jeremic, B, Shibamoto, Y, Acimovic, L, Milisavljevic, S. Initial versus delayed accelerated hyperfractionated radiation therapy and concurrent chemotherapy in limited small-cell lung cancer: a randomized study. *J Clin Oncol.* 1997;15:893–900.
55. Qiao, TK, Zhou, DA, Xin, L, Shu, L, Wu, W. [Concurrent RT combined with carboplatin and etoposide in limited stage small cell lung cancer]. *Zhonghua Jie He He Hu Xi Za Zhi.* 2004;27:237–239.
56. Schild, SE, Stella, PJ, Geyer, SM, et al. Phase 2 trial comparing chemotherapy plus once-daily or twice-daily RT in Stage III non-small-cell lung cancer. *Int J Radiat Oncol Biol Phys.* 2002;54:370–378.
57. Komaki, R, Allen, PK, Wei, X, et al. Prognostic factors identified in the long term survivors with limited small cell lung cancer. *J Clin Oncol* ASCO meeting. 2008;26: abstract 7552.
58. Eaton, W, Maurer, H, Glicksman. The relationship of infield recurrences to prescribed tumor dose in small cell carcinoma of the lung [abstract]. *Int J Radiat Oncol Biol Phys.* 1981;7:1223.
59. White, JE, Chen, T, McCracken, J, et al. The influence of radiation therapy quality control on survival, response and sites of relapse in oat cell carcinoma of the lung: preliminary report of a Southwest Oncology Group study. *Cancer.* 1982;50:1084–1090.
60. Mira, JG, Livingston, RB. Evaluation and RT implications of chest relapse patterns in small cell lung carcinoma treated with RT-chemotherapy: study of 34 cases and review of the literature. *Cancer.* 1980;46:2557–2565.
61. Liengswangwong, V, Bonner, JA, Shaw, EG, et al. Limited-stage small-cell lung cancer: patterns of intrathoracic recurrence and the implications for thoracic RT. *J Clin Oncol.* 1994;12:496–502.
62. Kies, MS, Mira, JG, Crowley, JJ, et al. Multimodal therapy for limited small-cell lung cancer: a randomized study of induction combination chemotherapy with or without thoracic radiation in complete responders; and with wide-field versus reduced-field radiation in partial responders: a Southwest Oncology Group Study. *J Clin Oncol.* 1987;5:592–600.
63. Brodin, O, Rikner, G, Steinholtz, L, Nou, E. Local failure in patients treated with RT and multidrug chemotherapy for small cell lung cancer. *Acta Oncol* (Stockholm, Sweden). 1990;29:739–746.
64. Graham, MV, Purdy, JA, Emami, B, et al. Clinical dose-volume histogram analysis for pneumonitis after 3D treatment for non–small cell lung cancer (NSCLC). *Int J Radiat Oncol Biol Phys.* 1999;45:323–329.
65. Emami, B, Lyman, J, Brown, A, et al. Tolerance of normal tissue to therapeutic irradiation. *Int J Radiat Oncol Biol Phys.* 1991;21:109–122.
66. Watkins, JM, Wahlquist, AE, Shirai, K, et al. Factors associated with severe acute esophagitis from hyperfractionated radiotherapy with concurrent chemotherapy for limited-stage small-cell lung cancer. *Int J Radiat Oncol Biol Phys.* 2009;74:1108–1113.
67. Videtic, GM, Belderbos, JS, Spring Kong, FM, Kepka, L, Martel, MK, Jeremic, B. Report from the International Atomic Energy Agency (IAEA) consultants' meeting on elective nodal irradiation in lung cancer: small-cell lung cancer (SCLC). *Int J Radiat Oncol Biol Phys.* 2008;72:327–334.
68. Sierocki, JS, Hilaris, BS, Hopfan, S, et al. cis-Dichlorodiammineplatinum(II) and VP-16–213: an active induction regimen for small cell carcinoma of the lung. *Cancer Treat Rep.* 1979;63:1593–1597.
69. Roth, BJ, Johnson, DH, Einhorn, LH, et al. Randomized study of cyclophosphamide, doxorubicin, and vincristine versus etoposide and cisplatin versus alternation of these two regimens in extensive small-cell lung cancer: a phase 3 trial of the Southeastern Cancer Study Group. *J Clin Oncol.* 1992;10:282–291.
70. Fukuoka, M, Furuse, K, Saijo, N, et al. Randomized trial of cyclophosphamide, doxorubicin, and vincristine versus cisplatin and etoposide versus alternation of these regimens in small-cell lung cancer. *J Natl Cancer Inst.* 1991;83:855–861.
71. McCracken, JD, Janaki, LM, Crowley, JJ, et al. Concurrent chemotherapy/RT for limited small-cell lung carcinoma: a Southwest Oncology Group Study. *J Clin Oncol.* 1990;8:892–898.
72. Noda, K, Nishiwaki, Y, Kawahara, M, et al. Irinotecan plus cisplatin compared with etoposide plus cisplatin for extensive small-cell lung cancer. *N Engl J Med.* 2002;346:85–91.
73. Lara, PN, Jr., Natale, R, Crowley, J, et al. Phase 3 trial of irinotecan/cisplatin compared with etoposide/cisplatin in extensive-stage small-cell lung cancer: clinical and pharmacogenomic results from SWOG S0124. *J Clin Oncol.* 2009;27:2530–2535.
74. Fox, W, Scadding, JG. Medical Research Council comparative trial of surgery and RT for primary treatment of small-celled or oat-celled carcinoma of bronchus. Ten-year follow-up. *Lancet.* 1973;2:63–65.
75. Shields, TW, Higgins, GA, Jr., Matthews, MJ, Keehn, RJ. Surgical resection in the management of small cell carcinoma of the lung. *J Thorac Cardiovasc Surg.* 1982;84:481–488.
76. Friess, GG, McCracken, JD, Troxell, ML, Pazdur, R, Coltman, CA, Jr., Eyre, HJ. Effect of initial resection of small-cell carcinoma of the lung: a review of Southwest Oncology Group Study 7628. *J Clin Oncol.* 1985;3:964–968.
77. Ichinose, Y, Hara, N, Ohta, M, Takamori, S, Kawasaki, M, Hata, K. Comparison between resected and irradiated small cell lung cancer in patients in stages I through IIIa. *Ann Thorac Surg.* 1992;53:95–100.
78. Chandra, V, Allen, MS, Nichols, FC, 3rd, Deschamps, C, Cassivi, SD, Pairolero, PC. The role of pulmonary resection in small cell lung cancer. *Mayo Clin Proc.* 2006;81:619–624.

79. Prager, RL, Foster, JM, Hainsworth, JD, et al. The feasibility of adjuvant surgery in limited-stage small cell carcinoma: a prospective evaluation. *Ann Thorac Surg.* 1984;38:622–626.
80. Shepherd, FA, Ginsberg, RJ, Patterson, GA, Evans, WK, Feld, R. A prospective study of adjuvant surgical resection after chemotherapy for limited small cell lung cancer. A University of Toronto Lung Oncology Group study. *J Thorac Cardiovasc Surg.* 1989;97:177–186.
81. Baker, RR, Ettinger, DS, Ruckdeschel, JD, et al. The role of surgery in the management of selected patients with small-cell carcinoma of the lung. *J Clin Oncol.* 1987;5:697–702.
82. Lad, T, Piantadosi, S, Thomas, P, Payne, D, Ruckdeschel, J, Giaccone, G. A prospective randomized trial to determine the benefit of surgical resection of residual disease following response of small cell lung cancer to combination chemotherapy. *Chest.* 1994;106:320S–323S.
83. Shepherd, FA, Ginsberg, R, Patterson, GA, et al. Is there ever a role for salvage operations in limited small-cell lung cancer? *J Thorac Cardiovasc Surg.* 1991;101:196–200.
84. Bleyer, WA, Poplack, DG. Prophylaxis and treatment of leukemia in the central nervous system and other sanctuaries. *Semin Oncol.* 1985;12:131–148.
85. Gregor, A. Prophylactic cranial irradiation in small-cell lung cancer: is it ever indicated? *Oncology* (Williston Park, N.Y). 1998;12:19–24.
86. Johnson, BE, Becker, B, Goff, WB, 2nd, et al. Neurologic, neuropsychologic, and computed cranial tomography scan abnormalities in 2- to 10-year survivors of small-cell lung cancer. *J Clin Oncol.* 1985;3:1659–1667.
87. Catane, R, Schwade, JG, Yarr, I, et al. Follow-up neurological evaluation in patients with small cell lung carcinoma treated with prophylactic cranial irradiation and chemotherapy. *Int J Radiat Oncol Biol Phys.* 1981;7:105–109.
88. Arriagada, R, Le Chevalier, T, Borie, F, et al. Prophylactic cranial irradiation for patients with small-cell lung cancer in complete remission. *J Natl Cancer Inst.* 1995;87:183–190.
89. Gregor, A, Cull, A, Stephens, R. Effects of prophylactic irradiation for patients with small cell lung cancer in complete response [abstract]. *Eur J Cancer Clin Oncol.* 1995;31a:s19.
90. Auperin, A, Arriagada, R, Pignon, JP, et al. Prophylactic cranial irradiation for patients with small-cell lung cancer in complete remission. Prophylactic Cranial Irradiation Overview Collaborative Group. *N Engl J Med.* 1999;341:476–484.
91. Le Pechoux, C, Dunant, A, Senan, S, et al. Standard-dose versus higher-dose prophylactic cranial irradiation (PCI) in patients with limited-stage small-cell lung cancer in complete remission after chemotherapy and thoracic RT (PCI 99–01, EORTC 22003–08004, RTOG 0212, and IFCT 99–01): a randomised clinical trial. *Lancet Oncol.* 2009;10:467–474.
92. Schild, SE, Stella, PJ, Brooks, BJ, et al. Results of combined-modality therapy for limited-stage small cell lung carcinoma in the elderly. *Cancer.* 2005;103:2349–2354.

demos
MEDICAL

RADIATION
MEDICINE ROUNDS

The Role of Radiotherapy for Extensive-Stage and Recurrent Small Cell Lung Cancer

Steven E. Schild[a]* and Walter J. Curran, Jr.[b]
[a]*Mayo Clinic, Scottsdale, AZ*
[b]*Emory University School of Medicine, Atlanta, GA*

ABSTRACT

Pathology and Natural History: Approximately two-thirds of all small cell lung cancer patients have extensive-stage disease (1). The anatomy of extensive-stage small cell lung cancer can vary from intrathoracic primary tumor and nodal disease which are only not encompassable by reasonable thoracic radiotherapy (RT) fields to extensive extra-thoracic metastases. The most common sites of extra-thoracic metastases are the liver, bone, brain, and adrenal glands.

Clinical Behavior, Evaluation, and Staging: The staging and workup for extensive-stage small cell lung cancer is identical to limited-stage disease. Most often in the recent past, extensive disease was treated with chemotherapy alone. The role of RT was solely for the palliation of symptoms that were not controlled by chemotherapy. While RT is still used widely for the palliation of symptoms from this disease, the role of RT has shifted and it is now part of frontline therapy for extensive disease. Recent evidence from phase III randomized trials have revealed proven survival advantages for both prophylactic cranial irradiation and thoracic RT in properly selected patients (2,3).

MANAGEMENT OF METASTATIC AND RECURRENT DISEASE

The initial management of most patients with newly diagnosed extensive-stage disease is four or more cycles of platinum-based chemotherapy. A recent Japanese trial compared irinotecan and cisplatin (IP) versus etoposide and cisplatin (EP) for extensive small cell lung cancer. The median survival was 12.8 months in the IP group compared with 9.4 months in the EP group (P = .002). At 2 years, the proportion of patients surviving was 19.5% in the IP group compared with 5.2% in the EP group. Severe or life-threatening myelosuppression was more frequent in the EP group, and severe or life-threatening diarrhea was more frequent in the IP group. They concluded that IP regimen is an effective treatment for metastatic small cell lung cancer (4). However, these findings were not confirmed in the phase 3 trial performed by the Southwest Oncology Group (SWOG), S0124 (5). The median survival times for IP and EP groups were 9.9 and 9.1 months, respectively (P = .71). Again, severe diarrhea was more common with the IP group (19% vs. 3%); severe neutropenia and thrombocytopenia were higher with the EP group (68% vs. 33% and 15% vs. 4%, respectively). This large North American trial failed to confirm the previously reported survival benefit observed with IP in Japanese patients. Both regimens

*Corresponding author, Department of Radiation Oncology, Mayo Clinic, 13400 E. Shea Blvd., Scottsdale, AZ 85259
E-mail address: sschild@mayo.edu

Radiation Medicine Rounds 1 (2010) 59–66.

DOI: 10.5003/2151–4208.1.1.59

produced comparable efficacy, with less hematologic but greater gastrointestinal toxicity with the IP regimen. Hanna et al. (6) reported similarly negative findings from another large phase 3 trial from the United States, Australia, and Canada. Both the EP and IP regimens in this study were modified compared with the JCOG regimens to improve delivery and reduce toxicity, and to be more consistent with dose and schedules given in the United States. As such, the combination of cisplatin and etoposide is still the regimen most often administered for small cell lung cancer. Novel targeted agents are the focus of much research, and it is hoped that newer agents will improve patient outcomes.

The Role of Non-CNS Radiotherapy for Extensive Small Cell Lung Cancer

Radiotherapy (RT) also has important utility for extensive-stage small cell lung cancer. One role for RT is to palliate bulky intrathoracic disease causing airway compromise, cough, hemoptysis, postobstructive pneumonia, or superior vena cava syndrome. This is often accomplished with a short regimen such as the administration of 30 Gy in 10 fractions to the gross tumor. This will improve symptoms in the majority of patients treated.

Although the role of thoracic RT is less clear in patients with extensive-stage small cell lung cancer, there appears to be a distinct survival benefit to delivering thoracic RT as part of the initial management of carefully selected patients with extensive disease. Jeremic et al. (2) reported the results of a randomized prospective study that evaluated chemotherapy with or without twice-daily thoracic RT in patients with extensive-stage small cell lung cancer. Patients initially received three cycles of carboplatin and etoposide. Those patients with a complete response at distant sites and a partial response or better in the chest were randomly assigned to receive either twice-daily thoracic RT (54 Gy in 36 fractions) plus concurrent carboplatin and etoposide followed by two cycles of the same chemotherapy or four cycles of the same chemotherapy without thoracic RT. All patients with a complete response at the distant sites also received prophylactic cranial irradiation (PCI). Patients who received thoracic RT had significantly better survival rate than those who did not (median survival time = 17 vs. 11 months and 5-year survival rate = 9.1% vs. 3.7%, respectively; P = .041). This study revealed the positive influence of a relatively aggressive course of thoracic RT on the survival of carefully selected extensive-stage small cell lung cancer patients. It appears that the cohort of patients who benefit are those in which the RT encompasses all known radiographically detectable residual disease within the body.

The hypothesis that aggressive RT can be added to chemotherapy to more effectively treat extensive-stage small cell lung cancer was evaluated further in a Mayo Clinic trial. Bonner et al. (7) performed a trial that explored the use of RT for both the thoracic component of disease and metastatic lesions in patients with extensive-stage small cell lung cancer. This study included an aggressive regimen of seven cycles of an alternating six-drug combination. The first cycle consisted of cyclophosphamide, doxorubicin, etoposide, vincristine, and lomustine. Subsequent cycles used a regimen of doxorubicin alternating with cisplatin. PCI and thoracic RT were given during the chemotherapy. Prophylactic cranial radiation was delivered in a split-course fashion during the first week of chemotherapy cycles 2 and 3 (1,700 cGy in 5 daily fractions, each of 340 cGy, during each week for a total of 3,400 cGy in 10 fractions). The thoracic radiation was delivered in a split-course fashion during the first week of chemotherapy cycles 5 and 6 (2,000 cGy in 5 daily fractions, each of 400 cGy, during each week for a total of 4,000 cGy in 10 fractions). After the seven cycles, patients received 600 cGy upper hemibody radiation followed by 800 cGy lower hemibody radiation each in a single fraction. Thirteen patients completed the initial seven cycles. Of the 20 patients, 2 (10%) had fatal hematologic complications after lower hemibody radiation. Three (15%) patients had severe peripheral neurologic toxicity, two (10%) had severe central nervous system toxicity, and one (5%) had severe cardiac toxicity. Of the 20 patients, 9 (45%) achieved a complete response. The median survival time was 11.5 months and 5-year overall survival rate was 16%.

There are valuable lessons to be learned from this data. First, it appeared that this combination of treatments was too toxic for further investigation of this regimen. The collective hematologic toxicity as the result of marrow suppression from six drugs combined with the thoracic RT, PCI, and sequential upper and lower hemibody RT resulted in 10% (2 of 20 patients) mortality due to hematologic toxicity. Irradiating the entire marrow led to excessive marrow suppression, toxicity, and mortality.

In addition, the regimen of 3,400 cGy in 340 cGy daily doses of PCI was subsequently found to be associated with an unacceptably high risk of leukoencephalopathy (8). Also, it appears best to administer the PCI after all other therapy because concurrent chemotherapy plus PCI further increases the risk of leukoencephalopathy.

However, in spite of the toxicity issues, the finding that there was a 16% 5-year survival was much better than generally reported in trials for patients with extensive-stage small cell lung cancer. Currently, hemibody RT is not used in many institutions. It appears quite possible that RT to the sites of initial disease or areas of residual disease that persist after chemotherapy could be helpful, as failures following chemotherapy alone frequently occur in the sites of original disease and RT may lower the risk of such recurrences. This may be a natural extrapolation from the study of Jeremic et al. (2) in that targeting all gross disease with RT may benefit patients in terms of survival.

The Centers for Medicare and Medicaid Services (CMS) recently approved Positron Emission Tomography (PET) scanning at the time of initial staging of small cell lung cancer. The use of PET combined with computed tomography (CT) scanning will allow us to better detect all areas of tumor within the patient and define target lesions. Incorporating PET scans into RT planning can be used to generate smaller, more precise tumor fields that may allow us to further decrease toxicity while treating all gross disease with radiation. Over time there will be further improved imaging techniques that will allow physicians to more precisely locate all sites of disease allowing physicians to focally irradiate all sites of disease. This approach may spare enough marrow to allow for the relatively safe delivery of aggressive multiagent chemotherapy while irradiating all radiographically detectable disease.

One could envision a future device similar in design to a tomotherapy unit that incorporates both diagnostic CT and PET to localize the disease precisely. This device could potentially also include megavoltage rotational intensity modulated RT to allow physicians to irradiate lesions while maximally sparing normal tissues. This could detect disease and also administer stereotactic body radiotherapy (SBRT). Thus allowing one to detect and treat all known radiographically visible disease with aggressive RT.

The Role of PCI

The administration of PCI is very important for the majority patients with extensive-stage small cell lung cancer. Slotman et al. (3) conducted a randomized trial (*EORTC* 08993–22993) of PCI in patients with extensive small cell lung cancer who had had any degree of response to chemotherapy (3). Patients between the ages of 18 and 75 years with extensive small cell lung cancer were randomly assigned to undergo PCI (irradiation group) or receive no further therapy (control group). The PCI included either 20 Gy in 5 or 8 fractions, 24 Gy in 12 fractions, 25 Gy in 10 fractions, or 30 Gy in 10 or 12 fractions. The primary endpoint was the time to symptomatic brain metastases. CT or magnetic resonance imaging of the brain was performed when any predefined key symptom suggestive of brain metastases was present. The two groups (each with 143 patients) were well balanced regarding baseline characteristics. Patients in the irradiation group had a lower risk of symptomatic brain metastases (hazard ratio, 0.27; $P < .001$). The cumulative risk of brain metastases within 1 year was 14.6% in the irradiation group and 40.4% in the control group. Irradiation was associated with an increase in median overall survival from 5.4 months to 6.7 months after randomization. The 1-year survival rate was 27.1% in the irradiation group and 13.3% in the control group ($P = .003$). Irradiation had side effects but did not have a clinically significant effect on global health status. The largest mean difference between the two arms was observed for fatigue and hair loss, which were greater in those who received PCI (9). The authors concluded that PCI reduces the incidence of symptomatic brain metastases and prolongs overall survival (3). They also concluded that PCI should be part of standard care for all patients with small cell lung cancer who have a favorable response to initial chemotherapy, and it should be part of the standard treatment in future studies involving these patients. While this trial provides a high level of evidence showing that PCI improves survival, it did not adequately evaluate which of the dose-fractionation regimens was optimal.

The optimal regimen would be the one that includes the following desirable characteristics: decreases brain metastases, increases survival, takes the least time from the patients' remaining life, decreases cost, and causes the least toxicity. An international consortium including the EORTC and RTOG studied dose-fractionation patterns in an international phase III trial. Le Pechoux (10) reported the results of this clinical trial that compared the effect of standard versus higher doses of PCI on the subsequent incidence of brain metastases. This trial included 720 patients with limited-stage small cell lung cancer in complete remission after chemotherapy and thoracic RT. Patients were randomly assigned to either standard (n = 360, 25 Gy in 10 daily fractions of 2.5 Gy) or high-dose PCI (n = 360, 36 Gy). The high-dose therapy was delivered using either conventional (18 daily fractions of 2 Gy) or accelerated hyperfractionated (24 fractions in 16 days with 2 daily sessions of 1.5 Gy separated by a minimum interval of 6 hours) regimens. All of the treatment schedules excluded weekend therapy. The primary endpoint was the incidence of brain metastases at 2 years. Analysis was by intention-to-treat. After a median follow-up of 39 months (range 0–89 months), 145 patients had brain metastases; 82 in the standard-dose group and 63 in the higher-dose group. There was no significant difference in the 2-year incidence of brain metastases between the standard PCI dose group and the higher-dose group at 29% and 23%, respectively (P = .18). The 2-year overall survival was 42% in the standard-dose group and 37% in the higher-dose group (P = .05). The lower overall survival in the higher-dose group was probably due to increased cancer-related mortality: 189 patients in the standard group versus 218 in the higher-dose group died of progressive disease. The most common acute toxic events were fatigue (106 [30%] patients in the standard-dose group vs. 121 [34%] in the higher-dose group), headache (85 [24%] vs. 99 [28%]), and nausea or vomiting (80 [23%] vs. 101 [28%]). They concluded that while there was a significant reduction in the total incidence of brain metastases observed after higher-dose PCI; there was also a significant increase in mortality. Therefore, the authors further concluded that PCI at 25 Gy in 10 fractions should be the standard of care for small cell lung cancer (10). While this trial did not address the effects of dose-fractionation for extensive-stage patients, it is still the most compelling data available regarding the radiation regimen used for PCI for small cell lung cancer patients. While the 25 Gy in 10 fraction regimen did not meet all the characteristics for the optimal regimen because there was a higher brain failure rate associated with its use compared to the higher dose regimens. In spite of this, the 25 Gy regimen was associated with better survival, decreased patient time required, and decreased health care costs. Thus, it appears that this regimen has the best data available supporting its use.

The use of the 25 Gy in 10 fraction regimen is also supported by the older toxicity data reported by Frytak et al. (8) in a study of the side effects of PCI. In this study, Mayo Clinic investigators found that only patients who receive PCI developed neurotoxicity. The incidence of neurotoxicity in long-term survivors (greater than or equal to 1.5 years) with respect to PCI total dose was 25% in those who received less than or equal to 3,000 cGy, 56% in those who received 3,200 cGy, and 36% in those who received 3,600 cGy. Most of these patients received 10 fractions; therefore, there were contributions to toxicity by both the daily and total doses received by the brain. In addition, all patients received chemotherapy concurrently with PCI (11). The risk of leukoencephalopathy appears most prominent if chemotherapy is given concurrently with the PCI (12). Fonseca et al. performed a retrospective analysis of patients with small cell lung cancer who received chemotherapy and thoracic radiation therapy. PCI was administered to patients who had limited disease or who had extensive disease that was subsequently down-staged to only residual chest disease after initial treatment. The total PCI dose was 3,200 cGy administered in 16 fractions of 200 cGy, given concurrently with systemic chemotherapy. Leukoencephalopathy developed in 5 of the 35 patients (14%) who received PCI. The most common signs and symptoms of leukoencephalopathy were intellectual changes, memory alterations, and motor abnormalities. The mean time to onset of symptoms after termination of irradiation was 1 year. This study revealed that even with what was thought to be a relatively safe regimen of PCI, the addition of concurrent chemotherapy appeared to increase the risk of developing leukoencephalopathy. Thus, it appears that PCI improves survival for patients with either limited or extensive disease. However, PCI is best administered after the other therapy is complete, as it is safest at that point with the least potential risk of leukoencephalopathy or exacerbating marrow suppression from chemotherapy. Twelve percent of the total marrow resides in the skull and as such, treatment of the whole brain can contribute to blood count problems (13).

Patients with brain metastases at diagnosis require cranial RT in their initial management, usually concurrently with the first or second cycle of chemotherapy. The whole-brain RT doses most commonly used for brain metastases range from 30.0 Gy in 10 fractions to 37.5 Gy in 15 fractions. The majority of which will receive effective palliation as a result of this treatment.

Patients with a very few or solitary brain metastases can be considered for other more aggressive treatment options such as radiosurgery. There is very little data addressing specialized therapy such as radiosurgery for small cell lung cancer patients. Sheehan performed a retrospective review of 27 patients with 47 recurrent small cell lung cancer brain metastases who underwent radiosurgery (14). Multivariate analyses were used to determine significant prognostic factors influencing survival. The overall median survival was 18 months after the diagnosis of brain metastases. In multivariate analyses, factors significantly affecting survival included tumor volume (P = .0042), preoperative Karnofsky Performance Scale score (P = .0035), and time between initial lung cancer diagnosis and development of brain metastasis (P = .0127). Postradiosurgical imaging of the brain metastases revealed that 62% decreased, 19% remained stable, and 19% eventually increased in size. One patient later underwent a craniotomy and tumor resection for a tumor refractory to radiosurgery and radiation therapy. New brain metastases were demonstrating on follow-up imaging in three patients. They concluded that radiosurgery for recurrent small cell lung carcinoma metastases provided effective local tumor control in the majority of patients. Early detection of brain metastases, aggressive treatment of systemic disease, and a therapeutic strategy including radiosurgery may be able to extend survival for carefully selected individuals. Thus, there may be a role for more aggressive treatments of brain metastases in selected patients with small cell lung cancer. The role of chemotherapy is clear in extensive small cell lung cancer. However, while chemotherapy is also able to cause responses in brain metastases, RT is the standard therapy for brain metastases due to small cell lung cancer (15).

One particular subgroup of extensive stage small cell lung cancer patients are those with radiographically detectable disease limited to the chest and the brain only. This group may benefit from the use of chemotherapy, whole-brain RT, and thoracic RT. Kochhar et al. (16) identified 30 such patients who initially received cisplatin-based chemotherapy and concomitant whole-brain RT consisting of 36 to 48 Gy. Subsequently, 22 patients also received thoracic RT. The median survival of the entire group was 14 months. The results of this study suggested that the outcome of extensive-disease patients with the brain as the sole site of distant metastases at initial diagnosis appeared similar to limited-disease patients. Of this cohort, patients who received thoracic RT tended to have a longer median survival (16 months) than those who did not receive thoracic RT or who received it at the time of local disease progression (12 months) (P = .3). This concept of treating extensive disease with chemotherapy and irradiating all known gross diseases was probably the reason for favorable results in the study of Kochhar et al. and the extraordinary 16% 5-year survival rate achieved in the Mayo Trial reported by Bonner et al. (7). Currently at least one cooperative cancer study group is planning a trial exploring this concept.

Sites of metastatic involvement may also require palliative RT for effective symptom management. These include painful or weight-bearing bony lesions, symptomatic adrenal metastases, or soft tissue masses. Lesions causing any debilitating symptoms can be considered for palliative RT. Since small cell lung cancer is frequently a chemotherapy-responsive disease, there is a greater tendency to rely on chemotherapy in the palliative management of metastases than for other solid tumors. It is important to recognize the potential benefits of properly integrating RT with chemotherapy.

Superior vena cava syndrome may also develop in patients with small cell lung cancer. This appears more frequent with this tumor histology than others due to a propensity to develop large bulky mediastinal adenopathy. Chan et al. (19) reported on 76 consecutive patients who had small cell lung cancer with superior vena cava syndrome. Their first analysis concerned a group of 50 patients who had superior vena cava syndrome at initial presentation. The second analysis concerned a group who had superior vena cava syndrome as a manifestation of persistent or recurrent disease. In the first analysis, 93% had significant improvement in symptoms of superior vena cava syndrome after chemotherapy compared with 94% after mediastinal radiation. In addition, a favorable response was almost universal despite a wide range of radiation fractionation patterns and total doses administered. Seventy percent remained free of superior vena cava syndrome before death. Thirty percent developed recurrence of superior vena cava syndrome symptoms from 1 to 16 months (median: 8) after beginning initial treatment. Those who received combined chemotherapy and radiation had a longer time to recurrence of superior vena

demos MEDICAL

RADIATION MEDICINE ROUNDS

Radiotherapy for the Palliation of Lung Cancer

Yolanda I. Garces*
Mayo Clinic, Rochester, MN

ABSTRACT

Natural History: The natural history of lung cancer has been described in the other chapters. Because lung cancer can commonly affect a variety of organs, radiotherapy (RT) can be used to alleviate many of the symptoms caused when lung cancer spreads to these organs (e.g., chest, liver, bone, brain).

Initial Evaluation of Patients: The staging and workup of patients with the localized disease often times unexpectedly finds metastatic disease. Previous chapters have detailed the staging and workup of patients at diagnosis. If metastatic disease is suspected either at initial diagnosis or during subsequent follow-up, it is important that a metastatic focus be biopsied to document similar histology and the extent of disease. This is especially true when only a single site or a limited number of sites of disease (oligometastatic) are found.

Therapy: RT doses for palliation can vary from a single fraction of 800 to 2,400 cGy up to 5,040 cGy in 28 fractions. Techniques are varied and can include simple opposed or en face fields or the more complex (e.g., stereotactic radiosurgery [SRS], stereotactic body radiotherapy [SBRT], or intensity modulated radiation therapy [IMRT]). This chapter will outline the role of RT in palliation of lung cancer patients. RT and radiation oncologists play an important role in the palliation of patients with lung cancer. A large percentage of lung cancer patients receive radiation therapy for palliation. RT can palliate many symptoms and disease processes such as chest symptoms, dyspnea, skeletal pain, brain metastases, and bone.

INTRODUCTION

Palliative or symptom modifying therapies should begin at diagnosis when treatment or disease modifying therapies are delivered (1). Satisfactory palliation provides patients with anticancer therapy, pain and/or symptom relief, a sense of control, less burden and strengthens relationships between patients and their caregivers including their physicians (2). Radiotherapy (RT) and radiation oncologists play in important role in the palliation of patients with lung cancer.

The majority of lung cancer patients are found to have metastatic disease at diagnosis. Regrettably, a large majority of patients who present with localized non–small cell lung cancer (NSCLC) or small cell lung cancer (SCLC) ultimately present

*Corresponding author, Department of Radiation Oncology, 200 1st St. SW, Rochester, MN 55905
E-mail address: garces.yolanda@mayo.edu

Radiation Medicine Rounds 1 (2010) 67–82.

DOI: 10.5003/2151–4208.1.1.67

with recurrent or metastatic disease. RT is used in approximately 55% of patients either at initial diagnosis or at the time of relapse (3). RT can be used for numerous indications and can effectively palliate a variety of symptoms including hemoptysis, dyspnea, and pain. It can also be used to alleviate symptoms from brain or bone metastases including spinal cord compression. The focus of this chapter is on palliation with RT. While equally important, this chapter will not focus on palliation by other means including chemotherapy (pain management) and other non-radiotherapeutic ablative (4) or bronchoscopic techniques (5). Furthermore, palliation of fatigue, anorexia, weight loss, or quality of life implications and caregiver support will not be reviewed in this chapter. Effective palliation often requires a multidisciplinary approach and starts at diagnosis of lung cancer (2).

■ RADIATION THERAPY FOR PALLIATION

Palliation of Symptomatic Disease

Overview

RT can be used to effectively palliate a variety of symptomatic sites. This can be seen in treating symptomatic chest disease (e.g., cough, hemoptysis, and chest pain) as well as bone pain and dyspnea. Numerous studies have been conducted in patients with lung cancer, and specific studies will be highlighted in the subsequent paragraphs to elucidate the role that RT has in treatment of patients with symptomatic chest disease.

Symptomatic Chest Disease

Countless studies have been conducted on palliation of lung cancer symptoms. These studies have also been the subject of numerous summaries, meta-analyses, and Cochrane reviews (6–8). No randomized trials comparing RT to supportive care have been conducted for stage IV disease. It is well known that the symptoms patients experience are subjective and that physicians tend to underestimate their patient's symptoms. Furthermore, medications may alter the symptoms that are being treated. For example, a trial assessing cough and dyspnea may be confounded by the use of narcotic medications that are used to treat pain, which will also improve cough and dyspnea symptoms. Finally, many studies that have been reported use a variety of different measures, definitions, and endpoints. All of the above make the comparison of different trials challenging (6,8). However, meta-analyses have been conducted.

Fairchild et al. (6) conducted a systematic review of randomized trial of thoracic RT (TRT) to assess high-dose versus low-dose radiation regimens. Not only did the authors want to review the impact of TRT on a variety of symptoms but also wanted to determine if they had any impact on overall survival. Unique to this review, as compared to those that preceded it, is that the biological equivalent dose (BED Gy10) was used to analyze the 13 trials as listed in Table 1.

As expected, the trials included in the systematic review used a variety of definitions of complete or partial response. Furthermore, the time point of assessments and the individual making the assessments (physician vs. patients' self-report) varied from trial to trial among those that recorded those particular symptoms. Despite these differences, symptoms were palliated for the vast majority of patients (hemoptysis [80.2%–81.2%], cough [48.2%–53.3%], and chest pain [64.8%–63.8%]) (6). No differences between the high-dose versus the low-dose arms were noted among the individual symptoms. However, overall symptom burden was reduced with the higher-dose arm as shown in Figure 1. In addition, the review found a statistically significant improvement in survival at 1 year for those randomized to the high-dose arm with a 35 Gy10 BED (which corresponds to 3,000 cGy in 10 fractions) as compared to the lower-dose arms. At 1 year, 26.5% versus 21.7% of the patients on the high-dose versus the low-dose arm were alive, respectively ($P = .002$; see Figure 2). There was a trend for a higher rate of dysphagia in the high-dose arms, and the survival difference was absent between the low-dose and high-dose arms at 2 years (6).

This meta-analysis in combination with other literature supports the use of TRT for relief of symptomatic chest disease to reduce overall symptom burden. We recommend the use of a high Gy10 BED dose equivalent (e.g., 3,000 cGy in 10 fractions) for those patients with a good performance status. For those patients with a poor performance status or limited life expectancy, one could use either 2,000 cGy in 5 fractions (9) or 1,700 cGy in 2 fractions (separated by 1 week) (10). See Table 2 for possible dose/fractionation recommendations.

TABLE 1 Dose/fractionation schema from Fairchild meta-analysis

			Lower-Dose Arm				Higher-Dose Arm			
Trial	**Year**	**Patient (No.)**	**Gy**	**Fractions (No.)**	**Duration**	**BED (Gy10)**	**Gy**	**Fractions (No.)**	**Duration**	**BED (Gy10)**
Simpson et al.[a]	1985	409	30	10	2 weeks	35.0	40	8	4 weeks	45.0
Teo et al.	1988	291	31.2	4	4 weeks	43.7	45	18	4.5 weeks	42.8
MRC 1991	1991	374	17	2	8 days	30.7	30	10	2 weeks[b]	35.0
MRC 1992	1992	235	10	1	1 day	24.8	17	2	8 days	30 7
Abratt et al.[c]	1995	84	35	10	2.5 weeks	40.1	45	15	4 weeks	45.0
MRC 1996	1996	509	17	2	8 days	30.7	39	13	2.5[d]	42.8
Rees et al.	1997	216	17	2	8 days	30.7	22.5	5	1 week	34.2
Nestle et al.[e]	2000	152	32	16 bid	10 days	36.0	60	30	6 weeks	45.9
Bezjak et al.	2002	230	10	1	1 day	24.8	20	5	1 week	29.6
Sundstrom et al.[a]	2004	421	17	2	8 days	30 7	50	25	5 weeks	39.4
Erridge et al.	2008	149	10	1	1 day	24.8	30	10	2 weeks	35.0
Kramer et al	2005	303	16	2	8 days[f]	28.0	30	10	2 weeks[f]	35.0
Senkus-Konefka et al.	2005	100	16	2	8 days	28.0	20	5	1 week	29.6

a Intermediate dose arm omitted; higher-dose arm was split course delivered 4 days/week with a 2-week break.
b Alternate schedule of 27 Gy in 6 fractions.
c Delivered 4 days/week.
d Alternate schedule of 36 Gy in 12 fractions.
e Interfraction interval ≥ 6 hours.
f Delivered 4 or 5 days/week.

Source: From Ref. 6. Reprinted with permission.

TABLE 2 Symptom, dose, and palliative radiotherapy goal

Symptom	Radiotherapy Dose (cGy)	Number of fractions[a]	Palliative Goal
Chest disease	3,000 4,500	10 15	Overall symptom burden and improved one year survival over lower dose regimens
	1,700	2[a]	Overall symptom burden for poor performance status patients
Skeletal pain	800 2,000[b]	1 5[b]	Pain relief in approximately 80% with complete response in 33%
	3,000	10	As above; used for patients where re-treatment would preferably be avoided
Dyspnea[c]	3,000	10	Relief of dyspnea (see Chest disease)

[a]Fractions separated by 1 week.
[b]2,000 cGy/5 fractions preferred over 800 cGy in 1 fraction for neuropathic pain (11).
[c]Thorough examination to determine etiology as dyspnea is often multifactorial.

lung cancer in the airway or indirectly by means of a pleural effusion or postobstructive pneumonia. Yet, others will have their dyspnea as a result of the cancer treatment itself (e.g., treatment related pneumonitis or chemotherapy toxicity resulting in lung damage and/or anemia) (24).

Treatment of dyspnea can involve nonpharmacologic therapies such as breathing control or paced breathing or even assisting with environmental situations (e.g., providing a cool and open room). Oxygen can be prescribed. There are also pharmacologic therapies that include the following: bronchodilators or corticosteroids, systemic corticosteroids, analgesics, anxiolytics/antidepressants, or opioid treatments. Furthermore, a variety of bronchoscopic techniques exist as well, which are beyond the scope of this chapter (5,25). Once the etiology has been determined, nonpharmacologic and pharmacologic therapies have been optimized, then patients with dyspnea can be offered brachytherapy or external beam RT.

Brachytherapy is a treatment alternative for select patients with endobronchial disease; however, a recent systematic review concluded that external RT is a better option than brachytherapy for palliation (26). The authors also concluded that additional randomized controlled clinical trials of brachytherapy as a boost following RT should be conducted. Brachytherapy involves the placement of radioactive seeds into an intraluminal location (e.g., trachea or bronchi). This can be accomplished by low-dose rate implant in which a patient is hospitalized to undergo RT, or it can be administered with remote afterloading high-dose rate implant, which can be done even as an outpatient. The technology for brachytherapy is rapidly improving and now includes computed tomography-based planning. Brachytherapy is performed together with a pulmonologist and is often delivered in combination with other therapies (e.g., maximal mechanical or laser debulking). It is difficult to treat extrinsic compression with this modality, as brachytherapy can only penetrate a short distance. Furthermore, the proximity to blood vessels, difficult locations, and prior RT can make brachytherapy a challenging and sometimes risky undertaking (26). Brachytherapy should be delivered by a well-experienced team of physicians for carefully selected patients. It is not commonly performed.

External beam RT can often be the cause of dyspnea, but paradoxically, it can also be a treatment for dyspnea. Again, a thorough evaluation of the etiology of the dyspnea should take place, and nonpharmacologic and pharmacologic therapies as well as invasive bronchoscopic techniques should be used if indicated. If these prove to be unsuccessful, then external beam RT can provide relief. Performance status, extent of disease, and prognosis would help determine the dose of radiation, but typically, doses used for symptomatic relief of chest disease (as described above) could be used for dyspnea. See Table 2.

Few empiric studies have been conducted on the treatment of dyspnea. Recently, the National Cancer Research Institute Palliative Care Breathlessness Subgroup presented a consensus statement on dyspnea and suggested multicenter interventional studies to concentrate on rational study designs for the treatment of dyspnea (24).

Brain Metastases From Lung Cancer

The majority of studies conducted among patients with brain metastases have included patients with metastases from a variety of primary cancers including lung cancer. Unfortunately, because of the high incidence of lung cancer, it often tends to be the most well-represented cancer on brain metastases studies. Further, because NSCLC is more common these studies have less patients with SCLC. The majority of stereotactic radiosurgery (SRS) trials exclude patients with SCLC. A variety of treatment options exist for patients with brain metastases from lung cancer. The subsequent paragraphs will focus on options for treatment of brain metastases from NSCLC and where there are exceptions for patients with SCLC these will be stated below. The options for patients with brain metastases include steroids, chemotherapy, surgery, SRS, whole-brain RT (WBRT) and/or a combination of these treatments (28). Treatment recommendations vary based on the extent of a patient's systemic disease, performance status, and age as well as number of metastases and prior and possibly even planned therapies.

Solitary/Single Brain Metastasis

Solitary brain metastases exist when truly no other known disease exists in the body besides the solitary brain metastasis. This could be either at initial diagnosis (which would be very rare) or after curative treatment for a known prior malignancy that has already been delivered. In contrast, a single brain metastasis could be present as a sole lesion in the brain, but there is known disease elsewhere in the body. One could surmise that the former group of patients will fare better in terms of long-term prognosis, and as such, treatment recommendations may vary for these different groups of patients. Because SCLC is radioresponsive, patients are not typically offered surgery or SRS and are treated with WBRT as described in the multiple brain metastases category below.

Surgery (either open surgical resection or SRS) is the main treatment for patients with solitary or single metastases to the brain. Typically, surgical resection is indicated for patients with brain tumors in operable locations especially when one is unable to gain a tissue diagnosis from another metastatic site. Surgical resection followed by WBRT has been compared with WBRT alone for primary treatment of patients with single brain metastasis (29–31). The most influential of these trials was conducted by Patchell and colleagues (29). The majority of patients on this randomized clinical trial had NSCLC. This study showed that patients who underwent surgery fared better than those who received WBRT alone, with a median survival of approximately 10 versus 4 months, respectively ($P < .01$) (29). Patients who underwent surgery were able to maintain better performance status and had less local recurrence in the brain as well. These same authors then asked another important question: Is the WBRT necessary?

Patchell's (32) second randomized clinical trial among patients with brain metastases involved surgery alone versus surgery followed by WBRT for patients with a single brain metastasis. WBRT decreased brain relapse rate from 70% to 18% ($P < .001$), and as a result, neurologic progression free (NPF) survival was improved. Median NPF survival was improved from 81 to 115 weeks with the addition of WBRT; $P = .03$. However, no difference was seen in overall survival or duration of functional independence (32). This study has resulted in a large number of patients and clinicians being very cautious about when to add WBRT after surgical resection; although, the authors did conclude that improvements in NPF survival was enough to continue to recommend the use of postoperative WBRT. Most experts conclude that after surgical resection that WBRT should remain the standard of care (33).

Oligometastatic Brain Disease (2–4 Metastases)

An intermediate group between those with solitary or single metastases and those with multiple metastases is a group of patients with 2–4 brain metastases. While craniotomy would likely not be recommended in this group of patients, SRS, with or without WBRT, might be a viable option. Some of the studies overlap with patients with solitary or single metastases as described above; however, a large number of these trials have also used SRS, with or without WBRT, for this group of oligometastatic patients.

This past year, a randomized phase 3 single institution trial was reported in abstract form (34). This trial was a randomized trial of SRS, with or without WBRT, in patients with 1 to 3 brain metastases, who were recursive partition analysis (RPA) class 1 or 2. The primary endpoint of the study was neurocognitive decline in 4 months as measured by the Hopkins Verbal Learning Test (HVLT). The study enrolled 58 patients (the majority of whom were NSCLC patients) over a 7-year time period and was halted by an independent data monitoring committee when they found that the WBRT arm had a decline in HVLT as compared with the non-WBRT arm (mean value 49% vs. 23%, respectively). The study was halted by an early stopping rule. Despite no obvious differences in patient's baseline demographics or clinical characteristics, the study also found a remarkable difference in survival between the SRS alone group as compared with the SRS plus WBRT group (median survival of 15.2 vs. 5.6 months, respectively; ($P = .003$). Furthermore, the local control and the brain tumor control at 1 year was lower in the SRS group as well, leading one to conclude that WBRT was detrimental to this group of patients on this study. However, 27 of the 30 patients on the SRS alone arm were able to undergo salvage therapies (craniotomy, WBRT, SRS, and/or chemotherapy) as compared with only 3 out of the 28 patients in the SRS plus WBRT arm due to rapid progression of systemic disease in the WBRT group. The authors suggest that SRS with salvage therapy should be the new standard of care.

The previously described study was a single institution trial and is not yet published in full manuscript form. Therefore, WBRT may be considered in patients wanting to improve neurologic progression-free survival extrapolating from the surgical data as well as data from a SRS with or without WBRT study (35). Ideally, a patient who is a candidate for SRS should be enrolled in the open cooperative group trials asking whether or not WBRT is necessary following SRS. The NCCTG study is actively accruing, and the EORTC study has completed accrual

(ClinicalTrials.gov identifier: NCT00377156 and NCT00002899, respectively). We await the results of these pivotal trials before we can state that SRS alone is the standard of care. We do offer WBRT to patients who have undergone SRS, with typical doses of WBRT being 3,000 cGy in 10 fractions to 3,750 cGy in 15 fractions. Patients with SCLC are often not eligible for the SRS studies and are often not offered surgery or SRS for initial treatment of brain metastases.

Multiple Brain Metastases

Patients with multiple brain metastases are typically treated with steroids (dexamethasone 16 mg/d, maximum dose) for approximately 4 weeks or less with a rapid taper (24). The Recursive Partitioning Analysis (RPA) study by the Radiation Therapy Oncology Group (RTOG) found three prognostic groups of patients with brain metastases with varying degrees of survival. Median survival was disappointingly 2 to 7 months for these various groups (36,37). A new classification system called the Graded Prognostic Assessment (GPA) is now being studied and may supplant the RPA classification system in the future. The GPA is felt to be simpler, as it involves the patient's age, Karnofsky performance status, number of metastases, and whether or not extracranial disease is present (38,39). Other prognostic classification system exist, but they are not used as often as the RPA or GPA and some are specific to patients undergoing SRS (40,41). SCLC tends to be very responsive to WBRT. The typical dose used for patients with multiple brain metastases from lung cancer is 3,000 cGy in 10 fractions.

Neurocognitive function or dysfunction is an area of active research in patients undergoing WBRT. The majority of studies have not shown a decline in neurocognitive function when appropriate fraction sizes are used, no brain disease progression is noted, and patients are not treated with concurrent chemotherapy (42,43). The rate of radiation-induced dementia following WBRT is thought to be low. However, the majority of patients will not live long enough to develop this toxicity, and few studies have truly conducted formal neurocognitive testing in which baseline assessments are performed. As described above, the NCCTG study of SRS, with or without WBRT, does have detailed neurocognitive testing. Another ongoing RTOG study is asking whether memantine can preserve cognitive function (specifically memory). Memantine is used for Alzheimer's disease and works by blocking NMDA glutamate receptors. This study is a randomized controlled phase 3 trial of placebo versus memantine among patients undergoing WBRT. This study is using a dose of 3,750 cGy in 15 fractions. The study is actively accruing patients (RTOG 0614; ClinicalTrials.gov identifier: NCT00566852).

Recurrent Brain Metastases

Patients can suffer with recurrent brain disease following WBRT. This is a challenging problem, especially if their systemic disease is still well-controlled and/or they have a good performance status. Often times, SRS is used as a salvage procedure. The RTOG conducted a study of salvage SRS for patients with recurrent brain metastases (or recurrent primary brain tumors) (44). A retrospective study by Chao (45) showed that the longer the interval between WBRT and the SRS, the better the prognosis. Occasionally, repeat WBRT is offered to these patients as well (46,47). The dose for whole-brain reirradiation is highly dependent on the previous dose of RT given. One could consider 3,000 cGy in 15 fractions or 2,000 cGy in 10 fractions.

Reirradiation following PCI is also possible but not widely reported. The PCI85 and PCI88 specified the reirradiation dose to be 5,000 cGy in 28 fractions for those who had not received PCI and 3,900 cGy in 22 fractions for those who had previously received PCI (typically 2,500 cGy in 10 fractions) (48). Their review reported patterns of failure after PCI but did not describe outcomes related to the WBRT or the reirradiation. As above, the reirradiation dose is highly dependent on the prior WBRT dose. One could consider 3,000 cGy in 15 fractions or 2,000 cGy in 10 fractions.

Chemotherapy and Brain Metastases

Although it is believed that most chemotherapy does not traverse the blood brain barrier, this notion is now being challenged. Studies have been conducted using chemotherapy (e.g., systemic chemotherapy, radiosensitizers, gadolinium targets, etc.) as an adjuvant to improve WBRT results (41,49–51). A very recent report shows that metoxafin gadolinium in combination with WBRT improves neurologic progression-free survival among patients with NSCLC as compared with WBRT alone, especially when delivered promptly after diagnosis (41). Other studies of chemotherapy for brain metastases are ongoing.

Spinal Cord Compression

Spinal cord compression can result due to epidural compression, intradural metastasis, or leptomeningeal compression. This section will focus on the more common epidural cord compression (ECC). This is defined as the indentation of the thecal sac in combination with the clinical symptoms at the corresponding vertebral body level of pain, weakness, numbness, and/or bowel or bladder sphincteric dysfunction. ECC requires clinical astuteness as well as prompt evaluation and treatment to avoid neurologic deterioration. ECCs are commonly located in the thoracic vertebral bodies. Synchronous lesions can occur in a large percentage of patients; therefore, magnetic resonance imaging (MRI) of the entire spine is recommended. Treatment for ECC includes steroids, RT, orthopedic or neurosurgery intervention, and/or a careful combination of these therapies. Ambulatory status prior to ECC, interval between diagnosis and development of the metastasis, and the rapidity of the development of symptoms are predictive of outcome (52). Patients with ECC from lung cancer tend to have worse outcomes (median survival of 1.5 months) as compared to those with ECC from other cancers (53).

Steroids

Dexamethasone is commonly begun at diagnosis of ECC. Although, the optimal dose is not known; commonly, a dosage of 16–96 mg/day is typically used. Most studies support the lower or moderate doses of steroids due to the adverse effects of high-dose of steroids (52).

Surgery

In the past, surgery was used predominantly for patients with spinal instability, bony collapse, intractable pain, and/or failure after other therapies (24). Improved surgical techniques, as well as a recent randomized trial of surgery with RT as compared with RT alone for ECC, has increased the importance of early surgical intervention to maintain the functional status in select patients (54). Therefore, multidisciplinary discussions and planning are important for patients with newly diagnosed ECC.

Patchell's (54) randomized trial of surgery with postoperative RT versus RT alone was an important study that reestablished surgery as an important treatment modality in select patients with ECC to maintain or improve functional outcomes. This study included 101 patients with a single site of ECC. Similar to other palliative treatment trials, patients with NSCLC comprised a larger percentage of the patients. The patients who underwent surgery followed by RT (3,000 cGy in 10 fractions) preserved their ambulatory rate and ability to walk for a greater length of time as compared with the primary RT patients: ambulatory rate 84% versus 57% ($P = .001$) and days walking 122 versus 13 days ($P = .003$), respectively. Furthermore, median survival time was longer in those patients undergoing surgery 126 versus 100 days for those not undergoing surgery; $P = .033$ (54). The authors are careful to conclude that surgery is not indicated for all patients with ECC but better used for well-selected patients with good prognosis, limited disease, and a short duration of neurologic symptoms.

RT

RT is most commonly used to alleviate the symptoms from ECC. Patients often times are not candidates for surgery, and RT becomes the treatment of choice. Patients are not candidates for surgery if multiple sites of cord compression exist, they are medically unfit, or their anticipated survival is limited. A dose of 3,000 cGy in 10 fractions is often employed, as it results in less re-treatment (see Skeletal Metastasis above). Typical volumes include the area of ECC including any paraspinal extension as well as one to two vertebral bodies above and below the index lesion. A recent secondary analysis of the Patchell study (55) has shown that age > 65 years might be an important poor prognostic factor and that these patients may be better served by primary RT over surgery followed by RT. For patients with an anticipated short life-expectancy, short-course RT can be recommended (e.g., 800 cGy in a single fraction) (56–59). Rades et al. (57) outlined clinical factors associated with survival and generated a scoring system related to patient survival. Using this scoring system, they were able to show that patients with a low score (<36) and poor prognosis should be treated with short-course RT and did not appear to benefit from long-course RT. This was in contrast to patients with a higher score (>36) and better prognosis. In this group, longer survival was associated with a more prolonged course of RT (30 Gy/10 or longer).

Invasive radiology procedures have also been used to treat some patients. Kyphoplasty and vertebroplasty are emerging as ways to strengthen the bone following radiation therapy (60).

ONGOING AND FUTURE RESEARCH

Oligometastatic Disease

Considerable interest exists in delivering ablative therapies to address patients with limited metastatic disease with a variety of localized therapies, which include RT (4). Many years ago, Hellman and Weichselbaum (61) first theorized about oligometastatic disease in that there might be a group of patients with limited metastatic disease that has not already become widely microscopically metastatic, whereby aggressive local therapies make clinical sense. While their initial description was in patients with breast cancer, many have extrapolated these findings into other cancers. The challenge is deciphering who has this limited oligometastatic disease at diagnosis or who has it at the time of subsequent relapse. A limited number of studies have been or are being conducted in this group of patients so that one can better select patients for aggressive local therapies.

The NCCTG, in cooperation with the Southwest Oncology Group, is conducting a randomized phase 2 trial of RT versus observation among patients with limited oligometastatic disease (N0724; Clinical. Trials.gov identifier: NCT00776100). The RT is delivered after patients undergo two to six cycles of standard chemotherapy and have stable or responsive disease in the chest as well as in one to three metastatic sites (which can include other intrathoracic lung metastases). The RT consists of 6,000 cGy in 30 fractions or 4,500 cGy in 15 fractions to the thoracic disease with 4,000 cGy in 20 fractions or 3,000 Gy in 10 fractions to the metastatic sites of disease. No concurrent chemotherapy is being administered. Any sites of complete response following chemotherapy are not given RT. This study recently opened and plans to accrue 98 evaluable patients.

Stereotactic Body Radiotherapy (SBRT)

SBRT involves the use of high doses of conformal RT to small volumes delivered in 2 to 5 fractions (SRS is single fraction and is most often used in the brain, see above). SRS and SBRT are not only being applied to patients with primary lung cancer, but they are also being used for patients with oligometastatic disease. With the advent of improving technology and thoughtful treatment planning, it is now possible to be more aggressive with the primary or metastatic site while sparing normal tissues. SBRT is being offered for patients with metastatic lung, spine, and/or liver disease. Numerous studies are ongoing with only a handful highlighted below.

SBRT Lung

For patients with limited metastatic disease or controlled other systemic disease, it is reasonable to consider SBRT for solitary or a few metastases (< 3 lesions). We consider biopsy of a prior metastatic disease or even possibly the lung metastasis prior to delivery of SBRT for lung lesions to ensure that the patient has metastases. Similar techniques and doses as described in the chapter for Radiotherapy for Early-Stage Non-Small Cell Carcinoma of the Lung (including SBRT) are used for patients with metastatic disease to the lung. Please see Figure 3A–C for example of a lung SBRT case treated to 6,000 cGy in 3 fractions (without heterogeneity correction).

Schefter et al. (62) reported results of a phase 1/2 trial of SBRT for patients with lung metastases. The study used a cohort of three study design for the phase 1 portion and determined that the maximum tolerated dose (MTD) was not reached as they had no dose-limiting toxicities (DLTs) at any of the three levels studied (4,800, 5,400, and 6,000 cGy all delivered in three fractions); therefore, 6,000 cGy in 3 fractions was their maximum dose. In addition, 13 patients from the phase 2 portion of the study were included in the safety analysis, and no DLTs were noted in this group (62). Local tumor control was recently reported with a total of 38 patients, and the authors found that the local control at 1 and 2 years was 100% to 96%, respectively. For those assessable, the median follow-up was 15 months (63).

SBRT Spine

SBRT can be delivered in a single fraction for patients with spine disease (SRS) or it can be delivered as a fractionated therapy (SBRT). SRS or SBRT spine is typically given to patients with oligometastatic disease who have disease that is amenable to SRS or SBRT or patients who have failed prior external beam RT (64,65). A recent single institution study demonstrated excellent local control with SRS; however, even patients with a single site of spine disease had poor outcomes due to systemic disease progression (66). The RTOG is conducting a phase 2/3 study of SBRT in patients with metastatic spine disease, in which the phase 2 portion is a single fraction of 1,600 cGy and the phase 3 portion of the study

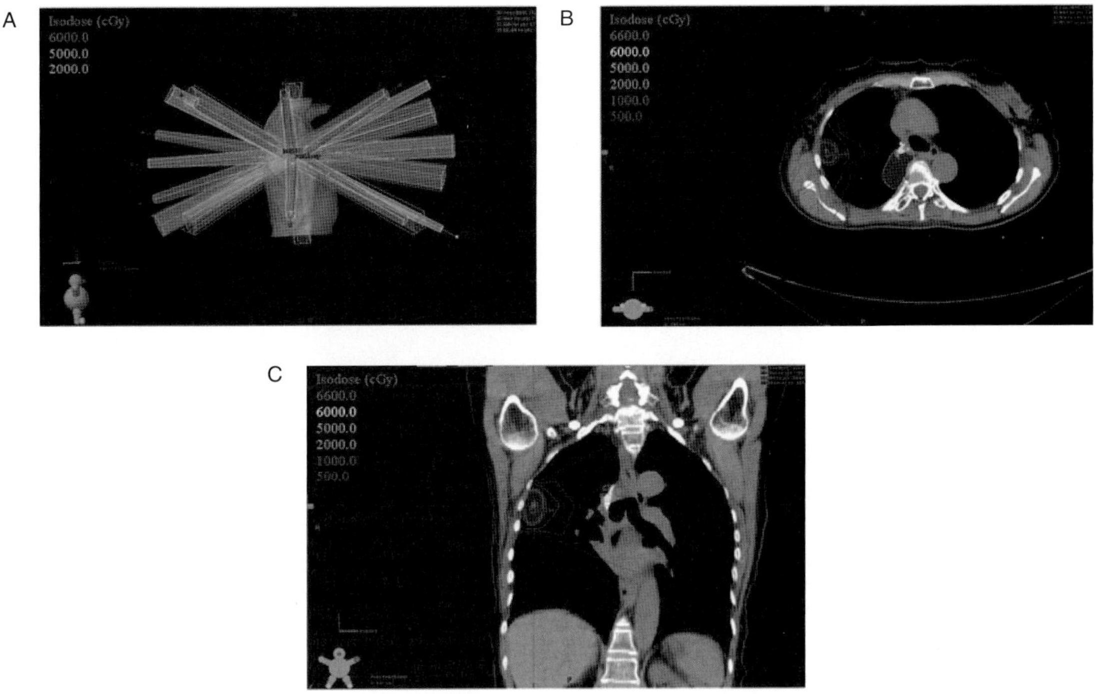

FIGURE 3 A. A beams eye view of a patient with a medically inoperable right lung cancer demonstrates multiple non-coplanar SBRT beams entering (and exiting) the patients external contour (shown in gray). B. A coronal computed tomography (CT) image shows the conformal dose around the lung cancer. C. An axial CT image shows the conformal dose around the lung cancer.

then compares this to external beam RT (800 cGy in a single fraction). (RTOG 0631; ClinicalTrials.gov identifier: NCT00922974.) See Figure 4 for an example of an SBRT plan (2,100 cGy in 3 fractions) to the thoracic spine in a patient with prior external beam RT.

SBRT Liver

SRS or SBRT for liver metastases is an emerging area as noninvasive ablative therapies improve. SRS or SBRT can be delivered to liver metastases in select patients who have oligometastatic disease and lesions that are 5 to 6 cm or less while sparing a specified volume of the liver, given its parallel functional structure. Mayo Clinic, Rochester, has a single arm study to determine the maximum tolerated dose, as well as to evaluate the safety of single fraction SBRT for patients with liver metastases. (MC0941: ClinicalTrials.gov identifier: NCT00938457.)

Rusthoven and colleagues (67) recently reported the final results of a multi-institutional phase 1/2 trial of SBRT for patients with liver metastasis (or metastases) provided that 700 cc of the liver would receive less than 1,500 cGy. The study enrolled 47 patients with 63 liver lesions, and 36 patients with 49 lesions were assessable for local control with a median follow-up of 16 months. The phase 1 portion of the study determined that the they did not reach an MTD and the upper-dose limit was 6,000 cGy in 3 fractions (68). The local control on the phase 1/2 study was 95% and 92% and 1 and 2 years, respectively. Median survival was 20.5 months, and the 2-year overall survival was 30% (67); however, a large percentage of patients had extrahepatic disease and prior chemotherapy. Minimal toxicity was noted (see Figure 5).

■ SUMMARY

In summary, RT can be used to effectively palliate many of the symptoms due to lung cancer. It is often used to treat the symptoms from the primary tumor or nodal metastases. This can range from tumor bleeding, blocking an airway, obstructing a major vessel (such as the superior vena cava), causing cough,

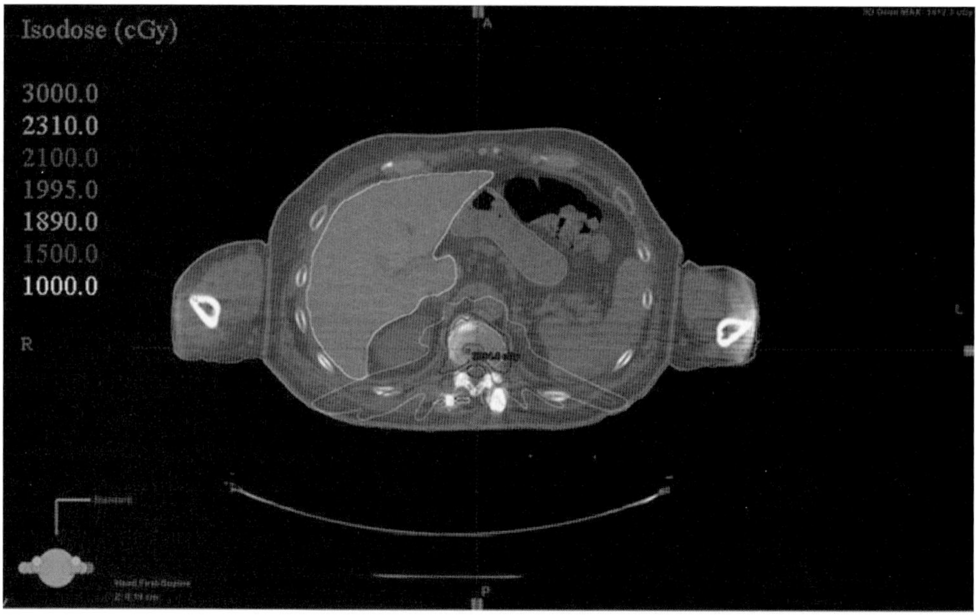

FIGURE 4 An axial CT image demonstrating the conformal SBRT isodose lines around a T11 vertebral body metastasis in a patient with a paraspinal carcinoma status post prior external beam radiotherapy. The plan was developed with intensity modulated radiation therapy to a dose of 2100 cGy in 3 fractions. The spinal cord is outlined in black. The planning target volume is in the light gray color wash.

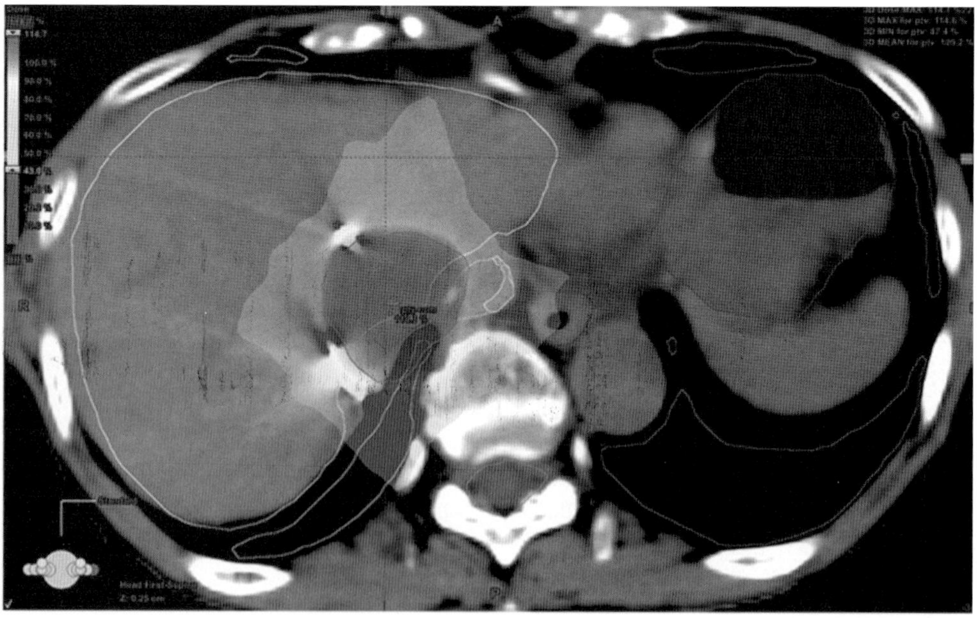

FIGURE 5 An axial CT image demonstrating the conformal SBRT isodose color washes around a liver metastasis in a patient with oligometastatic colorectal cancer with markers placed for four-dimensional treatment planning and delivery.

impairing swallowing and many other problems. Additionally, distant metastases can cause pain, fractures of bones, or impair neurologic function. Most focal symptoms related to tumor impinging or invading normal tissues can be effectively palliated with a short course of RT. Newer technologies have allowed us to pinpoint the therapy more precisely that should provide better outcomes with fewer side effects. In addition, it might be possible to render some patients with oligometastatic disease free of disease with the judicious use of RT to all known gross disease combined with systemic treatment.

REFERENCES

1. Cancer pain relief and palliative care. Report of a WHO Expert Committee. *World Health Organ Tech Rep Ser.* 1990;804:1–75.
2. Levy M, Carducci M, Weinstein S. Palliative care clinical practice guidelines in oncology. *J Natl Compr Canc Netw.* 2003;1(3):394–420.
3. Tyldesley S, Boyd C, Schulze K, Walker H, Mackillop WJ. Estimating the need for radiotherapy for lung cancer: an evidence-based, epidemiologic approach. *Int J Radiat Oncol Biol Phys.* 2001 Mar 15;49(4):973–985.
4. Timmerman RD, Bizekis CS, Pass HI, et al. Local surgical, ablative, and radiation treatment of metastases. *CA Cancer J Clin.* 2009;59(3):145–170.
5. Sminoff M, Kvale P. Advances in supportive and palliative care for lung cancer patients. In: Jeremic' B, ed. *Advances in Radiation Oncology in Lung Cancer.* Berlin: Springer; 2005:321–336.
6. Fairchild A, Harris K, Barnes E, et al. Palliative thoracic radiotherapy for lung cancer: a systematic review. *J Clin Oncol.* 2008;26(24):4001–4011.
7. Toy E, Macbeth F, Coles B, Melville A, Eastwood A. Palliative thoracic radiotherapy for non-small-cell lung cancer: a systematic review. *Am J Clin Oncol.* 2003;26(2): 112–120.
8. Lester J, MacBeth F. Palliative external beam thoracic radiotherapy. In: Jeremic' B, ed. *Advances in Radiation Oncology in Lung Cancer.* Berlin: Springer;2005:247–254.
9. Bezjak A, Dixon P, Brundage M, et al. Randomized phase III trial of single versus fractionated thoracic radiation in the palliation of patients with lung cancer (NCIC CTG SC.15). *Int J Radiat Oncol Biol Phys.* 2002; 54(3):719–728.
10. Macbeth FR, Bolger JJ, Hopwood P, et al. Randomized trial of palliative two-fraction versus more intensive 13-fraction radiotherapy for patients with inoperable non-small cell lung cancer and good performance status. Medical Research Council Lung Cancer Working Party. *Clin Oncol (R Coll Radiol).* 1996;8(3):167–175.
11. Roos DE, Turner SL, O'Brien PC, et al. Randomized trial of 8 Gy in 1 versus 20 Gy in 5 fractions of radiotherapy for neuropathic pain due to bone metastases (Trans-Tasman Radiation Oncology Group, TROG 96.05). *Radiother Oncol.* 2005;75(1):54–63.
12. Nieder C, Pawinski A, Haukland E, Dokmo R, Phillipi I, Dalhaug A. Estimating need for palliative external beam radiotherapy in adult cancer patients. *Int J Radiat Oncol Biol Phys.* 2009;76(1):207–211.
13. Townsend PW, Smalley SR, Cozad SC, Rosenthal HG, Hassanein RE. Role of postoperative radiation therapy after stabilization of fractures caused by metastatic disease. *Int J Radiat Oncol Biol Phys.* 1995;31(1):43–49.
14. Goudas L, Carr DB, Bloch R, et al. Management of cancer pain. *Evid Rep Technol Assess.* 2001;(35)(AHRQ Publication No. 02-E002).
15. Berenson JR. Recommendations for zoledronic acid treatment of patients with bone metastases. *Oncologist.* 2005; 10(1):52–62.
16. Rosen LS, Gordon D, Tchekmedyian S, et al. Zoledronic acid versus placebo in the treatment of skeletal metastases in patients with lung cancer and other solid tumors: a phase III, double-blind, randomized trial—the Zoledronic Acid Lung Cancer and Other Solid Tumors Study Group. *J Clin Oncol.* 2003;21(16):3150–3157.
17. Bauman G, Charette M, Reid R, Sathya J. Radiopharmaceuticals for the palliation of painful bone metastasis—a systemic review. *Radiother Oncol.* 2005; 75(3):258–270.
18. Liepe K, Kotzerke J. A comparative study of 188Re-HEDP, 186Re-HEDP, 153Sm-EDTMP and 89Sr in the treatment of painful skeletal metastases. *Nucl Med Commun.* 2007;28(8):623–630.
19. Ashamalla H, Cardoso E, Macedon M, et al. Phase I trial of vertebral intracavitary cement and samarium (VICS): novel technique for treatment of painful vertebral metastasis. *Int J Radiat Oncol Biol Phys.* 2009;75(3):836–842.
20. Chow E, Harris K, Fan G, Tsao M, Sze WM. Palliative radiotherapy trials for bone metastases: a systematic review. *J Clin Oncol.* 2007;25(11):1423–1436.
21. Wu JS, Wong R, Johnston M, Bezjak A, Whelan T. Meta-analysis of dose-fractionation radiotherapy trials for the palliation of painful bone metastases. *Int J Radiat Oncol Biol Phys.* 2003;55(3):594–605.
22. Sze WM, Shelley MD, Held I, Wilt TJ, Mason MD. Palliation of metastatic bone pain: single fraction versus multifraction radiotherapy--a systematic review of randomised trials. *Clin Oncol (R Coll Radiol).* 2003;15(6):345–352.
23. Dudgeon DJ, Kristjanson L, Sloan JA, Lertzman M, Clement K. Dyspnea in cancer patients: prevalence and associated factors. *J Pain Symptom Manage.* 2001; 21(2):95–102.
24. Kvale PA, Selecky PA, Prakash UB. Palliative care in lung cancer: ACCP evidence-based clinical practice guidelines (2nd edition). *Chest.* 2007;132(3)(suppl):368S–403S.
25. Prakash U. Chapter 22—Bronchoscopy. In: Mason R, Murray J, Broaddus V, Nadel J, eds. *Mason: Murray & Nadel's Textbook of Respiratory Medicine.* 4th ed. Philadelphia: Saunders; 2005:617–642.
26. Ung YC, Yu E, Falkson C, et al. The role of high-dose-rate brachytherapy in the palliation of symptoms in patients

with non-small-cell lung cancer: a systematic review. *Brachytherapy.* 2006;5(3):189–202.

27. Dorman S, Jolley C, Abernethy A, et al. Researching breathlessness in palliative care: consensus statement of the National Cancer Research Institute Palliative Care Breathlessness Subgroup. *Palliat Med.* 2009;23(3): 213–227.
28. Eichler AF, Loeffler JS. Multidisciplinary management of brain metastases. *Oncologist.* 2007;12(7):884–898.
29. Patchell RA, Tibbs PA, Walsh JW, et al. A randomized trial of surgery in the treatment of single metastases to the brain. *N Engl J Med.* 1990;322(8):494–500.
30. Noordijk EM, Vecht CJ, Haaxma-Reiche H, et al. The choice of treatment of single brain metastasis should be based on extracranial tumor activity and age. *Int J Radiat Oncol Biol Phys.* 1994;29(4):711–717.
31. Mintz AH, Kestle J, Rathbone MP, et al. A randomized trial to assess the efficacy of surgery in addition to radiotherapy in patients with a single cerebral metastasis. *Cancer.* 1996;78(7):1470–1476.
32. Patchell RA, Tibbs PA, Regine WF, et al. Postoperative radiotherapy in the treatment of single metastases to the brain: a randomized trial. JAMA. 1998;280(17): 1485–1489.
33. Brown PD, Asher AL, Farace E. Adjuvant whole brain radiotherapy: strong emotions decide but rational studies are needed. *Int J Radiat Oncol Biol Phys.* 2008;70(5): 1305–1309.
34. Chang E, Meyers C, Wefel J, Hess K. Phase III randomized clinical trial of radiosurgery with or without whole brain irradiation in patients newly diagnosed with 1 to 3 brain metastases. *Int J Radiat Oncol Biol Phys.* 2008;72(1)(suppl):LB.
35. Aoyama H, Shirato H, Tago M, et al. Stereotactic radiosurgery plus whole-brain radiation therapy vs stereotactic radiosurgery alone for treatment of brain metastases: a randomized controlled trial. *JAMA.* 2006;295(21): 2483–2491.
36. Gaspar L, Scott C, Rotman M, et al. Recursive partitioning analysis (RPA) of prognostic factors in three Radiation Therapy Oncology Group (RTOG) brain metastases trials. *Int J Radiat Oncol Biol Phys.* 1997;37(4):745–751.
37. Gaspar LE, Scott C, Murray K, Curran W. Validation of the RTOG recursive partitioning analysis (RPA) classification for brain metastases. *Int J Radiat Oncol Biol Phys.* 2000;47(4):1001–1006.
38. Sperduto CM, Watanabe Y, Mullan J, et al. A validation study of a new prognostic index for patients with brain metastases: the Graded Prognostic Assessment. *J Neurosurg.* 2008;109(suppl):87–89.
39. Sperduto PW, Berkey B, Gaspar LE, Mehta M, Curran W. A new prognostic index and comparison to three other indices for patients with brain metastases: an analysis of 1,960 patients in the RTOG database. *Int J Radiat Oncol Biol Phys.* 2008;70(2):510–514.
40. Nieder C, Mehta MP. Prognostic indices for brain metastases—usefulness and challenges. *Radiat Oncol.* 2009;4:10.
41. Mehta MP, Shapiro WR, Phan SC, et al. Motexafin gadolinium combined with prompt whole brain radiotherapy prolongs time to neurologic progression in non-small-cell lung cancer patients with brain metastases: results of a phase III trial. *Int J Radiat Oncol Biol Phys.* 2009;73(4):1069–1076.
42. Li J, Bentzen SM, Renschler M, Mehta MP. Regression after whole-brain radiation therapy for brain metastases correlates with survival and improved neurocognitive function. *J Clin Oncol.* 2007;25(10):1260–1266.
43. Meyers CA, Smith JA, Bezjak A, et al. Neurocognitive function and progression in patients with brain metastases treated with whole-brain radiation and motexafin gadolinium: results of a randomized phase III trial. *J Clin Oncol.* 2004;22(1):157–165.
44. Shaw E, Scott C, Souhami L, et al. Single dose radiosurgical treatment of recurrent previously irradiated primary brain tumors and brain metastases: final report of RTOG protocol 90–05. *Int J Radiat Oncol Biol Phys.* 2000;47(2):291–298.
45. Chao ST, Barnett GH, Vogelbaum MA, et al. Salvage stereotactic radiosurgery effectively treats recurrences from whole-brain radiation therapy. *Cancer.* 2008;113(8): 2198–2204.
46. Wong WW, Schild SE, Sawyer TE, Shaw EG. Analysis of outcome in patients reirradiated for brain metastases. *Int J Radiat Oncol Biol Phys.* 1996;34(3):585–590.
47. Sadikov E, Bezjak A, Yi QL, et al. Value of whole brain re-irradiation for brain metastases—single centre experience. *Clin Oncol (R Coll Radiol).* 2007;19(7):532–538.
48. Arriagada R, Le Chevalier T, Riviere A, et al. Patterns of failure after prophylactic cranial irradiation in small-cell lung cancer: analysis of 505 randomized patients. *Ann Oncol.* 2002;13(5):748–754.
49. Suh JH, Stea B, Nabid A, et al. Phase III study of efaproxiral as an adjunct to whole-brain radiation therapy for brain metastases. *J Clin Oncol.* 2006;24(1):106–114.
50. Lind JS, Lagerwaard FJ, Smit EF, Senan S. Phase I study of concurrent whole brain radiotherapy and erlotinib for multiple brain metastases from non-small-cell lung cancer. *Int J Radiat Oncol Biol Phys.* 2009;74(5):1391–1396.
51. Tsao MN, Lloyd NS, Wong RK, Rakovitch E, Chow E, Laperriere N. Radiotherapeutic management of brain metastases: a systematic review and meta-analysis. *Cancer Treat Rev.* 2005;31(4):256–273.
52. George R, Jeba J, Ramkumar G, Chacko AG, Leng M, Tharyan P. Interventions for the treatment of metastatic extradural spinal cord compression in adults. *Cochrane Database Syst Rev.* 2008;(4):CD006716.
53. Loblaw DA, Laperriere NJ, Mackillop WJ. A population-based study of malignant spinal cord compression in Ontario. *Clin Oncol (R Coll Radiol).* 2003;15(4):211–217.
54. Patchell RA, Tibbs PA, Regine WF, et al. Direct decompressive surgical resection in the treatment of spinal cord compression caused by metastatic cancer: a randomized trial. *Lancet.* 2005;366(9486):643–648.
55. Chi JH, Gokaslan Z, McCormick P, Tibbs PA, Kryscio RJ, Patchell RA. Selecting treatment for patients with

malignant epidural spinal cord compression-does age matter?: results from a randomized clinical trial. *Spine (Phila Pa 1976).* 2009;34(5):431–435.
56. Maranzano E, Trippa F, Casale M, et al. 8 Gy single-dose radiotherapy is effective in metastatic spinal cord compression: results of a phase III randomized multicentre Italian trial. *Radiother Oncol.* 2009;doi:10.1016/j.radon.2009.05.012.
57. Rades D, Dunst J, Schild SE. The first score predicting overall survival in patients with metastatic spinal cord compression. *Cancer.* 2008;112(1):157–161.
58. Rades D, Lange M, Veninga T, et al. Preliminary results of spinal cord compression recurrence evaluation (score-1) study comparing short-course versus long-course radiotherapy for local control of malignant epidural spinal cord compression. *Int J Radiat Oncol Biol Phys.* 2009;73(1):228–234.
59. Rades D, Rudat V, Veninga T, et al. A score predicting posttreatment ambulatory status in patients irradiated for metastatic spinal cord compression. *Int J Radiat Oncol Biol Phys.* 2008;72(3):905–908.
60. Gofeld M, Bhatia A, Burton AW. Vertebroplasty in the management of painful bony metastases. *Curr Pain Headache Rep.* 2009;13(4):288–294.
61. Hellman S, Weichselbaum R. Oligometastases. *J Clin Oncol.* 1995;13(1):8–10.
62. Schefter TE, Kavanach BD, Raben D, et al. A phase I/II trial of stereotactic body radiation therapy (SBRT) for lung metastases: initial report of dose escalation and early toxicity. *Int J Radiat Biol Phys.* 2006;66(4):S120–S127.
63. Rusthoven KE, Kavanagh BD, Burri SH, et al. Multi-institutional phase I/II trial of stereotactic body radiation therapy for lung metastases. *J Clin Oncol.* 2009; 27(10):1579–1584.
64. Ryu S, Fang Yin F, Rock J, Zhu J, et al. Image-guided and intensity-modulated radiosurgery for patients with spinal metastasis. *Cancer.* 2003;97(8):2013–2018.
65. Ryu S, Jin R, Jin JY, et al. Pain control by image-guided radiosurgery for solitary spinal metastasis. *J Pain Symptom Manage.* 2008;35(3):292–298.
66. Amdur RJ, Bennett J, Olivier K, et al. A prospective, phase II study demonstrating the potential value and limitation of radiosurgery for spine metastases. Am *J Clin Oncol.* 2009;32(5):515–520.
67. Rusthoven KE, Kavanagh BD, Cardenes H, et al. Multi-institutional phase I/II trial of stereotactic body radiation therapy for liver metastases. *J Clin Oncol.* 2009; 27(10):1572–1578.
68. Schefter TE, Kavanagh BD, Timmerman RD, Cardenes HR, Baron A, Gaspar LE. A phase I trial of stereotactic body radiation therapy (SBRT) for liver metastases. *Int J Radiat Oncol Biol Phys.* 2005;62(5):1371–1378.
69. Gaspar LE, Chansky K, Albain KS, et al. Time from treatment to subsequent diagnosis of brain metastases in stage III non-small-cell lung cancer: a retrospective review by the Southwest Oncology Group. *J Clin Oncol.* 2005;23(13):2955–2961.
70. Lester JF, MacBeth FR, Coles B. Prophylactic cranial irradiation for preventing brain metastases in patients undergoing radical treatment for non-small-cell lung cancer: a Cochrane review. *Int J Radiat Oncol Biol Phys.* 2005;63(3):690–694.
71. Sun A, Bae K, Gore E, et al. A phase III comparison of prophylactic cranial irradiation (PCI) versus observation in patients with locally advanced non–small cell lung cancer (LA-NSCLC). Initial analysis of primary and secondary endpoints: RTOG 0214. WCLC—13th World Conference on Lung Cancer, abstract C6, August 2009; San Francisco.
72. Topkan E, Yildirim BA, Selek U, Yavuz MN. Cranial prophylactic irradiation in locally advanced non-small cell lung carcinoma: current status and future perspectives. *Oncology.* 2009;76(3):220–228.
73. Slotman B, Faivre-Finn C, Kramer G, et al. Prophylactic cranial irradiation in extensive small-cell lung cancer. *N Engl J Med.* 2007;357(7):664–672.
74. Auperin A, Arriagada R, Pignon JP, et al. Prophylactic cranial irradiation for patients with small-cell lung cancer in complete remission. Prophylactic Cranial Irradiation Overview Collaborative Group. *N Engl J Med.* 1999;341(7):476–484.
75. Le Pechoux C, Dunant A, Senan S, et al. Standard-dose versus higher-dose prophylactic cranial irradiation (PCI) in patients with limited-stage small-cell lung cancer in complete remission after chemotherapy and thoracic radiotherapy (PCI 99–01, EORTC 22003–08004, RTOG 0212, and IFCT 99–01): a randomised clinical trial. *Lancet Oncol.* 2009;10(5):467–474.
76. Grosshans DR, Meyers CA, Allen PK, Davenport SD, Komaki R. Neurocognitive function in patients with small cell lung cancer: effect of prophylactic cranial irradiation. *Cancer.* 2008;112(3):589–595.

demos MEDICAL

RADIATION MEDICINE ROUNDS

Radiotherapy as Adjuvant Therapy and Salvage Therapy After Resection of Non–Small Cell Lung Cancer

Jonathan B. Ashman*
Mayo Clinic, Phoenix, AZ

ABSTRACT

Although distant metastatic disease is the predominant pattern of failure in lung cancer, local recurrence after surgery or radiotherapy can be a significant clinical problem. Post-operative adjuvant radiation therapy remains controversial but should be considered for patients with N2 disease. In patients who have not received prior radiation therapy, thoracic radiation is widely used for palliative symptom relief for locally recurrent and progressive disease. However, for patients with limited disease and good performance status, thoracic radiation with aggressive, curative doses is indicated for local recurrence after surgery. Brachytherapy has also been well-described as an effective technique for endobronchial disease. Even in the setting of recurrent disease after primary radiation, several series have confirmed the benefit and safety of repeat thoracic radiation. Therefore, radiation therapy has multiple indications in the management of appropriately selected patients with locally recurrent lung cancer.

INTRODUCTION

Local Recurrence after Surgery for Early-Stage Disease

In order to understand the role of local therapy in the management of recurrent lung cancer, the importance of local and regional recurrence (LRR) must be put into context. Distant metastatic disease (DM) is the dominant and most lethal pattern of failure in lung cancer. However, especially in non–small cell lung cancer (NSCLC), LRR after initial surgery or radiation therapy causes morbidity and mortality in a significant number of patients. Typically, LRRs are treated in the palliative setting, but curative regimens also can be considered in selected patients. In general, LRR rates of between 5% and 80% have been reported in the literature. The retrospective nature of most case series is one important factor, but heterogeneity also is related to patient-specific factors such as the extent of surgery, pathologic stage, and the use of adjuvant therapy.

Several retrospective series have reported rates of LRR after surgery for early stage disease. Pairolero et al. (1) reported outcomes at Mayo Clinic after surgery for 346 patients initially treated between 1972 and 1978. Patients with pathologic T1 N0 M0, T2 N0 M0, and T1 N1 M0 were followed with physical examination, sputum cytology, and chest x-ray. Thirty-nine percent of patients developed additional disease: 45% DM, 25% new primary, 20% LRR, and 10% DM plus LRR. Interestingly, while the rate of overall disease recurrence was highest during the first year of follow-up and then declined with time, the rate of LRR remained constant over the first 4 years.

*Corresponding author, Department of Radiation Oncology, Mayo Clinic, 5777 E. Mayo Blvd., Phoenix, AZ 85054
E-mail address: ashman.jonathan@mayo.edu

Radiation Medicine Rounds 1 (2010) 83–100.

DOI: 10.5003/2151–4208.1.1.83

At 2 years from detection of recurrence, 23.4% of patients had survived after isolated LRR compared to only 8.9% with DM.

The Ludwig Lung Cancer Study Group analyzed the patterns of failure for 1,012 patient with resected stages I and II NSCLC (2). Patients were entered onto studies between 1977 and 1983. Overall, 42% of patients developed objective evidence of failure. The site of first failure was intrathoracic in approximately one-half of these patients, with recurrence at the bronchial resection line occurring in more than one-quarter of this subset. Intrathoracic recurrence was reduced in patients who underwent pneumonectomy or bilobectomy.

During a similar time span of treatment, Martini et al. (3) reported a series of 598 patients treated surgically for pathologic stage I NSCLC at Memorial Sloan-Kettering Cancer Center. Lobectomy was performed in 85% of cases, pneumonectomy in 4%, and wedge or segmentectomy in 11%. Mediastinal staging was performed in 94% of cases. Recurrence was observed in 27% of patients, and, of these patients, 20% experience LR and 8% regional recurrence. In this series, only 5% of patients who underwent mediastinal lymph node dissection developed LRR, and most cases of LRR were seen in the patients treated with wedge resection or segmentectomy.

Several other smaller series reported similar results for early-stage patients. Al-Kattan et al. (4) performed a retrospective analysis of 123 patients treated in the United Kingdom between 1987 and 1988. All of the patients underwent complete resection for stage I lung cancer. Of the patients, 96 were treated with lobectomy and 27 with pneumonectomy. The rate of LRR was 15%. Virgo and colleagues (5) analyzed 182 patients who underwent surgical resection with curative intent between 1982 and 1992 at the St. Louis Department of Veterans Affairs Medical Center. Patients were included if they had stage I–IIIA disease, but "most" of the patients were reported to have had stage I lesions. The LRR rate was found to be 13%. Choi et al. (6) reported a more modern series from Korea of 482 stages I and II patients treated surgically between 1995 and 2000. Isolated LRR was identified in 19% of the patients, and combined LRR and DM occurred in another 11% of the patients.

The rate of LRR in patients undergoing sublobar resections has also been the subject of several reports. Researchers at M.D. Anderson Cancer Center reviewed 358 patients with stage I–III disease who had undergone complete resection for NSCLC (7). Patients were excluded if they had superior sulcus tumors or mixed small cell or neuroendocrine pathology. While 25% of the patients developed DM, 9% of the patients developed LRR only and an additional 4% developed LRR together with DM. Patients who underwent wedge or segmental resections were almost twice as likely to have LRR as were patients undergoing lobectomy. Patients with LRR only had a median survival of 33.9 months compared to approximately 19 months for patients with DM (P = nonsignificant).

A recent series from Germany by Sienel and colleagues (8) analyzed 87 stage IA patients who all underwent a sublobar resection between 1987 and 2003. One-quarter of the patients overall developed LRR, but the incidence was significantly higher in patients who underwent wedge resection compared to segmentectomy (55% vs. 16%). The rate of DM was not significantly different, but survival was poorer in the wedge resection group. Even in patients with primary tumors less than 2 cm in size, there was a 40% recurrence rate among the patients in the wedge resection cohort compared with 11% in the segmentectomy cohort, and the survival difference persisted between groups.

In a prospective randomized trial, the Lung Cancer Study Group also found a significantly higher rate of recurrence for patients for patients undergoing more limited procedures (9). All patients underwent mediastinal node sampling and were deemed T1 N0 at the time of intraoperative randomization. A tripling of the rate of LRR was found for patients undergoing wedge resections or segmentectomy compared with lobectomy.

Not all series have shown a higher recurrence rate with sublobar resections. Okada et al. (10) reported a nonrandomized, prospective study from three Japanese institutions over a period of 10 years from 1992 to 2001. The cohort contained 567 patients with node-negative, peripheral tumors <2 cm (305 patients in the sublobar resection group; 262 patients in the lobectomy group). With a median follow-up of over 70 months, LRR was detected in only 4.9% of patients in the sublobar resection group and 6.9% of patients in the lobectomy group (P = nonsignificant).

Adjuvant Radiation After Surgery

LRR after surgery potentially presents a more clinically significant concern for patients with locally advanced disease. Especially in the setting of N2 disease, the use of postoperative thoracic radiation therapy (TRT) continues to be an area of controversy. To better understand patterns of failure and potential risk factors, a detailed retrospective analysis of patients with pathologic N2 disease was performed in two studies by Sawyer and colleagues (11) at Mayo Clinic. In the initial report, 224 patients were included who underwent surgery between 1987 and 1993. The surgical procedures were segmentectomy in 33 patients, lobectomy in 115 patients, and removal of >1 lobe or pneumonectomy in 76 patients. Postoperative TRT was delivered in 88 patients, and 26 patients also received chemotherapy. In patients who had surgery alone, the 4-year actuarial freedom from LRR was only 60%, and 4-year freedom from LRR as the site of first recurrence was 50%. Indeed, in patients with more than a single involved N2 lymph node, only 20% were free from LRR at 4 years. Adjuvant TRT was quite effective in controlling LRR. Regardless of the number of involved N2 nodes, the 4-year freedom from LRR after TRT was increased to approximately 80%. The authors extended their findings using regression tree analysis to further stratify this same cohort of N2 patients into risk groups (12). Prognostic factors for LRR included involvement of N1 lymph nodes, T stage, involvement of the superior or inferior mediastinum or both, and whether that involvement was in accordance to the location of the primary tumor. The 4-year actuarial freedom from LRR for the low-risk, medium-risk, and high-risk groups was 70%, 40%, and zero, respectively. These studies demonstrated that the risk of LRR after surgery for N2 patients is high and that postoperative TRT can significantly reduce LRR. In addition, the data suggested a significant impact of adjuvant TRT on overall survival, especially in the medium-risk and high-risk N2 populations. The 4-year actuarial survival for high-risk patients who received adjuvant TRT was 37% compared with 4% for patients who did not receive TRT ($P = 0.0002$).

The importance of determining the relationship of LRR on survival spurred several randomized trials to define a role for TRT in the postoperative setting. These trials provide additional insight into the rate of LRR both after surgery alone and after adjuvant TRT. An excellent overview of these data is provided in a recent review by Krupitskaya and Loo (13). Many of these trials included patients with node-positive disease. Surgery alone resulted in a rate of LRR between 16% and 47%. The impact of adjuvant postoperative TRT varied quite dramatically across the studies, with rates of LRR between 1% and 42%. However, the importance of LRR and postoperative TRT on survival remained unclear. The data from the PORT Meta-analysis Trialists Group suggested a decrement in survival for adjuvant TRT for early-stage patients but a trend toward improvement in survival after adjuvant TRT for stage III or N2 patients (14). A criticism of this analysis was the inclusion of trials using outdated radiation techniques, which likely increased the risk for treatment-related mortality. To address these concerns, Lally and colleagues (15) performed a retrospective analysis of the Surveillance, Epidemiology, and End Results (SEER) database. Patients with stage II or III disease treated between 1988 and 2002 were included in the analysis and evaluated for outcome with respect to use of adjuvant TRT. This time period was selected because treatment was likely to have been delivered using modern, linear accelerator-based techniques. Consistent with the prior meta-analysis, adjuvant TRT in patients with either N0 or N1 disease resulted in a decrement in survival. However, a survival benefit was observed with the use of adjuvant TRT in patients with N2 disease. This benefit was statistically significant for both overall survival and disease-specific survival and on both univariate and multivariate analysis.

Additional insight regarding adjuvant TRT delivered with modern techniques in the setting of a prospective trial was learned from the recent Adjuvant Navelbine International Trialist Association (ANITA) study (16). The primary design of this trial was to test adjuvant chemotherapy after completely resected stage IB-IIIA NSCLC. Between 1994 and 2000, 840 patients were randomized after surgery to either observation or cisplatin plus vinorelbine chemotherapy. However, a subgroup of node-positive patients also received adjuvant TRT in a nonrandomized fashion. In a subsequent analysis, the rates of LRR were reported for patients receiving surgery alone, surgery plus chemotherapy, surgery plus adjuvant TRT, or surgery plus chemotherapy plus adjuvant TRT (17). For patients who received neither chemotherapy nor postop TRT, the rate of isolated LRR in patient with N0, N1, and N2 disease was 18%, 21%, and 29%, respectively. Chemotherapy appeared to reduce the rate of LRR even in the absence of TRT. Again for N0, N1, or N2 patients, isolated LRR with postoperative chemotherapy was 10.4%, 13.4%, and 18.6%, respectively. These recurrence rates were similar to those for postoperative

TRT in the absence of chemotherapy. Patients with N1 or N2 disease appeared to benefit from the combination of chemotherapy and adjuvant TRT with isolated LRR rates of 8% and 6.3%, respectively. With regards to overall survival, TRT appeared to benefit only those N1 patients who did not get chemotherapy. For patients with N2 disease, postoperative TRT improved the survival rate regardless of the use of adjuvant chemotherapy. Indeed, for N2 patients who received adjuvant chemotherapy, the addition of TRT approximately doubled the median survival from 23.8 months to 47.4 months.

Taken together, the data from these retrospective and prospective studies suggest that a subset of high risk N2 patients may benefit from postoperative TRT. Two phase 3 trials are being planned; one in the United States and the other in Europe. A joint American College of Surgical Oncologists Group (ACOSOG) and Radiation Therapy and Oncology Group (RTOG) trial includes patients with resected N2 disease who receive chemotherapy and are randomly assigned to receive either TRT versus no radiotherapy. This is the Adjuvant Mediastinal Observation or Radiotherapy Evaluation (AMORE) Trial. The European trial is entitled the Lung Adjuvant Radiotherapy Trial (Lung ART) and will compare three-dimensional (3D) conformal PORT versus no PORT for N2 patients who have had complete resection irrespective of chemotherapy. These trials should better define the role of adjuvant radiotherapy for resected N2 patients.

■ TREATMENT OF LOCAL RECURRENCE

Re-operation for Postoperative Recurrence

There is little data with regard to surgical salvage of patients with LRR. One early study by Gabler and Leibig (18) evaluated 12 patients who underwent re-operation for ipsilateral LRR. Eleven patients had a pneumonectomy and one patient had a wedge resection. Three of the patients survived over a long-term period, and the patients who lived greater than 30 days after the second surgery had a median survival of 18 months. A more modern study of iterative resections was reported from Italy by Voltolini and colleagues (19). Representing just 1.1% of all patients who had undergone primary surgical resection between 1978 and 1998, 12 patients were identified who underwent a re-operation for LRR. Ten patients were treated with pneumonectomy, one patient with lobectomy, and one patient with wedge resection. Five-year survival was 15.5% and median survival was 26 months. Thus, it appears possible to successfully salvage a small percentage of patients who fail resection with further surgical interventions.

TRT for Postoperative Recurrence

For patients who did not receive adjuvant postoperative radiation as part of their primary management, salvage TRT is logical for LRR. The intent of such salvage TRT may be curative or palliative. Without randomized trials, only single institution series are available (Table 1). Green and Kern were among the first in the modern era to describe their experience treating locally recurrent lung cancer (20). They reported on 46 patients treated with TRT for postoperative LRR and no evidence of DM between 1963 and 1976. Mediastinal or hilar recurrences were observed in 36 patients. Radiation doses were generally delivered with aggressive regimens, and 34 patients received doses ≥ 4,000 cGy. Subjective response was observed in 63% of patients, which correlated well with an objective response in 61% of patients. Favorable responses were more common among patients in the higher dose group than in those patients who received lower doses (70% vs. 33%, P value not stated). The median survival was 11 months, and 2-year survival was 10%. The median survival was 19 months for those patients both who received ≥ 4,000 cGy and who had a favorable response.

Shortly thereafter, Kopelson and Choi (21) reported their series from Harvard. Between 1962 and 1979, 24 patients were treated with TRT for LRR of lung cancer after surgery. All of the patients had non-small cell histology, no prior history of TRT, and no DM. The median time interval from surgery to recurrence was 15 months (range 4–39 months). Chemotherapy was only used in two patients who developed DM subsequent to TRT. Radiotherapy techniques varied over the time period, and doses ranged from 1,865 cGy to 6,200 cGy. One patient received three courses of TRT for bronchial stump recurrences. The median survival was almost 12 months, and two patients were long-term survivors. Symptoms were palliated either completely or partially 80% of the time. Approximately one-half of the patients developed LRR after TRT.

TABLE 1 External beam thoracic radiation therapy for postoperative local recurrence

1st Author (Ref)	Number of Patients	Dose (Gy)	Median Survival (months)	Notes
Green (20)	46	25–65	11	MS = 19 months in patients with favorable response to high dose
Kopelson (21)	24	18–62	11	2 long-term survivors
Law (22)	14	51–60	32	5 long-term survivors
Shaw (23)	37	12–75	13.7	5-year survival = 4%
Curran (24)	37	56 (median)	12	Survival similar between patients with recurrent or primary disease
Yano (25)	32	50–60	19	MS = 27 months in responding patients
Kagami (26)	32	47.5–65	14	4 long-term survivors
Leung (27)	45	20–60	10	MS = 16 months for high dose patients
Emami (28)	52	16–75	8.5	MS = 12 months for patients recurring greater than 24 months after surgery
Jeremic (29)	61	30–60	13	MS = 38 months for recurrence only at bronchial stump
Kelsey (30)	29	46–74	17	Local control = 62%; 2-year survival = 38%
Cai (31)	54	>59.4 in 63%	19.8	MS equivalent between stage I–III patients with recurrent or primary disease

mo = months; MS = median survival.

One of the first studies to report the particularly favorable outcome of isolated LRR at the bronchial stump was by Law et al. (22) from London. They reviewed the records of 1,000 patients who had undergone surgical resection for lung cancer between 1966 and 1975, and 17 patients were identified with bronchial stump recurrence. Of these patients, the recurrence was confined only to the bronchial stump in six patients, and all received additional radiation therapy. Two were treated with radioactive gold grains and four received external beam doses of 5,000 to 6,100 cGy in standard fractionation. Five of these six patients survived >5 years without evidence of disease.

The Mayo Clinic experience was reported by Shaw et al. (23) and included 37 patients treated with definitive intent TRT between 1976 and 1985. Total doses ranged from 1,200 cGy to 7,500 cGy, and the most frequent dose regimen was 4,000 cGy in 10 fractions with a split course. Radiographic responses were assessed by chest x-ray, and 54% of the patients had a complete or partial response while only 6% progressed. Symptomatic response was observed in 48% of the patients, and the remainder had stable symptoms. The median survival was 13.7 months. Survival was 30% at 2 years and 4% at 5 years. Only one patient did not have evidence of treatment failure. Approximately two-thirds of patients developed local failure and one-half the patients developed DM. In this cohort, there was no difference in survival with the addition of chemotherapy to salvage TRT. The authors' conclusion was that more aggressive local therapy was necessary.

At approximately the same time as the Mayo study, Curran and colleagues (24) reported a series from Fox Chase Cancer Center. The outcomes of 37 patients with NSCLC treated with salvage TRT for LRR after surgery were compared with those of 759 patients treated with primary TRT for unresected disease. Over 80% of patients in each cohort had stage III disease at the time of TRT. Radiation doses were generally higher than in the Mayo Clinic series. The median dose for patients with recurrent and primary disease was 5,600 cGy and 5,900 cGy, respectively. Despite the more aggressive doses, median survival for patients with recurrent disease was 12 months and the 2-year survival rate was 22%. There was no statistical difference in this rate of survival compared with patients treated with primary TRT. Both groups were found to have a 30% 2-year freedom from local-regional progression. Patients with bronchial stump recurrence had a median survival of 36 months compared with only 9 months for patients with nodal or chest wall recurrences. These results were interpreted as justification for aggressive salvage of select patients with LRR and good performance status.

Yano et al. (25) reported a series from Japan describing 32 patients with isolated LRR recurrences after surgical resection. Within this cohort, 17 had previously been treated with adjuvant chemotherapy and 6 had been treated with adjuvant radiotherapy. Hilar and mediastinal recurrences were the most common sites of recurrence. Treatment of recurrent disease included TRT in 29 patients and chemotherapy in 12 patients. The total radiation dose was between 5,000 cGy and 6,000 cGy in standard fractionation. The median survival was 19 months, and 2-year survival was 38%. Sixteen patients achieved a complete or partial response to therapy, and these patients had a significantly longer median survival compared to nonresponders (27 months vs. 6 months, $P < .01$). Response to TRT was the only significant prognostic factor on multivariate analysis.

A second Japanese series reported by Kagami and colleagues (26) included another 32 patients with LRR who had undergone surgical resection for lung cancer between 1981 and 1991. All of the patients were treated with salvage TRT, and an aggressive radiation regimen was undertaken with doses ranging from 4,750 cGy to 6,500 cGy in 250 cGy fractions delivered 4 days per week. Twenty-five patients received doses of 6,000 cGy or more. Clinical improvement was achieved in 17 or 19 symptomatic patients. Response was assessed by bronchoscopy, chest x-ray, and chest computed tomography (CT). An objective response rate of 65% was observed, and a complete response was achieved in 7 of 25 patients treated to doses of 6,000 cGy or more. Despite these encouraging initial responses, approximately two-thirds of patients ultimately relapsed, and only 4 patients survived more than 5 years. Median survival was 14 months, and 2-year survival was 28.1%.

Leung and colleagues (27) reported their experience from Australia with 45 patients treated with salvage TRT for LRR after surgery between 1984 and 1990. Seventeen of these patients with performance status 0–1, weight loss <10%, and no evidence of DM were treated with 6,000 cGy TRT in 6 weeks. The remaining 28 patients were treated with palliative fractionation schedules. For the entire cohort, the median survival was 10 months, and the 2-year survival was 27%. However, the patients treated with curative intent had a median survival of 15.6 months. The disease-free interval between surgery and first relapse was not a significant prognostic factor for survival. Similar to the study of Curran et al. (24), no significant difference in survival was identified between the 17 patients who were treated with curative doses of TRT at the time of recurrence compared to 211 patients treated with similar doses of TRT as primary treatment.

A large series was reported by Emami and colleagues (28) from the Mallinckrodt Institute including 52 patients who were treated with definitive surgery between 1975 and 1988 and then presented for salvage TRT without evidence of DM. TRT was delivered using standard fractionation over a range of doses from 1,620 cGy to 7,500 cGy, and 35 patients received doses of 5,000 cGy or greater. The median survival was 8.5 months, and the 2-year survival was 18%. Patients who had complete or partial responses to TRT had improved survival, and response to TRT was significantly related to higher doses. Local control was obtained in approximately one-half of the patients after TRT. In this series, the disease-free interval between surgery and LRR was a significant prognostic factor. The median survival for patients recurring less than 6 months after surgery was 4.8 months compared to 12 months for patients recurring greater than 24 months after surgery. The disease-free interval itself was significantly related to initial surgical stage.

The largest experience in the literature was reported by Jeremic et al. (29). The authors identified 61 patients who had been treated between 1982 and 1993 with LRR after complete resections and no DM. At the discretion of the treating physician, patients were treated with either radical TRT doses between 5,500 cGy and 6,000 cGy in standard fractionation or a palliative dose of 3,000 cGy in 10 fractions. Patients treated with palliative intent were more likely to have initial-stage IIIA disease and to have weight loss >5% prior to salvage TRT. The median survival was 13 months, and the 2-year survival was 28%. Survival was significantly better for patients treated with curative intent compared with palliative intent: median survival 18 months versus 7 months, and 2-year survival 36% versus 11% ($P < .0001$). No patient treated with palliative intent was alive at 3 years. Salvage TRT resulted in an improvement in symptoms for both groups, but was significantly more frequent in the high-dose TRT group (72% vs. 42%, P = .029). Both groups still experienced high local failure rates (50% vs. 74%, P = .083). Factors that influenced survival among patients treated with curative intent included female sex, initial surgical stage, and recurrent stage. In addition, patients with only bronchial stump recurrence did significantly better than those patients who relapsed in the nodes or chest wall. The median survival for the 15 patients with isolated bronchial stump recurrence was 38 months, and the 2- and 5-year survival was 73% and 33%, respectively.

Two more modern series have been published addressing the role of salvage TRT. Kelsey et al. (30) reported the experience of Duke University of 29 patients treated with surgical resection between 1991 and 2003. One patient had been treated with adjuvant postoperative chemotherapy, but none had been treated with postoperative TRT. At the time of relapse, all patients had CT and bone scan imaging, and 15 patients also had Positron Emission Tomography (PET). All of the patients were treated with curative intent to a median dose of 6,600 cGy. Most were treated with standard fractionation, but six received accelerated hyperfractionation and three received 250 cGy fractions. Chemotherapy was added in 15 patients, either neoadjuvantly in 7 patients or concurrently in 8 patients. The median survival was 17 months, and the 2-year survival was 38%. Local control was achieved at 2 years in 62% of patients. No prognostic factors influencing survival could be readily identified, which was most likely related to the small sample size.

The most recent series has been reported from the University of Michigan (31). Cai and colleagues describe 661 patients treated with TRT for lung cancer between 1992 and 2004. Of these patients, 54 patients received TRT at the time of relapse after surgery and 607 received TRT as primary treatment. Stage IV patients comprised a greater percentage of patients in the newly diagnosed cohort. This difference may be reflected in the finding that 63% of recurrent patients received definitive doses of radiotherapy (>5,940 cGy) compared with only 47% of the newly diagnosed patients. There were no differences in the use of chemotherapy between cohorts. When only patients with stage I–III at the time of TRT were considered, there were 46 patients in the recurrent cohort and 408 patients in the newly diagnosed cohort. For patients treated at the time of recurrence, the median survival was 13.8 months, and the 5-year survival was 8.9%. This was not significantly better than the median survival and the 5-year survival for patients with primary disease (12.6 months and 9.7%, respectively). Stratification for stage, histology, gender, or use of chemotherapy did not reveal significant differences between patients with recurrent or newly diagnosed disease. However, survival was better for patients with recurrent disease compared to patients with newly diagnosed disease in the subgroups either treated palliative TRT doses or among patients <60 years of age. Univariate and multivariate analyses were used to look for prognostic factors only with the 46 recurrent patients with stage I–III disease. Stage, histology, gender, age, TRT dose, and time from surgery to recurrence were not significant. Chemotherapy use was the only factor associated with improved survival.

These data are striking in the consistency with prior studies dating back decades despite advances in imaging and treatment. Patients with LRR after surgery still have a poor prognosis overall. However, outcomes with TRT are comparable and, in some scenarios, superior to newly diagnosed patients of similar stage. Together the data argue strongly for use of TRT in the management of recurrent lung cancer after surgery and for aggressive, definitive doses for selected patients. Patients with bronchial stump recurrence may be especially good candidates for aggressive local treatment as they appear to have a better prognosis. Jeremic et al. (32) reviewed the literature in 2002 specifically with regards to the use of high-dose TRT for bronchial stump recurrence. A median survival of 30 months and a 2-year survival rate of 55% were reported. In addition, as is the case with locally advanced NSCLC patients, patients with recurrences are at high risk for failure with TRT alone and probably would benefit from the addition of chemotherapy to the radiation therapy.

Brachytherapy for Endobronchial Recurrence After Thoracic Radiation

Brachytherapy represents an alternative or complementary treatment strategy for locally recurrent lung cancer. It has the advantages of delivering high doses very precisely, short treatment courses, and low risks of acute toxicities. High dose rate brachytherapy (HDR-BT) has been the principle technique described for endobronchial treatment, especially in the setting of recurrent disease after TRT (33).

TABLE 2 High dose rate brachytherapy after prior thoracic radiation therapy

1st Author (Ref)	Number of Patients	Dose (Gy)	Number of Fractions	Median Survival (months)	Symptom Relief (%)	Toxicity
Seagren (34)	20	10	1	9	94	PH in 5 cases
Sutedja (35)	31	10	3	7	71	PH in 10 cases; fistula in 2 cases
Bedwinek (36)	32	6	3	6.5	76	PH in 12 cases
Speiser (37)	151	7.5	3	6.2	80	PH in 7%; Bronchitis 12%
Nori (38)	32	4–5	3–4	7.5	100	No severe reported
Ornadel (39)	109	15	1	12	50–90	PH 11% @ 1 yr
Hernandez (40)	29	7.5–10	3	5.5	24–69	PH in 1 cases
Kelly (41)	175	15	2	6	66	PH 9% @ 1 yr

PH = pulmonary hemorrhage.

Several of the most influential studies are reviewed here and described in Table 2.

One of the earliest reports was from Seagren et al. (34) in 1985. These authors describe 20 patients previously treated with TRT to at least 5,000 cGy who presented with symptomatic endobronchial recurrence. Patients were treated between 1982 and 1983 to a dose of 1,000 cGy in a single fraction. Two patients received an additional course of HDR-BT for progressive disease. Laser therapy was performed in four patients. The median interval from primary TRT to HDR-BT was 9 months (range 3–21 months). The median survival from HDR-BT was 9 months, and one patient had long-term survival greater than 2 years. Symptomatic relief was achieved in 94% of patients, and six patients had complete resolution of symptoms. Twelve patients had a recurrence of symptoms at a mean interval of 4.3 months. Toxicity was reported as minimal without long-term complications appreciated such as fistula or bronchitis. Five patients (28%) died of massive hemoptysis. All of these patients were known to have active endobronchial disease, and, therefore, the authors favored tumor progression rather than treatment effect as the most likely cause of death.

Sutedja et al. (35) conducted a phase 2 trial of HDR-BT for patients with endobronchial recurrence of NSCLC after TRT. Thirty-one patients were entered over approximately 1 year from 1988 to 1989. Fourteen patients were treated with laser resection prior to HDR-BT. The dose of brachytherapy was 1,000 cGy per fraction prescribed at 1 cm from the source and delivered every 2 weeks to a maximum of three treatments. Twenty-two patients had a partial response, and nine patients had no response. The median survival of responders was 7 months, but it was only 3 months for nonresponders. The cause of death was attributed to local disease progression in 16 patients, fatal hemorrhage in 10 patients, and fistula in 2 patients. Of the 10 patients who developed hemorrhage, 7 also had laser resection.

Bedwinek and colleagues (36) reported their experience with endobronchial HDR-BT for recurrent disease after TRT in 1992. Thirty-eight patients were analyzed with inclusion criteria similar to those from Seagren et al. The dose was 600 cGy per fraction prescribed to 1 cm from the center of the source in 3 weekly fractions. Four patients underwent a second course of three-fraction HDR-BT for a second relapse. Nine patients had endobronchial laser ablation prior to brachytherapy. The median survival from HDR-BT was 6.5 months. Partial or complete symptom relief was achieved in 76% of patients. The median duration of symptom relief was 5 months (range 2–14 months). Among the 27 patients who underwent repeat bronchoscopy, 82% had partial or complete objective regression of disease. The strongest predictor of symptom relief was extrabronchial disease measuring <5 cm. There were no cases of fistula, pneumothorax, bronchial stenosis, or bronchitis. However, fatal pulmonary hemorrhage occurred 32% of patients at a median interval of 10 weeks post-brachytherapy. Causation could not be definitively assigned to either tumor progression or treatment-related complication. However, a potential risk factor was location of the tumor, because all of the cases occurred in patients with tumors located in the right mainstem bronchus, right upper lobe, or left upper lobe. It was noted that tumors in these location would have a close proximity to the pulmonary artery.

With the high complication rate reported by Bedwinek et al. and Seagren et al., several more studies were published to add additional institutional experiences to the literature. Speiser and Spratling (37) provided a detailed analysis in their 1993 report. They included 151 patients treated with HDR-BT between 1987 and 1991 for recurrent disease after prior TRT. Patient selection for HDR-BT required symptomatic, endobronchial disease of the proximal airways. The dose was 750 cGy per fraction prescribed to a depth of 1 cm from the source for 3 weekly fractions. Selected patients also had endobronchial laser ablation. The median survival from retreatment was 6.2 months. Hemoptysis and postobstructive pneumonia were relieved in essentially all patients by first post-brachytherapy follow-up, and dyspnea and cough were relieved in more than 80% of patients. Acute complications from the procedures were rare. Long-term complications included radiation bronchitis and stenosis in 12% of patients. Fatal hemoptysis occurred in 7.3% of patients, but all of these patients had documented recurrent or residual disease.

Nori and colleagues (38) described a series of 32 patients treated with HDR-BT after TRT. Seventeen of these patients had LRR at mean interval of 6 months after TRT and a median prior dose of TRT of 5,000 cGy (range 4,000–5,000 cGy). The HDR-BT dose was 400 cGy to 500 cGy per fraction prescribed to 1 cm from the source and delivered in 3 or 4 weekly fractions. For locally recurrent patients, the median follow-up after brachytherapy was 8 months, and the median survival was 7.5 months. All of the patients had a symptomatic response, and 70% had local control at 6 months. Complications were described as minimal, and there were no cases of hemorrhage or fistula.

Ornadel et al. (39) reported a large prospective series from England. A total of 117 patients were treated between 1991 and 1995, and, of these, 109 had lung cancer. Prior treatment included TRT in 92 patients and laser ablation in 51 patients. The HDR-BT was delivered as a single fraction of 1,500 cGy prescribed to 1 cm from the source. Three patients received two HDR-BT treatments at intervals of 1, 6, and 14 months. One patient received three treatments separated by 3 and 4 months. The median survival was 12 months. Hemoptysis was palliated in approximately 90% of patients, and cough and dyspnea improved in approximately one-half of the patients. Patients with greater initial dyspnea scores were more likely to die within 2 months of treatment. Eleven patients suffered fatal hemoptysis, with an actuarial risk of 11% at 1 year and 20% at 2 years. Prior laser therapy was significantly associated with this complication.

A prospective trial of HDR-BT for persistence or recurrence of endobronchial disease after TRT was reported from Canada (40). Hernandez et al. studied 29 patients treated between 1992 and 1994. Four patients had small cell histology. The median interval from TRT to HDR-BT was 12.9 months (range 1–21.3 months). Three patients underwent laser debulking of tumor at least 4 weeks prior to brachytherapy. The mean single fraction dose was 805 cGy (range 750–1,000 cGy) prescribed to a depth of 1 cm from the source. Twenty-six of the patients completed the planned 3 fractions delivered at 2-week intervals. The median survival from study entry was 5.5 months. Of the patients who underwent repeat bronchoscopy, 11 patients (42%) had improvement in bronchial obstruction, and only two patients (8%) had progression of disease. Hemoptysis was improved in 69% of patients. One patient developed nonfatal, massive hemoptysis that occurred within 2 hours of brachytherapy.

The 10-year experience of M.D. Anderson Cancer Center using HDR-BT for patients with relapsed or persistent endobronchial lung cancer was reported by Kelly and colleagues (41) in 2000. The series included 175 patients treated between 1988 and 1997, and 160 of these patients had previously received TRT. A subset of these patients had been previously reported by Delclos et al. (42) Most of the patients had NSCLC, but 5% of the patients had small cell histology. Most of the patients were treated with 1,500 cGy per fraction prescribed to a distance of 6 mm from the source and received 2-weekly fractions. This dose was calculated to be approximately 840 cGy at 1 cm from the source. Twenty patients received laser ablation, and 17 patients had chemotherapy. The median survival was 6 months. An objective response rate was 78% on the basis of repeat bronchoscopy. Symptom improvement was observed in 66% of patients. The mean duration of response was 3.8 months. Patients who had a symptomatic response had a median survival of 7 months compared with only 4 months in patients courses of TRT was 16 months (range 5–60 months). Reirradiation dose was delivered with standard fractionation to a dose of 5,000 cGy for 18 patients and 6,000 cGy for 1 patient. The spinal cord was not included in the reirradiation field. The median survival was 7.1 months, and the 2-year survival was 11%. Five patients did not complete the full course of repeat TRT. Improved survival was associated with better performance status, and the median survival for patients with performance status 0–1 was 12.6 months. Improved survival also was associated with a longer disease-free interval from initial treatment. Patients with >18 months between courses of TRT had a median survival of 11.5 months, while patients with <12 months interval had a median survival of only 2.1 months. The response rate was 43% among patients who completed full dose reirradiation, and seven of eight patients were successfully palliated by repeat TRT. Only one patient developed grade 3 pneumonitis.

A third, more recent paper from Japan reported the largest case series to date. Ebara et al. (54) describe 44 patients treated between 1990 and 2004. The cohort was generally high functioning prior to reirradiation with 38 patients ECOG PS 0–1. Histology was small cell in nine patients. The median time between courses of TRT was 12.6 months (range 5.8–47.2 months). Radiation fields were defined conventionally using an x-ray simulator. The median dose was 6,000 cGy for initial TRT and was 4,000 cGy for repeat TRT. The median cumulative dose was 10,200 cGy with a range of 8,000 to 13,000 cGy. Chemotherapy was used during the initial therapy for 25 patients and during the reirradiation for 16 patients. The median survival of the whole group was 6.5 months. When only patients with local disease were analyzed, median survival was 7.1 months, and 2-year survival was 31.3%. Symptoms were well controlled, and 74% of all symptoms resolved or improved with repeat TRT. Similar to the findings from Gressen et al. (51), hemoptysis and pain were more readily controlled than cough and dyspnea. Grade 2 and 3 pneumonitis each was observed in three patients within 3 months of reirradiation. However, no other severe toxicities were documented with a median follow-up of 6.5 months.

The most recent study on reirradiation has been reported by Cetingoz and colleagues (55) from Turkey. The authors describe 38 patients who underwent repeat TRT between 1992 and 2006. All of the patients initially had nonmetastatic NSCLC, and all but two patients were stage III. Nevertheless, the intent of initial treatment was palliative in 84% of patients. Doses of initial TRT ranged between 2,880 cGy and 6,720 cGy (median 3,000 cGy) and delivered in 200 to 320 cGy fractions. The median interval between courses of TRT was 35 weeks (range 4–189 weeks). At the time of reirradiation, all of the patients had documented radiological progression, six patients had evidence of DM, and 36 patients were symptomatic. The intent of repeat TRT was palliative in all of the patients. The median dose was 2,500 cGy (range 500–3,000 cGy), and the median fraction size was 300 cGy (range 200–1,000 cGy). Nine patients received chemotherapy prior to reirradiation, and one patient received chemotherapy concurrently with reirradiation. The median survival was 3 months, and only one patient was alive beyond 2 years. An interval free from local recurrence of greater than 35 weeks was the only significant prognostic factor for survival on univariate and multivariate analysis. Partial or complete symptomatic response was observed in 78% of patients and was seen at higher frequency in patients with central tumors compared with peripheral tumors (90% vs. 75%, $P = .01$). Toxicity was not described in great detail in this series. There was one case of acute grade 3 esophagitis, but no reported late grade 3 or 4 cases of pneumonitis. The rate of grade 2 pneumonitis was not reported.

Two prospective series of repeat TRT for lung cancer are reported in the literature. Wu et al. (56) conducted a Chinese phase 1–2 trial using 3D-conformal techniques. Eligibility criteria included Karnofsky Performance Status (KPS) of at least 70 and an interval between TRT courses of 6 months or greater. Between 1999 and 2001, 23 patients were enrolled in the study. Six patients had initially been treated with palliative intent. Seven patients had small cell histology. The median dose delivered for the first course of TRT was 6,600 cGy (range 3,000–7,800 cGy). The median dose delivered for reirradiation was 5,100 cGy (range 4,600–6,000 cGy) and delivered using conventional fractionation. The dose to the spinal cord was restricted to less than 2,500 cGy at the second course of TRT. The median interval between courses of TRT was 13 months (range 6–42 months). The number of patients receiving chemotherapy was not directly stated, but the median number of chemotherapy cycles was one. No acute grade 3 or greater toxicity was observed, but 22% of patients developed grade 2 pneumonitis. With a median follow-up of 15 months, the median survival was 14 months, and

2-year survival was 21%. Seven patients were still alive at the last follow-up, and five were disease-free. Two patients developed symptomatic late pulmonary fibrosis. No data regarding palliation of symptoms were provided in this report.

Kramer et al. (57) reported a second prospective trial from Europe in which they specifically investigated a hypofractionated treatment regimen of 1,600 cGy in two 800 cGy fractions separated by 1 week. Between 1991 and 1999, 28 patients with NSCLC were enrolled on the protocol. Initial TRT doses ranged from 3,600 cGy to 6,000 cGy. The spinal cord was excluded in the reirradiation plans, and the dose to the contralateral lung was minimized. The median survival was 5.6 months, and only three patients remained alive at 1 year postreirradiation. All of these patients had a recurrence-free interval of greater than 1 year between courses of TRT. Improvement in symptoms was achieved in 71% of patients. Superior vena cava syndrome and hemoptysis were successfully palliated in all symptomatic patients. The authors emphasized that palliation of symptoms was achieved for greater than 50% of the patient's remaining lifespan in 22 of 25 cases. One patient developed grade 2 esophagitis. One treatment-related death occurred from bronchopulmonary fistula. This patient suffered from recurrent hemoptysis and had been initially treated with brachytherapy, then 8 months later with repeat TRT on the protocol, and then 2 months later with laser vaporization.

Stereotactic body radiotherapy has become an exciting technique that offers the possibility of safely delivering radiobiologically potent high doses per fraction. Tumor targeting is maximized and toxicity is limited by utilizing new delivery systems and image guidance. Only one report has specifically addressed using SBRT techniques to deliver repeat TRT for NSCLC. Poltinnikov et al. (58) report the Thomas Jefferson University early experience with 17 patients treated with stereotactic techniques between 1999 and 2003. All of the patients had been treated with at least 5,000 cGy and concurrent chemotherapy during their initial treatment course. Concurrent chemotherapy was delivered in five patients at the time of reirradiation. The median time interval between courses of TRT was 13 months (range 2–39 months). Margins from the gross tumor volume (GTV) to the planning treatment volume (PTV) were kept to 5 mm, and daily pretreatment CT was done for image-guidance. The median dose was 3,200 cGy delivered in 400 cGy fractions prescribed to the 90% isodose line. The median survival time from reirradiation was 5.5 months (range 2.5–30 months), and one patient was alive and disease-free for 2.5 years after completion of a second course of SBRT reirradiation. Of the 13 patients who presented with symptoms, 11 had partial or complete symptom relief. All of these patients had pain and/or dyspnea. Only one patient developed grade 2 pneumonitis, and this patient had previously undergone a pneumonectomy. No grade 3 or higher toxicities were observed.

■ CONCLUSION

Although DM is the dominant pattern of failure in lung cancer, LRR occurs frequently and is often symptomatic. The use of immediate postoperative adjuvant TRT remains controversial. The risks of adjuvant therapy appear to outweigh the benefits in early-stage disease with N0 or N1 lymph node status. However, for patients with N2 disease, the risk of LRR is significant and current evidence provides support for postoperative TRT in selected cases. Trials are planned to more definitively address the role of adjuvant radiotherapy for resected N2 patients. If TRT is not used initially and LRR develops after primary surgery, TRT is the standard treatment. In selected patients, especially with bronchial stump recurrence, radical treatment with curative radiation doses is indicated and can result in long-term survival. Indeed, several studies found that patients treated with aggressive salvage TRT have comparable survival to those unresectable patients treated with primary TRT. In the setting of endobronchial disease, HDR-BT is a reasonable treatment option and multiple studies support its use either alone or in combination with laser resection. Initial concerns of serious complications such as massive hemoptysis have limited the enthusiasm for its use but have not consistently been reported in modern studies. However, care should be taken with tumors in the mainstem or upper lobe bronchi. Even when recurrences occur after prior TRT, reirradiation with either external beam TRT or HDR-BT can provide symptomatic relief and improve quality of life. Despite concerns over the potential toxicity of reirradiation, the short-term palliative benefits appear to outweigh the risks of delayed morbidity in this population of patients with very limited survival. Consistent with this belief, several studies of repeat TRT have demonstrated

55. Cetingoz R, Arican-Alicikus Z, Nur-Demiral A, Durmak-Isman B, Bakis-Altas B, Kinay M. Is re-irradiation effective in symptomatic local recurrence of non small cell lung cancer patients? A single institution experience and review of the literature. *J Buon.* 2009;14(1):33–40.
56. Wu KL, Jiang GL, Qian H, et al. Three-dimensional conformal radiotherapy for locoregionally recurrent lung carcinoma after external beam irradiation: a prospective phase I-II clinical trial. *Int J Radiat Oncol Biol Phys.* 2003;57(5):1345–1350.
57. Kramer GW, Gans S, Ullmann E, van Meerbeeck JP, Legrand CC, Leer JW. Hypofractionated external beam radiotherapy as retreatment for symptomatic non-small-cell lung carcinoma: an effective treatment? *Int J Radiat Oncol Biol Phys.* 2004;58(5):1388–1393.
58. Poltinnikov IM, Fallon K, Xiao Y, Reiff JE, Curran WJ, Jr., Werner-Wasik M. Combination of longitudinal and circumferential three-dimensional esophageal dose distribution predicts acute esophagitis in hypofractionated reirradiation of patients with non-small-cell lung cancer treated in stereotactic body frame. *Int J Radiat Oncol Biol Phys.* 2005;62(3):652–658.

demos MEDICAL

RADIATION MEDICINE ROUNDS

Surgery for Non–Small Cell Lung Cancer

Sandra C. Tomaszek and Dennis A. Wigle*
Mayo Clinic, Rochester, MN

ABSTRACT

Pathology and Natural History: In the United States and worldwide, non–small cell lung cancer is the leading cause of cancer-related death. Surgical resection is currently the most effective treatment for localized tumors, and the only treatment approach with significant cure rates.

Staging: Thorough preoperative staging is essential for any treatment approach. For surgical resection, patients need to be carefully selected with respect to potential operative risk factors on the basis of underlying comorbidities. Minimally invasive approaches to lung resection have the potential for offering curative surgery to patients unable to tolerate standard open thoracotomy.

INTRODUCTION

Lung cancer continues to be a substantial health care problem with an estimated 219,440 newly diagnosed men and women and an estimated 159,390 patients dying of the disease in 2009, based on statistics from the National Cancer Institute Surveillance Epidemiology and End Results (SEER) program (1). Surgical resection for non–small cell lung cancer (NSCLC) remains the best chance for cure. If the tumor is unresectable, chemotherapy and/or radiation therapy are used, either as a neoadjuvant approach to achieve resectability of the tumor, or as a definite treatment (2,3).

For surgically resected NSCLC, the pathologic tumor node metastases (TNM) stage is the most important prognostic factor. The histologic cell type seems to be less important, according to an analysis of 9,137 surgically managed cases selected from the international staging database of the International Association for the Study of Lung Cancer (IASLC) (3). The IASLC proposed a revision of the current TNM classification system in 2008 and developed the forthcoming 7th edition of the International Union Against Cancer and American Joint Committee on Cancer TNM Classification of Malignant Tumors based on the international staging database of 67,725 cases of NSCLC (4).

The overall 5-year survival in surgically managed patients according to the forthcoming TNM classification system is illustrated in Table 1.

PREOPERATIVE STAGING IN NSCLC

Thorough clinical staging is essential in patients with NSCLC. It is the foundation of appropriate

*Corresponding author, Division of General Thoracic Surgery, 200 1st St. SW, Rochester, MN 55905
E-mail address: wigle.dennis@mayo.edu

Radiation Medicine Rounds 1 (2010) 101–112.

DOI: 10.5003/2151–4208.1.1.101

TABLE 1 Survival in surgically resected NSCLC (3)

Stage (7th Ed.)	Overall 5-year survival rate (%)
IA	66
IB	56
IIA	43
IIB	35
IIIA	23

treatment for the individual patient by surgical and/or nonsurgical options. Various staging modalities are currently used in clinical practice, including both invasive and noninvasive techniques. In many instances these approaches complement one another.

Noninvasive Techniques

A computed tomography (CT) scan is commonly obtained as a baseline evaluation of the clinical T-status, assessing the location and size of the tumor as well as potential chest wall or great vessel involvement. It is furthermore a helpful tool to evaluate the mediastinal lymph nodes and extrathoracic structures (N- and M-status) for potential metastatic disease. For the latter purpose, however, superior techniques have become available in the past years. Preoperative whole-body positron emission tomography with computed tomography (PET-CT) has become a mainstay of preoperative staging in NSCLC to identify patients with mediastinal and extrathoracic disease (5,6).

When PET scans are obtained for extrathoracic staging, specific imaging of the brain is not routinely obtained by most surgeons for early-stage disease unless medical history and/or physical examination of the patient suggest potential metastatic involvement. Typically PET scanning or a combination of CT scan of the abdomen with bone scan and/or brain imaging are used in most major North American centers.

Invasive Techniques

A bronchoscopy can be obtained either within the scope of preoperative staging or at the time of surgery for an assessment of the airway for potential tumor involvement. The current gold standard for mediastinal staging is surgical cervical mediastinoscopy. Endobronchial ultrasound (EBUS) and transesophageal endoscopic ultrasound (EUS) are novel technologies playing an enlarging role in mediastinal staging for NSCLC. They offer the opportunity to biopsy enlarged lymph nodes suspicious of metastatic involvement prior to surgery, including lymph nodes in the aortopulmonary window commonly not accessible by mediastinoscopy. These less invasive techniques have shown reasonable sensitivity, however, in some cases: inferior negative predictive values compared with surgical cervical mediastinoscopy (7).

■ OPERATIVE RISK STRATIFICATION

In addition to preoperative staging, an evaluation of the overall health status of the patient is necessary to determine whether the patient is a suitable operative candidate. With mortality ranging between 2% and 20% and morbidity rates as high as 40% depending on the extent of resection, proper case selection and careful pre- and perioperative management are essential to minimize complications.

Even though postoperative complications, particularly pulmonary and cardiovascular complications, occur more frequently in older patients compared with the younger population, surgical resection is still a feasible and safe procedure associated with a reasonable quality of life if patients are selected carefully (8–11). The smoking status of the patient should be obtained and smoking cessation programs offered for active smokers at the time of their diagnosis. Patients who experience angina pectoris or similar symptoms in the past or those with known underlying cardiovascular disease should be risk-stratified by functional tests to evaluate whether the patient may tolerate general anesthesia and an extensive surgical procedure.

Pulmonary Function Tests with vital capacity (VC), forced expiratory volume in one second (FEV1) and Carbon Monoxide Diffusion Capacity (DLCO) are obtained preoperatively to evaluate the extent of surgical resection the patient might tolerate. According to recently published guidelines by the European Society of Thoracic Surgeons (ESTS) and the European Respiratory Society (ERS) patients with FEV1 and DLCO of below 80% should undergo formal cardiopulmonary exercise testing with peak VO2 measurements, and FEV1- and DLCO- values of less than 30% predicated as being high-risk indicators (12). In these patients it may be advantageous to undergo preoperative pulmonary rehabilitation as an attempt to improve pulmonary function.

SURGICAL APPROACHES

Surgical resection of NSCLC traditionally has been performed by means of an open thoracotomy. For early stage lung cancer, lobectomy is the preferred method of resection with a posterolateral incision to enter the pleural space being regarded as the gold standard.

In cases of locally advanced disease, more centrally located tumors may require a bilobectomy, sleeve lobectomy, or even pneumonectomy. The first successful one-stage pneumonectomy for lung cancer was performed in 1933, and rapidly this became the procedure of choice for resectable lung cancer. Frequency of pneumonectomies has declined over the past years, however, and it is now reserved for tumors unresectable by less invasive approaches such as lobectomy or sleeve lobectomy.

A less extensive surgical resection is the anatomic segmental resection, which is defined as the removal of one or more bronchopulmonary segments of an individual lobe through ligation and division of bronchovascular structures. This is distinct from a limited pulmonary resection or a so-called wedge resection, where portions of lobes are excised by cautery, stapling devises, or laser ablation. Originally it was described as a technique to resect irreversibly damaged lung tissue, such as in bronchiectasis, yet preserving functioning lung parenchyma. Its implementation for patients with lung cancer is controversial, as discussed in more detail below. A limited pulmonary resection (wedge resection) is typically used for excisional biopsies of indeterminate lesions. For lung cancer, careful patient selection is required as this type of resection should be limited to patients with severely compromised pulmonary function not tolerating lobectomy or segmental resection.

In the past years minimally invasive approaches have emerged for segmental and wedge resections as well as for lobectomies, in an attempt to reduce the associated morbidity of the procedure and hence providing patients with a better quality of life.

Minimally Invasive Surgery

Video-assisted thoracoscopic surgery (VATS) as a minimal invasive oncologic surgical procedure has been introduced at the beginning of this century, followed by robot-assisted surgery in recent years. The role of minimally invasive surgery as a tool for surgical thoracic oncology has been subject to much debate in past years. The main concern with minimally invasive approaches to date has been the ability to demonstrate equivalent oncologic results as that achieved by conventional open thoracotomy. One possibility that exists is the potential for an inadequate lymph node dissection at operation, leading to an understaging of patients in comparison to conventional open thoracotomy techniques. Another point of criticism is that a thorough bimanual lung palpation possible during open thoracotomy to rule out further lung nodules is not feasible via the minimally invasive VATS or robotic approach.

Advocates of the minimally invasive approach point out that, in comparison with the open approach, minimally invasive lobectomies have the potential advantage of decreased postoperative pain and a shorter hospital length of stay (13–15). Other proposed advantages of a thoracoscopic approach include decreased blood loss, fewer postoperative complications, preserved pulmonary function, decreased inflammatory response, and a more rapid return to preoperative activity (16–21). A potential shorter postoperative recovery time may allow adjuvant treatment application at a shorter postoperative interval with better compliance and treatment completion rates, if adjuvant chemo- or radiation therapy is indicated (22,23).

Furthermore, there is a need for technological advances to permit surgery with enhanced safety in an increasingly elderly population (24,25) due to a rising percentage of the elderly in our society with an ever-increasing life expectancy (26). According to the SEER database of the National Cancer Institute, the median age at diagnosis of lung cancer between 2002 and 2006 was 71 years of age. Of the patients, 29.1% were between 75 and 84, while 7.7% were over 85 years old (1). Cattaneo and colleagues (14) showed in their retrospective, matched case-control series that VATS lobectomies in septuagenarians are associated with fewer complications and shorter hospitalization compared with open thoracotomies. Another retrospective study conducted by Mun and colleagues (27) showed that VATS lobectomy used for early-stage lung cancer also is a safe procedure in octogenarians with good results with proper patient selection. Likewise in patients with underlying pulmonary disease or diminished pulmonary function, VATS lobectomies can be performed safely (28,29).

VATS

VATS was first described by several groups in the early 1990s, being performed for the management of pleural effusion or pneumothorax, exploration of the chest, and limited resection of lung nodules (30–35). In subsequent years it has achieved broad application in clinical practice as a minimally invasive tool for multiple indications (16–20,22,36–43). Following the experience of these early years, techniques for VATS lobectomy as an oncologic resection emerged, with multiple large retrospective series demonstrating safety as well as feasibility of this approach (17–19,22,44–47). The Cancer and Leukemia Group B 39802 trial of 127 patients evaluated and confirmed the technical feasibility and safety of the approach for small lung cancers prospectively (40). Although the existing retrospective data suggest equivalent oncologic outcomes in comparison with lobectomy using a conventional open thoracotomy, prospective studies are needed and ongoing to confirm this hypothesis, as this procedure has evolved into the common practice of many large thoracic centers. Recently, the feasibility of VATS segmentectomy for selected peripheral, early-stage lung carcinomas has also been reported with acceptable 5-year survival (48).

The ACCP evidence-based clinical practice guidelines by Scott and colleagues (49) for the treatment of stage I and II NSCLC considers VATS lobectomy as an acceptable alternative to open thoracotomy.

Surgical Technique

For VATS lobectomy an epidural catheter may be placed before surgery for pain management, but more frequently intravenous patient controlled analgesia (PCA) is used following surgery after placement of intraoperative intercostal nerve blocks. A standard thoracoscopy is then performed with three 10 mm incisions: an anterior port is positioned between the latissimus dorsi and pectoralis major muscles in the 4th or 5th intercostal space, a posterior port adjacent to the scapula in the 5th or 6th intercostal space, and a camera port is placed in the anterior axillary line in the 7th or 8th intercostal space (Figure 1). An exploratory thoracoscopy is performed through these working ports. Subsequently, the surgeon proceeds with the VATS lobectomy by extending the anterior thoracoscopy incision to create a 3–5 cm muscle sparing access incision to allow for removal of the lobectomy specimen. During surgical resection, rib-spreading or rib retractors are avoided. After pulmonary resection, hilar and mediastinal lymphadenectomy, or lymph node sampling is performed.

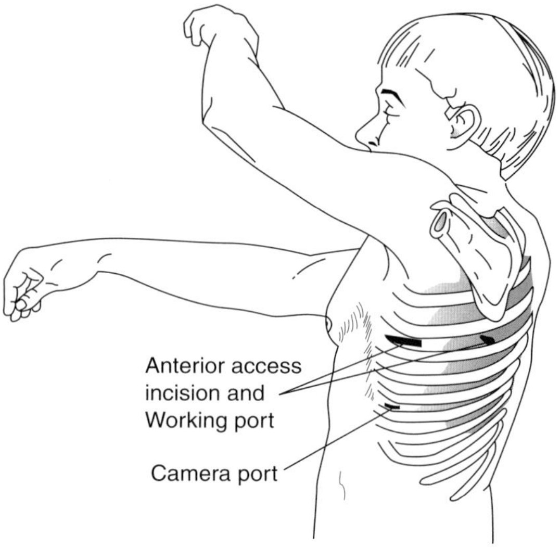

FIGURE 1 VATS lobectomy incisions. Adapted from the original figure provided by Mayo Clinic, Section of Illustration and Design, Rochester, USA.

Robotic-Assisted Surgery

Robotic-assisted surgery was introduced to the specialty of thoracic surgery in order to overcome some of the limitations of VATS. Potential benefits include improvement of the limited maneuverability of instruments and providing superior imaging by means of three-dimensionality through a high-resolution binocular view of the surgical field (50). First described for advanced thoracoscopic procedures (51), it soon was used for lobectomy. An early report by Park and colleagues (50) proved the safety and feasibility of this novel technique for lobectomy in early stage lung cancer. These data were confirmed by Gharagozloo and co-workers (52) in 2008. To date, no data are available with respect to morbidity and mortality of robotic-assisted lobectomy when compared to VATS or conventional open lobectomy. Furthermore, techniques continue to evolve and need further clinical investigation for proof of oncologic adequacy in comparison to conventional open approaches. At present no specific recommendations for the use of robotic-assisted lobectomy in NSCLC can be made.

Surgical Technique

The da Vinci Surgical System is the robotic system most commonly used worldwide. It incorporates three arms, of which two are dissection arms and one is the camera port. Newer versions have a fourth arm that can be used for retraction. The robotic device is usually set up at the head of the patient, who is positioned on the operating table in the lateral decubitus position. The surgeon is operating the robot by means of a console separate from the operative field, while the assistant surgeon is physically present at the operative field. The incisions for the ports are positioned similarly to those for VATS lobectomy, and the dissection of the hilum and resection of the lobe are performed correspondingly.

Controversies

Extension of Resection

Lobectomy is regarded the gold standard for the treatment of NSCLC. This is based on the findings from a randomized trial by the Lung Cancer Study Group (LCSG) in 1995, showing that there is a lower local recurrence rate after lobectomy compared with sublobar resection in early stage NSCLC (53). In fact, the study suggested an almost three-fold increase in the incidence of locoregional recurrence in patients treated by resections smaller than lobectomy (21/122 = 17%) compared with lobectomy (8/125 = 6.4%)(P = 0.008). Survival was not significantly different between the two treatment arms (P = .08, two-tailed P value). Furthermore the claimed advantage of limited resection by conservation of lung tissue appeared not evident in the assessment of long-term pulmonary function after resection.

In recent years, however, discussions about the role of sublobar resection in the definitive treatment of lung cancer have increased, as its potential advantages include surgical management options for the elderly population or individuals with significant cardiopulmonary comorbidities. Several retrospective studies have shown comparable oncologic results to sublobar resection for stage I NSCLC when compared with lobectomy (54–56). Therefore, the need for an updated randomized trial investigating this alternative approach has evolved. The Cancer and Leukemia Group B (CALGB) 140503 study is a currently enrolling phase 3, randomized trial comparing lobectomy to sublobar resection of peripheral tumors of 2 cm or less in size.

Mediastinal Lymph Node Dissection

The accurate assessment of lymph node involvement is recognized as an essential component of staging and treatment in NSCLC. To date there is no evidence-based consensus on the extent of mediastinal lymph node assessment during surgery.

As described in the guidelines for intraoperative lymph node staging published by the ESTS in 2006, systematic nodal dissection involves complete removal of all the mediastinal tissue containing lymph nodes within anatomic landmarks, while sampling represents removal of one or more lymph nodes guided by preoperative or intraoperative findings thought to be representative (57). The prospective, randomized American College of Surgeons Oncology Group (ACOSOG) Z0030 trial of >1,000 patients compared lymph node sampling with lymph node dissection, finding that both approaches are safe surgical procedures. No increase in morbidity or mortality was found from lymph node dissection, and therefore the authors concluded that there seemed no benefit from limiting a mediastinal lymph node dissection (58). Data on potential differences in long-term survival have not been published yet. Retrospective studies, however, reported that mediastinal lymph node dissection may provide a longer disease-free survival when compared with lymph node sampling (59,60). A prospective, three-center study of 206 patients found sampling to be inaccurate in 88% of patients, when conducting nodal sampling followed by systematic nodal dissection in all patients (61). Ultimately, considering the limited data available to date, complete mediastinal nodal dissection should remain the standard of care in NSCLC.

Specific Surgical Considerations

Intraoperative Tumor Spillage

Transgression of the tumor with intraoperative spillage of tumor cells theoretically can lead to pleural implants and local recurrence. If such tumor spillage occurs, the hemithorax should be abundantly irrigated with large quantities of saline. Whether cell lysing agents (e.g., hypertonic saline, water, absolute alcohol, or chemotherapeutic agents) have any role to play in such irrigations remains unknown.

Positive Resection Margins

Bronchial, vascular and close-proximity margins should always be monitored by frozen-section analysis at the time of surgery and re-resection to negative margins is advised if positive margins are identified. A 2-cm bronchial resection margin is considered ideal, but any negative margin, no matter the distance from the tumor, is ultimately accepted. Currently no data are available, whether a larger margin is superior with respect to disease-free survival or local recurrence rates.

If no negative margin is feasible due to anatomic restrictions or inability of the patient to tolerate more extensive resection, most surgeons advocate postoperative radiation to potentially minimize local-regional recurrence.

EARLY-STAGE NSCLC

Stage I

According to the 7th edition of TNM classification, stage IA comprises patients with tumors <2 cm (T1a) and tumors >2 cm but < 3 cm (T1b), while T2a lesions of <5 cm in size are considered as stage IB if there is no lymph node involvement (4).

Commonly patients with these early-stage lesions are detected on routine chest radiographs or CT scans of the chest and upper abdomen performed for unrelated medical conditions. Most are discrete peripheral lesions. Surgical therapy is the management of choice in an otherwise healthy patient without mediastinal lymph node involvement. The role of prethoracotomy mediastinoscopy is still controversial in the case of a negative CT scan. However, systematic lymph node sampling or dissection is carried out at the time of surgery to ensure that no hilar or mediastinal nodal metastases are present.

As discussed earlier, sublobar resection of peripheral lesions is associated with increased local recurrence rates and, therefore, this type of resection should be reserved for patients with significantly limited lung reserve at the time of resection. Isolated lesions located more centrally typically require a lobectomy or pneumonectomy for adequate resection.

Patients with tumors confined to the lung parenchyma without evidence of regional lymphatic metastases or extension to chest wall, diaphragm, or pleura have a 5-year disease-free survival rate of 66% for stage IA and 56% for stage IB when treated by primary surgical resection (Table 1) (3). No adjuvant treatment is recommended for patients with stage IA disease following complete resection. There is a measurable benefit for adjuvant chemotherapy particularly for patients with selected stage IB and those with greater stages of disease.

Of the 20% to 30% of patients who have recurrences following resection for stage I disease, the majority have relapses at distant sites, with more than 20% being solitary brain metastases. Close follow-up for the detection of solitary recurrences or second primaries is consequently advised.

LOCALLY ADVANCED NSCLC

Stage II

This stage comprises a heterogeneous group of tumors including stage IIA (T2aN1 and T2bN0) and stage IIB (T3N0) NSCLCs. Complete surgical resection of these tumors may be still feasible, as this group includes larger tumors in size invading structures like chest wall, pleura, or pericardium, which are closer than 2 cm from the carina yet do not invade it, or tumors associated with obstructive pneumonitis. Adjuvant platinum-based chemotherapy has now been shown to provide survival benefit following surgery for stage II patients (62).

ADVANCED STAGE NSCLC

Unfortunately, the majority of lung cancers are at advanced stage at presentation. Greater than 60% of patients present with stage III or stage IV disease. Advanced NSCLCs involve tumors >7 cm with nodal metastases or tumors of any size invading the mediastinum, heart, great vessels, vertebral body, trachea or carina, esophagus, as well as those with another tumor nodule in a different ipsilateral lobe.

Survival in advanced stage NSCLC is poor, with surgery playing a minor role in these tumors, as they usually are not amenable to primary surgical resection. Typical treatment approaches involve neoadjuvant chemoradiotherapy with surgery as part of a trimodality approach or definitive chemoradiation.

Stage III

Stage IIIA includes all tumors staged as T3,N1-N2 as well as T4,N0-N1, while T3,N3 and T4,N2–3 are stage IIIB lung cancers (4).

Patients with N1 NSCLC represent a heterogeneous population with an overall worse prognosis compared with no lymph node involvement. Surgical resection by means of lobectomy remains the mainstay of treatment in T1,N1 and T2,N1 tumors (63,64). Recent data have solidified the role of adjuvant chemotherapy for these tumors, though randomized data does exist contesting this treatment approach.

NSCLCs with distant metastases being absent, but present mediastinal lymphatic metastases are classified as stage III disease (N2 disease). Many of these locally advanced tumors are amenable to surgical or combined modality therapy that includes surgery. These patients may benefit from trimodality treatment consisting of neoadjuvant chemoradiation therapy followed by surgery if response to treatment is observed, with improved survival rates (65). The North American Intergroup Trial 0139 (RTOG 9309) evaluated the outcome of surgery after induction chemoradiation therapy in patients with stage IIIA (N2) NSCLC. Complete study results published this year failed to demonstrate a survival advantage for resection after radiotherapy. Concerns remain, however, with this study as to whether or not an inordinately high mortality rate for pneumonectomy diluted the potential survival benefit for patients undergoing chemoradiation therapy followed by lobectomy. This trial has unfortunately not resolved the issue of how best to treat the patient with good performance status and limited or single-station N2 disease (66).

In some patients involvement of the mediastinal lymph nodes is diagnosed at the time of thoracotomy after initial negative preoperative staging, which is referred to as occult N2-diesease. This is an infrequent occurrence, ranging from approximately 6% (67,68) to 15% to 18% (69–71) in patients clinically staged N2-negative. In a study conducted by Lee and colleagues (72), the prevalence of histologically confirmed N2 disease is stated as 6.5% in clinical T1 patients and 8.7% in clinical T2 patients with a CT-negative and PET-negative mediastinum. The risk for occult N2-disease seems to increase with the size of the tumor (69,73). Veeramachaneni and colleagues (69) reported a three-fold increase in occult nodal disease with every 1 cm increase in tumor size.

Many patients with limited N2 disease can benefit from effective management by primary surgery. For example, overall 5-year survival of 46% has been reported in patients with pT1 and N2 disease incidentally discovered during mediastinal lymph node dissection (68). A series by Martini and colleagues (74) describing 706 patients seen at Memorial Sloan-Kettering from 1974 to 1981 with mediastinal lymph node metastases found that only 151 (21%) were completely resectable. The overall 5-year survival rate of this group was 30% (75).

Supraclavicluar or contralateral mediastinal lymph node metastases (N3) are considered by most investigators to be absolute contraindication to surgery because long-term survival with surgery is rare and anecdotal. However, the Southwest Oncology Group has completed a phase 2 induction chemotherapy and radiotherapy program followed by surgery for this group of patients. The early results of this trial suggested a complete resection rate similar to that seen with induction therapy for N2 disease (76). Long-term results, including survival rates, in patients treated for N3 disease by this aggressive fashion have been reported. None of the patients with N3 disease due to contralateral mediastinal involvement survived 5 years. The only survivors were two patients with preoperatively proven scalene node involvement. At the time of surgery, no attempt was made to remove the cervical lymph nodes. At the present time, however, the standard of care for patients with proven N3 involvement is chemotherapy and radiation without surgery.

Stage IV

With the 7th edition of the TNM classification, pleural effusion and nodules in the contralateral lung are classified as M1a, while distant metastases are M1b. Metastatic sites frequently include the contralateral lung, brain, adrenal glands, skeletal system, and liver.

The most common extrathoracic metastases are skeletal metastases, followed by metastases to the brain, adrenal glands, and the liver with a median survival of 8 months and 5-year survival rates of <1%. Some metastatic sites are associated with worse survival than others.

One metastatic lesion is an independent predictor of prolonged survival compared with multiple lesions, which should be taken into account when treatment decisions are made (77). The role of surgery in NSCLC with distant solitary metastases remains controversial. Retrospective studies suggest a survival benefit for patients with NSCLC and synchronous solitary metastasis who undergo resection (78,79).

The American College of Chest Physicians (ACCP) published evidence-based clinical practice guidelines for lung cancer in September 2007 (80). These guidelines recommend resection or radiosurgical ablation of brain metastases in addition to resection of the primary lung cancer if no other sites of metastases are found and if the primary NSCLC is resectable and staged N0 or N1, followed by whole-brain radiation therapy (WBRT). Isolated adrenal metastases should be considered for resection if the primary NSCLC is resectable and staged N0 or N1 without any further sites of metastases. For metachronous presentations of an isolated adrenal metastasis, a resection of the metastasis is recommended when the disease-free interval is >6 months and complete resection of the primary NSCLC has been achieved. For bone metastases, the ACCP guidelines do not recommend any particular surgical treatment in disease metastatic to the skeletal system; a non-surgical approach is preferred. Ultimately, prospective, randomized controlled trials are warranted to determine if there is a survival advantage in adding surgical resection to patients with limited metastatic NSCLC.

There might be a role in neoadjuvant approaches, as they may enrich the patient population who may most benefit from a surgical approach to limited metastatic disease (81). Our bias is that patients who rapidly progress on systemic therapy would likely not benefit from surgical resection and should not be subjected to the possible morbidity that may arise from surgery. There is also a subset of patients who undergo surgical resection and are found to have solitary metastatic disease. In addition, it remains to be evaluated whether it is beneficial for the patient to proceed with resection if solitary metastases are noted at the time of primary surgery, or whether the added risk of potential morbidity and mortality outweighs this benefit.

■ PALLIATION

For surgery to be effective and potentially curative in controlling lung cancer, the resection must be complete. The role of surgery for the palliation of patients with unresectable tumors is debatable. Specific situations, such as an unremitting lung abscess distal to an obstructing tumor, massive hemoptysis, or painful invasion of the chest wall have led surgeons to consider palliative or incomplete resections in the hope of improving the patient's symptoms. With an ongoing improvement in radiation and chemotherapeutic treatment approaches, however, this is rarely employed in the modern era.

■ SUMMARY

Surgery is the standard of care for the treatment of early-stage and selected locally advanced NSCLC. Multimodality approaches are recommended in large tumors or if mediastinal lymph node involvement is apparent at the time of diagnosis. For advanced or metastatic tumors, the role of surgery in general is unproven but deserves more study. Specific patient subgroups with advanced disease may benefit from surgery as part of multimodality approaches.

■ REFERENCES

1. National Cancer Institute. Surveillance Epidemiology and End Results (SEER) web site. Available at: http://seer.cancer.gov (Accessed July 20, 2009).
2. Caglar HB, Baldini EH, Othus M, et al. Outcomes of patients with stage III nonsmall cell lung cancer treated with chemotherapy and radiation with and without surgery. *Cancer.* 2009;115(18):4156–4166.
3. Chansky K, Sculier JP, Crowley JJ, et al. The International Association for the Study of Lung Cancer Staging Project: prognostic factors and pathologic TNM stage in surgically managed non-small cell lung cancer. *J Thorac Oncol.* 2009;4(7):792–801.
4. Goldstraw P, Crowley J, Chansky K, et al. The IASLC Lung Cancer Staging Project: proposals for the revision of the TNM stage groupings in the forthcoming (seventh) edition of the TNM Classification of malignant tumours. *J Thorac Oncol.* 2007;2(8):706–714.
5. Maziak DE, Darling GE, Inculet RI, et al. Positron emission tomography in staging early lung cancer: a randomized trial. *Ann Intern Med.* 2009;151(4):221–228,W-48.
6. Fischer B, Lassen U, Mortensen J, et al. Preoperative staging of lung cancer with combined PET-CT. *N Engl J Med.* 2009;361(1):32–39.
7. Medford AR, Bennett JA, Free CM, et al. Mediastinal staging procedures in lung cancer: EBUS, TBNA and mediastinoscopy. *Curr Opin Pulm Med.* 2009;15(4):334–342.
8. Ferguson MK, Parma CM, Celauro AD, et al. Quality of life and mood in older patients after major lung resection. *Ann Thorac Surg.* 2009;87(4):1007–1012.

9. Schulte T, Schniewind B, Walter J, et al. Age-related impairment of quality of life after lung resection for non-small cell lung cancer. *Lung Cancer.* 2009;[Epub ahead of print]
10. Voltolini L, Rapicetta C, Ligabue T, et al. Short- and long-term results of lung resection for cancer in octogenarians. *Asian Cardiovasc Thorac Ann.* 2009;17(2):147–152.
11. Okami J, Higashiyama M, Asamura H, et al. Pulmonary resection in patients aged 80 years or over with clinical stage I non-small cell lung cancer: Prognostic factors for overall survival and risk factors for postoperative complications. *J Thorac Oncol.* 2009;[Epub ahead of print]
12. Brunelli A, Charloux A, Bolliger CT, et al. The European Respiratory Society and European Society of Thoracic Surgeons clinical guidelines for evaluating fitness for radical treatment (surgery and chemoradiotherapy) in patients with lung cancer. *Eur J Cardiothorac Surg.* 2009; 36(1):181–184.
13. Landreneau RJ, Hazelrigg, SR, Mack MJ, et al. Postoperative pain-related morbidity: video-assisted thoracic surgery versus thoracotomy. *Ann Thorac Surg.* 1993; 56(6):1285–1289.
14. Cattaneo SM, Park BJ, Wilton AS, et al. Use of video-assisted thoracic surgery for lobectomy in the elderly results in fewer complications. *Ann Thorac Surg.* 2008; 85(1):231–235.
15. McKenna RJ Jr., Mahtabifard A, Pickens A, et al. Fast-tracking after video-assisted thoracoscopic surgery lobectomy, segmentectomy, and pneumonectomy. *Ann Thorac Surg.* 2007;84(5):1663–1667.
16. Kirby TJ, Mack MJ, Landreneau RJ, et al. Lobectomy—video-assisted thoracic surgery versus muscle-sparing thoracotomy. A randomized trial. *J Thorac Cardiovasc Surg.* 1995;109(5):997–1001.
17. McKenna RJ Jr., Houck W, Fuller CB. Video-assisted thoracic surgery lobectomy: experience with 1,100 cases. *Ann Thorac Surg.* 2006;81(2):421–425.
18. Solaini L, Prusciano F, Bagioni P, et al. Long-term results of video-assisted thoracic surgery lobectomy for stage I non-small cell lung cancer: a single-centre study of 104 cases. *Interact Cardiovasc Thorac Surg.* 2004;3(1):57–62.
19. Solaini L, Prusciano F, Bagioni P, et al. Video-assisted thoracic surgery (VATS) of the lung: analysis of intraoperative and postoperative complications over 15 years and review of the literature. *Surg Endosc.* 2008;22(2):298–310.
20. Giudicelli R, Thomas P, Lonjon T, et al. Major pulmonary resection by video assisted mini-thoracotomy. Initial experience in 35 patients. *Eur J Cardiothorac Surg.* 1994;8(5):254–258.
21. Landreneau RJ, Hazelrigg, SR, Mack MJ, et al. Postoperative pain-related morbidity: video-assisted thoracic surgery versus thoracotomy. *Ann Thorac Surg.* 1993;56(6):1285–1289.
22. Nicastri DG, Wisnivesky JP, Litle VR, et al. Thoracoscopic lobectomy: report on safety, discharge independence, pain and chemotherapy tolerance. J *Thorac Cardiovasc Surg.* 2008;135(3):642–647.
23. Peterson RP, Pham D, Burfiend WR, et al. Thoracoscopic lobectomy facilitates the delivery of chemotherapy after resection for lung cancer. *Ann Thorac Surg.* 2007; 83:1245–1249.
24. Dominguez-Ventura A, Allen MS, Cassivi SD, et al. Lung cancer in octogenarians: factors affecting morbidity and mortality after pulmonary resection. *Ann Thorac Surg.* 2006;82(4):1175–1179.
25. Dominguez-Ventura A, Cassivi SD, Allen MS, et al. Lung cancer in octogenarians: factors affecting long-term survival following resection. *Eur J Cardiothorac Surg.* 2007;32(2):370–374.
26. Lutz W, Sanderson W, Scherbov S. The coming acceleration of global population ageing. *Nature.* 2008;451(7179): 716–719.
27. Mun M, Kohno T. Video-assisted thoracic surgery for clinical stage I lung cancer in octogenarians. *Ann Thorac Surg.* 2008;85(2):406–411.
28. Demmy TL, Nwogu C. Is video-assisted thoracic surgery lobectomy better? Quality of life considerations. *Ann Thorac Surg.* 2008;85(2):S719–S728.
29. Shaw JP, Dembitzer FR, Wisnivesky JP, et al. Video-assisted thoracoscopic lobectomy: state of the art and future directions. *Ann Thorac Surg.* 2008;85(2):S705–S709.
30. Allen MS, Deschamps C, Jones DM, Trastek VF, Pairolero PC. Video-assisted thoracic surgical procedures: the Mayo experience. *Mayo Clin Proc.* 1996;71(4):351–359.
31. Allen MS, Deschamps C, Lee RE, Trastek VF, Daly RC, Pairolero PC. Video-assisted thoracoscopic stapled wedge excision for indeterminate pulmonary nodules. *J Thorac Cardiovasc Surg.* 1993;106(6):1048–1052.
32. Hazelrigg SR, Nunchuck SK, LoCicero J 3rd. Video assisted Thoracic Surgery Study Group data. *Ann Thorac Surg.* 1993;56(5):1039–1043.
33. Lewis RJ, Caccavale RJ, Sisler GE, et al. One hundred consecutive patients undergoing video-assisted thoracic operations. *Ann Thorac Surg.* 1992;54(3):421–426.
34. Miller DL, Allen MS. Set-up and present indications: video-assisted thoracic surgery. Semin *Thorac Cardiovasc Surg.* 1993;5(4):280–283.
35. Coltharp WH, Arnold JH, Alford WC Jr., et al. Videothoracoscopy: improved technique and expanded indications. *Ann Thorac Surg.* 1992;53(5):776–778.
36. Boffa DJ, Allen MS, Grab JD, et al. Data from The Society of Thoracic Surgeons General Thoracic Surgery database: the surgical management of primary lung tumors. *J Thorac Cardiovasc Surg.* 2008;135(2):247–254.
37. Congregado M, Merchan RJ, Gallardo G, et al. Video-assisted thoracic surgery (VATS) lobectomy: 13 years' experience. *Surg Endosc.* 2008;22(8):1852–1857.
38. Kirby TJ, Rice TW. Thoracoscopic lobectomy. *Ann Thorac Surg.* 1993;56(3):784–786.
39. Sakuraba M, Miyamoto H, Oh S, et al. Video-assisted thoracoscopic lobectomy vs. conventional lobectomy via open thoracotomy in patients with clinical stage IA non-small cell lung carcinoma. *Interact Cardiovasc Thorac Surg.* 2007;6(5):614–617.
40. Swanson SJ, Herndon JE 2nd, D'Amico TA, et al. Video-assisted thoracic surgery lobectomy: report of CALGB 39802—a prospective, multi-institution feasibility study. *J Clin Oncol.* 2007;25(31):4993–4997.

41. Whitson BA, Andrade RS, Boettcher A, et al. Video-assisted thoracoscopic surgery is more favorable than thoracotomy for resection of clinical stage I non-small cell lung cancer. *Ann Thorac Surg.* 2007;83(6):1965–1970.
42. Lewis RJ, Caccavale RJ, Sisler GE, et al. Video-assisted thoracic surgical resection of malignant lung tumors. *J Thorac Cardiovasc Surg.* 1992;104(6):1679–1685.
43. McKenna RJ Jr. Lobectomy by video-assisted thoracic surgery with mediastinal node sampling for lung cancer. *J Thorac Cardiovasc Surg.* 1994;107(3):879–881.
44. Tomaszek SC, Cassivi SD, Shen KR, et al. Clinical outcomes of video-assisted thoracoscopic lobectomy. *Mayo Clin Proc.* 2009;84(6):509–513.
45. Alam N, Flores RM. Video-assisted thoracic surgery (VATS) lobectomy: the evidence base. *JSLS.* 2007;11(3):368–374.
46. Sawada S, Komori E, Yamashita M, et al. Comparison in prognosis after VATS lobectomy and open lobectomy for stage I lung cancer. *Surg Endosc.* 2007;21(9):1607–1611.
47. Rocco G, Internullo E, Cassivi SD, et al. The variability of practice in minimally invasive thoracic surgery for pulmonary resections. *Thorac Surg Clin.* 2008;18(3):235–247.
48. Watanabe A, Ohori S, Nakashima S, et al. Feasibility of video-assisted thoracoscopic surgery segmentectomy for selected peripheral lung carcinomas. *Eur J Cardiothorac Surg.* 2009;35(5):775–780.
49. Scott WJ, Howington J, Feigenberg S, et al. Treatment of non-small cell lung cancer stage I and stage II: ACCP evidence-based clinical practice guidelines. 2nd ed. *Chest.* 2007;132(3)(suppl):234S–242S.
50. Park BJ, Flores RM, Rusch VW. Robotic assistance for video-assisted thoracic surgical lobectomy: technique and initial results. *J Thorac Cardiovasc Surg.* 2006;131(1): 54–59.
51. Morgan JA, Ginsburg ME, Sonett JR, et al. Advanced thoracoscopic procedures are facilitated by computer-aided robotic technology. *Eur J Cardiothorac Surg.* 2003;23(6):883–887.
52. Gharagozloo F, Margolis M, Tempesta B. Robot-assisted thoracoscopic lobectomy for early-stage lung cancer. *Ann Thorac Surg.* 2008;85(6):1880–1885.
53. Ginsberg RJ, Rubinstein LV. Randomized trial of lobectomy versus limited resection for T1N0 non-small cell lung cancer. Lung Cancer Study Group. *Ann Thorac Surg.*1995;60(3):615–622.
54. Pettiford BL, Schuchert MJ, Santos R, et al. Role of sublobar resection (segmentectomy and wedge resection) in the surgical management of non-small cell lung cancer. *Thorac Surg Clin.* 2007;17(2):175–190.
55. Schuchert MJ, Pettiford BL, Keeley S, et al. Anatomic segmentectomy in the treatment of stage 1 non-small cell lung cancer. *Ann Thorac Surg.* 2007;84(3):926–932.
56. Martin-Ucar AE, Nakas A, Pilling JE, et al. A case-matched study of anatomical segmentectomy versus lobectomy for stage 1 lung cancer in high-risk patients. *Eur J Cardiothorac Surg.* 2005;27(4):675–679.
57. Lardinois D, De Leyn P, Van Schil P, et al. ESTS guidelines for intraoperative lymph node staging in non-small cell lung cancer. *Eur J Cardiothorac Surg.* 2006;30(5):787–792.
58. Allen MS, Darling GE, Pechet TT, et al. Morbidity and mortality of major pulmonary resections in patients with early-stage lung cancer: initial results of the randomized, prospective ACOSOG Z0030 trial. *Ann Thorac Surg.* 2006;81(3):1013–1019.
59. Su X, Wang X, Long H, et al. Mediastinal lymph node dissection affects survival in patients with stage I non-small cell lung cancer. *Thorac Cardiovasc Surg.* 2008;56(4):226–230.
60. Lardinois D, Suter H, Hakki H, et al. Morbidity, survival, and site of recurrence after mediastinal lymph-node dissection versus systematic sampling after complete resection for non-small cell lung cancer. *Ann Thorac Surg.* 2005;80(10):268–274.
61. Massard G, Ducrocq X, Kochetkowva EA, et al. Sampling or node dissection for intraoperative staging of lung cancer: a multicentric cross-sectional study. *Eur J Cardiothorac Surg.* 2006;30(10):164–167.
62. Jang RW Le Maître A, Ding K, et al. Quality-adjusted time without symptoms or toxicity analysis of adjuvant chemotherapy in non-small cell lung cancer: an analysis of the National Cancer Institute of Canada Trials Group JBR.10 trial. *J Clin Oncol.* 2009;27(26):4268–4273.
63. Ferguson MK, Little AG, Golomb HM, et al. The role of adjuvant therapy after resection of T1 N1 M0 and T2 N1 M0 non-small cell lung cancer. *J Thorac Cardiovasc Surg.* 1986;91(3):344–349.
64. Marra A, Hillejan L, Zaboura G, et al. Pathologic N1 non-small cell lung cancer: correlation between pattern of lymphatic spread and prognosis. *J Thorac Cardiovasc Surg.* 2003;125(3):543–553.
65. Steger V, Walles T, Kosan B, et al. Trimodal therapy for histologically proven N2/3 non-small cell lung cancer: mid-term results and indicators for survival. *Ann Thorac Surg.* 2009;87(6):1676–1683.
66. Albain KS, Swann RS, Rusch VW, et al. Radiotherapy plus chemotherapy with or without surgical resection for stage III non-small-cell lung cancer: a phase III randomised controlled trial. *Lancet.* 2009;374(9687):379–386.
67. Meyers BF, Haddad F, Siegel BA, et al. Cost-effectiveness of routine mediastinoscopy in computed tomography- and positron emission tomography-screened patients with stage I lung cancer. *J Thorac Cardiovasc Surg.* 2006;131(4):822–829.
68. Defranchi SA, Cassivi SD, Nichols FC, et al. N2 disease in T1 non-small cell lung cancer. *Ann Thorac Surg.* 2009;88(3):924–928.
69. Veeramachaneni NK, Battafarano RJ, Meyers BF, et al. Risk factors for occult nodal metastasis in clinical T1N0 lung cancer: a negative impact on survival. *Eur J Cardiothorac Surg.* 2008;33(3):466–469.
70. Al-Sarraf N, Aziz R, Gately K, et al. Pattern and predictors of occult mediastinal lymph node involvement in non-small cell lung cancer patients with negative mediastinal uptake on positron emission tomography. *Eur J Cardiothorac Surg.* 2008;33(1):104–109.
71. Carnochan FM, Walker WS. Positron emission tomography may underestimate the extent of thoracic disease in lung cancer patients. *Eur J Cardiothorac Surg.* 2009;35(5):781–784.

72. Lee PC, Port JL, Korst RJ, Liss Y, Meherally DN, Altorki NK. Risk factors for occult mediastinal metastases in clinical stage I non-small cell lung cancer. *Ann Thorac Surg.* 2007;84(1):177–181.
73. Gajra A, Newman N, Gamble GP, et al. Impact of tumor size on survival in stage IA non-small cell lung cancer: a case for subdividing stage IA disease. *Lung Cancer.* 2003;42(1):51–57.
74. Martini N, Flehinger BJ, Zaman MB, et al. Results of resection in non-oat cell carcinoma of the lung with mediastinal lymph node metastases. *Ann Surg.* 1983;198(3):386–397.
75. Martini N, Flehinger BJ. The role of surgery in N2 lung cancer. *Surg Clin North Am.* 1987;67(5):1037–1049.
76. Rusch VW, Albain KS, Crowley JJ, et al. Surgical resection of stage IIIA and stage IIIB non-small-cell lung cancer after concurrent induction chemoradiotherapy. A Southwest Oncology Group trial. *J Thorac Cardiovasc Surg.* 1993;105(1):97–104.
77. Oh Y, Taylor S, Bekele BN, et al. Number of metastatic sites is a strong predictor of survival in patients with nonsmall cell lung cancer with or without brain metastases. *Cancer.* 2009;115(13):2930–2938.
78. Modi A, Vohra HA, Weeden DF. Does surgery for primary non-small cell lung cancer and cerebral metastasis have any impact on survival? *Interact Cardiovasc Thorac Surg.* 2009;8(4):467–473.
79. Mercier O, Fadel E, Mussot S, et al. Is surgery required for patients with isolated adrenal metastasis of non-small cell lung carcinoma? *Presse Med.* 2007;36(12pt1):1743–1752.
80. Shen KR, Meyers BF, Larner JM, et al. Special treatment issues in lung cancer: ACCP evidence-based clinical practice guidelines. 2nd ed. *Chest.* 2007;32(3)(suppl): 290S–305S.
81. Cartei G, Binato S, Sacco C, et al. Simplified gemcitabine and platin regimen in patients with advanced or metastatic non-small cell lung cancer (NSCLC) to be proposed as neoadjuvant therapy. *Ann Oncol.* 2006;17(suppl 5): v47–v51.

demos MEDICAL

RADIATION MEDICINE ROUNDS

Systemic Therapy for Lung Cancer

Harshita R. Paripati* and Helen J. Ross
Mayo Clinic, Scottsdale, AZ

ABSTRACT

Pathology/natural history: Lung cancer is the leading cause of cancer related deaths in both men and women. It is broadly classified into two main categories—non–small cell lung cancer (85%) and small cell lung cancer (15%), which differ in histology, clinical behavior, treatment and prognosis. Non small cell lung cancer is further classified into adenocarcinoma, including bronchioalveolar subtype, squamous cell carcinoma, and large cell carcinoma. The major risk factor for both non small cell and small cell lung cancer is cigarette smoking. Small cell lung cancer is a highly aggressive malignancy that usually presents with metastatic disease or micrometastases even when apparently localized at diagnosis. It is almost exclusively a disease of smokers. The risk of lung cancer increases with the number of cigarettes smoked per day and with duration of exposure. Women may have a higher risk of developing lung cancer at the same level of nicotine exposure. Other risk factors include asbestos, radon, arsenic, chromium and nickel.

Genetic susceptibility plays an important role in development of lung cancer. Several oncogenes and tumor suppressor genes have been implicated in the pathogenesis of lung cancer. K-ras mutations are commonly seen in non-small cell lung cancer. They are usually present in smokers and confer a poor prognosis. ALK mutations are also seen in adenocarcinoma, but are usually seen in non-smokers or light smokers, and are associated with resistance to EGFR TKIs. PTEN loss is also frequently seen in lung cancer and may be associated with resistance to EGFR TKIs. Genes implicated in the pathogenesis of small cell lung cancer include c-myc and RB (Retinobastoma) gene. P53 mutations and alterations in FHIT are seen both in non-small cell lung cancer and small cell lung cancer.

EGFR (epidermal growth factor receptor) belongs to the erbB family of growth factor receptors and is overexpressed in almost 70% of non-small cell lung cancers. EGFR mutations lead to activation of cell survival signals and provide a therapeutic target. They are most commonly seen in women, Asians, non-smokers and patients with adenocarcinoma.

Clinical behavior/evaluation/staging: The most common presenting systemic symptoms of lung cancer are weight loss, anorexia, and fatigue. Local symptoms include cough, dyspnea, hemoptysis and occasionally chest pain. Paraneoplastic syndromes are commonly associated with small cell lung cancer but are also seen in non-small cell lung cancer. Some commonly seen paraneoplastic syndromes are hypercalcemia (usually with squamous cell carcinoma), SIADH and Eaton-Lambert myasthenic syndrome associated with small cell lung carcinoma.

*Corresponding author, Division of Hematology/Oncology, Mayo Clinic, 13400 E. Shea Blvd., Scottsdale, AZ 85259
E-mail address: paripati.harshita@mayo.edu

Radiation Medicine Rounds 1 (2010) 113–140.

DOI: 10.5003/2151–4208.1.1.113

demosmedpub.com/rmr

Staging for NSCLC is based on the TNM staging system. The 7th edition of the TNM staging system for NSCLC was recently published. Changes in the 7th edition include reclassification of tumors >7cm as T3 instead of T2, additional pulmonary nodules in the same lobe as T3, same lung as T4 and reclassification of pleural effusions from T4 to M1a. Staging for small cell lung cancer is based on the Veterans' Affairs Lung Study Group (VALCSG) system and is classified into limited stage and extensive stage disease depending on whether the disease can be encompassed within a single hemithorax radiation port.

Therapy:

NSCLC: Early stage NSCLC is best treated by surgical resection, preferably lobectomy. Patients with resected Stage II disease and selected patients with Stage IB disease should receive adjuvant chemotherapy with four cycles of platinum based therapy. Patients with Stage III disease should optimally be treated with combined chemoradiation therapy.

The treatment of Stage IV disease is primarily chemotherapy and targeted therapy, with the goal of treatment being palliation and prolongation of survival. Factors to be taken into account include the patient's performance status, co-morbidities, histology and smoking history. Recently, molecular factors such as EGFR mutation status have been found to play an important role and may impact primary treatment in select patients. In general, the standard of care for first line chemotherapy in advanced NSCLC is a platinum based doublet for 4–6 cycles of therapy. Cisplatin is preferred over Carboplatin. In patients with adenocarcinoma, pemetrexed with a platinum agent is preferred; in patients with squamous cell carcinoma, gemcitabine with a platinum agent is optimal therapy. Elderly patients with good performance status should receive platinum based doublet therapy unless otherwise contraindicated. Bevacizumab is the only targeted agent to be approved for use with chemotherapy (carboplatin and paclitaxel) in the first line setting, and can be used in suitable patients. It is anticipated that other targeted agents such as erlotinib and cetuximab may be approved in the first line setting in the near future.

The approved agents for second line therapy include docetaxel, erlotinib and pemetrexed. Pemetrexed has now been approved as a first line agent in patients with adenocarcinoma. The issue of maintenance therapy remains unresolved; recent studies of erlotinib as maintenance have shown promise.

Small cell lung cancer: The treatment of choice for limited stage disease is concurrent chemoradiation therapy with cisplatin and etoposide. Twice a day radiation is associated with a survival advantage and is preferred in patients who can tolerate it although alternate radiation dosing and fractionation are under study. Patients with a good response after chemoradiation should receive prophylactic cranial irradiation (PCI), which reduces the risk of developing brain metastases and improves survival. Extensive stage disease is usually incurable and the treatment of choice is chemotherapy with cisplatin and etoposide for four to six cycles. PCI improves survival in these patients as well and for patients who respond completely; radiation to the primary site should be considered as it also improves survival. Patients who relapse within 3 months after first line therapy have a poor prognosis and are considered refractory. Patients who relapse 3 months after first line therapy may be treated with second line therapy with topotecan.

INTRODUCTION

Lung cancer is the leading cause of cancer-related deaths in both men and women worldwide (1). In the United States, it is estimated that 219,440 men and women (116,090 men and 103,350 women) will be diagnosed with and 159,390 will die of cancer of the lung and bronchus in 2009 (2). Annual deaths due to lung cancer in women exceed those caused by breast, cervical, and uterine cancers combined; in men, the number of deaths from lung cancer is larger than deaths caused by colorectal and prostate cancers combined. Bronchogenic carcinoma refers to all cancers arising in the airways or pulmonary parenchyma. About 95% of lung cancers are classified as either non–small cell lung (NSCLC) or small cell lung cancers (SCLC). The remaining 5% are unclassified and rare tumors. Non–small cell cancers are further classified on the basis of histology as will be discussed later in this chapter. In the United States, the most common form of lung cancer was squamous cell cancer until the late 1980s and has now been replaced by adenocarcinoma, which is increasing in incidence and is seen in both smokers and nonsmokers. The incidence of squamous cell cancer, large cell cancer, and SCLC has been decreasing over the past several years.

Risk Factors

The common risk factors for lung cancer are listed in Table 1. The most important cause of lung cancer is smoking, accounting for approximately 85% to 90% of all cases (3). Numerous epidemiologic studies, both retrospective and prospective have established the role of nicotine as a causative agent in lung cancer.

The first evidence of an epidemiologic association between tobacco use and lung cancer was reported in the 1950s (4–6). The risk of lung cancer among smokers increases with the number of cigarettes smoked per day and with the duration of smoking history, with a stronger effect for duration of smoking when compared with number of cigarettes smoked per day (7,8). Based on overwhelming epidemiological data, the U.S. Surgeon General issued a report in 1964 stating that smoking was a definite cause of cancers of the lung and larynx and chronic bronchitis in both men and women (9). The risk of lung cancer decreases with cessation of smoking (10). The greater the number of years of abstinence, the lower the risk of developing lung cancer; however, this risk never becomes equal to that of never-smokers (11).

The composition of cigarettes has changed significantly over the past few decades (3). There has been a shift toward "low tar" or "light" cigarettes. These designations are misleading; they are not associated with decreased risks when compared with other cigarettes and are now subject to regulation by the Food and Drug Administration. Tar and nicotine yields are measured with a smoking machine according to a standardized protocol established by the Federal Trade Commission (FTC) that specifies such details as puff volume, the frequency of puffing, and the length to which the cigarette is to be smoked (12). The low tar and nicotine numbers measured on the FTC machines are artificial and do not take into account the compensatory changes in smoking patterns (13).

TABLE 1 Risk factors for lung cancer

- Smoking
- Environmental toxins-asbestos, radon , arsenic, heavy metals
- Radiation therapy: breast cancer and Hodgkin's disease survivors
- Genetic susceptibility
- Dietary: beta carotene supplementation
- Prior lung damage: fibrosis, COPD, alpha 1 anti-trypsin deficiency

In recent years, data suggest that women may be more susceptible to the carcinogenic effects of smoking than men. This is based on possible hormonally related differences in carcinogen metabolism and the higher expression of estrogen receptor beta in females. Other risk factors include exposure to occupational or environmental agents including asbestos, radon, arsenic, chromium, and nickel (3). Asbestos is a well-known occupational carcinogen. Lung cancer is associated with the principal commercial forms of asbestos, and the risk of lung cancer increases with increased exposure to asbestos (14,15). Asbestos and cigarette smoking synergistically increase the risk of lung cancer. Radon is a chemically inert gas that is a decay product of uranium. Underground miners exposed to high levels of radon have a significantly elevated risk of developing lung cancer. Radon is also an indoor air pollutant and can cause lung cancer in the general population from residential exposure. Mitigation is fairly straightforward but does require knowledge of radon levels.

Genetic susceptibility in lung cancer has been long postulated on the basis of the fact that exposure to carcinogens in cigarette smoke and other environmental agents causes cancer in relatively few individuals compared with the population exposed. Carcinogens such as polycyclic aromatic hydrocarbons in tobacco are metabolized by the enzymes of the cytochrome p450 system (3). These metabolites form reactive intermediates that bind to DNA and cause genetic injury. Polymorphisms in enzymes of the cytochrome p450 system, in particular, CYP1A1 and CYP2D6 are thought to cause increased risk of lung cancer (16). Other enzyme polymorphisms that can contribute to increased risk include glutathione S-transferase, which detoxifies reactive metabolites of polycyclic aromatic hydrocarbons (17). Impaired DNA repair capacity may also explain some genetic susceptibility to lung cancer (18).

Dietary factors that have been studied in relation to lung cancer risk include retinol, β carotenoids, and Vitamin C. Although some data suggest that dietary β carotene may have a protective effect, three very large randomized double-blind placebo-controlled studies not only did not show a protective effect (19–21), but indeed showed that β carotene supplementation was associated with an increased risk of lung cancer in smokers.

TABLE 4 TNM elements included in stage groups

	Descriptors, % of all			
Stage Groups	T	N	M	Patients, %[a]
IA	T1a,b	N0	M0	15
IB	T2a	N0	M0	13
IIA	T1a,b	N1	M0	2
	T2a	N1	M0	4
	T2b	N0	M0	4
IIB	T2b	N1	M0	2
	T3	N0	M0	14
IIIA	T1–3	N2	M0	20
	T3	N1	M0	6
	T4	N0,1	M0	2
IIIB	T4	N2	M0	1
	T1–4	N3	M0	3
IV	TAny	NAny	M1a,b	14

[a]Percentage of patients in IASLC database according to best stage (rounded to nearest integer).

Source: From Ref. 41.

TABLE 5 Summary of clinical features

Local
- Dyspnea
- Cough
- Hemoptysis
- Chest pain
- Hoarseness (Recurrent laryngeal nerve involvement)
- Superior vena cava syndrome
- Pancoast syndrome

Systemic
- Fever (low-grade)
- Weight loss
- Anorexia
- Fatigue

Paraneoplastic syndromes
- Hypercalcemia (squamous cell ca)
- SIADH (small cell ca)
- Hypertrophic pulmonary osteoarthropathy
- Eaton-Lambert syndrome
- Cushing's syndrome
- Neurological-optic neuritis, cerebellar degeneration, limbic encephalopathy, autonomic neuropathy

tumor. Cancer need not be widespread to produce paraneoplastic syndromes. Indeed, some of these syndromes may precede diagnosis of localized disease. Hypercalcemia is one of the most common paraneoplastic syndromes. It is most commonly associated with NSCLC, specifically squamous cell carcinoma. It may be caused by bone metastases; however, the paraneoplastic syndrome is caused by ectopic production of parathyroid hormone-related peptide. It is treated with hydration and bisphosphonates. Eaton-Lambert myasthenic syndrome is most commonly seen in SCLC and causes proximal muscle weakness, which improves with repetitive activity, in contrast to myasthenia gravis. The treatment of paraneoplastic syndromes is to treat the underlying cancer; however, some of these conditions are irreversible.

■ SYSTEMIC THERAPY FOR NSCLC

Therapy

Optimal treatment of NSCLC may include surgical resection, radiation, and/or chemotherapy and is determined by several factors—stage, histological subtype, the patient's performance status, comorbidities, and suitability for resection for early-stage disease. Recent data suggest that molecular profiling may also have an important role in determining type of treatment, and this will be reviewed later.

Early-Stage NSCLC: (Stages I and II)

Only about 15% of patients diagnosed with NSCLC present with localized disease (42). Surgery is the recommended treatment for patients with stages I and II disease, who are suitable candidates. Patients who are not candidates for surgery should receive potentially curative radiation therapy. The 5-year survival rate for patients with localized disease is approximately 53% (42).

Lobectomy is preferred to pneumonectomy whenever feasible, due to high rates of morbidity and mortality associated with pneumonectomy (43). Pulmonary function testing is part of the routine preoperative testing and should include both exercise testing and DLCO. In patients who cannot tolerate lobectomy, a more limited surgery such as segmentectomy or wedge resection can be done. However, this is controversial and should be avoided for patients with tumors >3 cm in size due to high risk of recurrence. The now-defunct Lung Cancer Study Group conducted a trial in which 276 patients with peripheral T1N0 (stage IA) NSCLC were randomly assigned to either lobectomy or a more limited procedure (i.e., wedge resection, segmentectomy). Limited pulmonary resection did not improve perioperative morbidity, mortality, or late postoperative pulmonary function, but was associated with a higher death and recurrence rates leading the LCSG to conclude that lobectomy should be the surgical procedure of choice for patients with peripheral T1 N0 NSCLC (44). With improved surgical and perioperative techniques, limited resections have come under study again recently and may be a reasonable option for carefully selected patients (45–47). Videoscopic resections (VATS) are usually preferred when feasible as they are associated with less postoperative pain and shorter hospital stays (48–50). VATS should be performed only by surgeons with specific expertise. VATS and standard thoracotomy appear to have similar survival and recurrence rates for stage I lung cancer (51–53). VATS resection may also improve tolerance of postoperative adjuvant chemotherapy (54,55).

In good performance status (PS) patients with stage II disease and probably in selected patients with larger stage I tumors who have undergone complete resection, adjuvant chemotherapy improves survival. The International Adjuvant Lung Cancer trial (56) randomized 1,867 patients with completely resected stage I, II, or III NSCLC to three to four cycles of cisplatin-based chemotherapy or observation with a primary endpoint of overall survival and a median follow-up of 56 months. Patients who received chemotherapy had a better overall survival (44.5% vs. 40.4 % at 5 years [469 deaths vs. 504]; hazard ratio for death [HR] = 0.86; 95% confidence interval [CI] = 0.76 to 0.98; $P < .03$) and improved disease-free survival (39.4% vs. 34.3% at 5 years [518 events vs. 577]; HR = 0.83; 95% CI = 0.74 to 0.94; $P < .003$) compared with the observation arm. No data have shown a survival benefit with adjuvant chemotherapy for unselected stage IA patients and many studies suggest a detriment. Thus chemotherapy should not be given routinely to those patients (57). Nevertheless, the 5-year survival for patients with resected stage IA NSCLC remains relatively low at about 70%, and efforts to identify appropriate adjuvant therapy and the population who may benefit are actively underway.

ANITA (Adjuvant Navelbine International Trialist Association) was a randomized controlled trial comparing adjuvant vinorelbine plus cisplatin to observation in 840 patients with completely resected stages IB–IIIA NSCLC (58). After a median follow-up of 76 months, median survival was 65.7 months (95% CI 47.9–88.5) in the chemotherapy group and 43.7 (35.7–52.3) months in the observation group. Adjusted risk for death was significantly reduced in patients on the chemotherapy arm (HR = 0.80 [95% CI 0.66–0.96]; $P = .017$). Overall survival at 5 years improved by 8.6% in the chemotherapy group, and was maintained at 7 years (8.4%). The benefit for chemotherapy was noted in stages II and III patients but not in stage I in a planned post hoc subset analysis.

Adjuvant chemotherapy with carboplatin and paclitaxel versus observation in stage IB patients was evaluated in the CALGB 9633 trial (59). This trial was initially reported as positive, but a second interim analysis with longer follow-up showed no differences in survival at 5 years (the primary endpoint of the trial). However, the progression-free survival (a secondary endpoint) remained significantly superior at 5 years in the chemotherapy arm and overall survival was improved over control at 3 years. A post hoc subset analysis showed a 5-year survival benefit in patients with tumors ≥4cm in diameter. This trial has been criticized as underpowered and for its use of non-cisplatin containing chemotherapy. Patients with tumors larger than 5 cm are now classified as stage IIA based on the current staging system, and adjuvant chemotherapy would be recommended for these patients.

The neoadjuvant or adjuvant chemotherapy in patients with operable NSCLC trial (NATCH) randomized patients with early stage NSCLC to surgery alone, neoadjuvant carboplatin/paclitaxel followed by surgery or surgery followed by adjuvant carboplatin/paclitaxel (60). The primary objective was to determine whether three cycles of neoadjuvant or adjuvant chemotherapy improved disease-free survival (DFS) compared to surgery alone. Results showed that neoadjuvant therapy was associated with improved survival when compared with surgery alone (5-year survival rates 53% vs. 41%; $P = .02$); adjuvant chemotherapy was associated with only a trend toward improved survival compared with surgery alone, which was not statistically significant. It should be noted that only 51% of patients received planned treatment in the adjuvant arm compared with 90% of patients in the preoperative arm.

Most positive studies of adjuvant chemotherapy have employed cisplatin-based chemotherapy. The lung adjuvant cisplatin evaluation (LACE) meta-analysis confirmed an overall survival benefit in the 5% range with cisplatin containing adjuvant chemotherapy (57) and cisplatin-based chemotherapy is preferred over carboplatin for patients without contraindications. Trials incorporating targeted agents concurrently or in sequence with chemotherapy are in progress.

Locally Advanced NSCLC: (Stage III)

Optimal treatment of most patients with stage III disease is chemoradiotherapy. Most patients with stage III disease are unresectable; although, surgery for patients with isolated positive N2 nodes can be considered after neoadjuvant chemotherapy or chemoradiotherapy. Patients with malignant pleural effusions or pleural involvement are now classified as stage IV (previously stage IIIB) and these patients are treated with chemotherapy alone. Chemoradiotherapy is superior to radiotherapy alone for good PS patients with unresectable stage III NSCLC. CALGB 8433 and RTOG 88–08 were two large randomized clinical trials comparing chemoradiation to radiotherapy alone in patients with stage III NSCLC. In the CALGB study (61), patients with stage III NSCLC received either cisplatin (100 mg/m^2 intravenously on days 1 and 29) and vinblastine (5 mg/m^2 intravenously weekly on days 1, 8, 15, 22, and 29) followed by radiation therapy with 60 Gy in 30 fractions beginning on day 50 (CT-RT group) or radiation therapy with 60 Gy alone beginning on day 1 (RT group) for a maximum duration of 6 to 7 weeks. Median survival after 7 years of follow-up was 13.7 months in the CT-RT group and 9.6 months in the RT group (P = .012). These results were confirmed by Sause et al. (62) in RTOG 88–08 in which patients were randomized to 2 months of chemotherapy with cisplatin, vinblastine followed by 60 Gy of radiation at 2.0 Gy per fraction or 1.2 Gy per fraction delivered twice daily to a total dose of 69.6 Gy, or radiation only at 2.0 Gy per fraction once daily to 60 Gy. Median survival for radiation only was 11.4 months; for chemotherapy and radiation, 13.2 months; and for hyperfractionated irradiation, 12 months. A statistical improvement in survival was achieved in the chemoradiation group but not in the hyperfractionated radiation group. In both of these studies, 5-year survivals were approximately doubled by the addition of chemotherapy compared with radiation alone.

Concurrent chemoradiation has been shown to be superior to sequential chemoradiation. Furuse et al. (63) conducted a phase 3 study of concurrent versus sequential radiotherapy in combination with mitomycin, vindesine, and cisplatin in patients with stage III NSCLC (63). The concurrent group demonstrated an improvement of median survival of 3 months over that of the sequentially treated patients (16.5 vs. 13.3 months), and the 5-year survival rates with concurrent therapy were 15.8% versus 8.9% with sequential therapy.

RTOG 94–10 (64) was a three-arm phase 3 trial in which 610 patients were randomized to sequential chemoradiation versus two concurrent chemoradiation therapy arms (one with standard once-daily radiation and the other with hyperfractionated twice a day radiation). The median survival was superior for patients who received concurrent chemoradiation compared with sequential treatment (17.0 vs. 14.6 months, P = .04). Hyperfractionated radiation did not result in improved survival compared with the sequential arm (15.2 vs. 14.6 months; P = .296). The 4-year survival for patients in the concurrent chemotherapy and daily standard radiation arm was 21% versus 12% with sequential chemotherapy followed by radiation (P = .046). The incidence of acute nonhematological toxicities was higher in the concurrent arms; however, late toxicities were similar for patients in all three arms. These studies established concurrent chemoradiation therapy as standard treatment in patients with unresectable stage III NSCLC.

In patients with nonbulky stage III disease with no involvement of mediastinal lymph nodes (T4N0, T3, or T4N1), surgery may be attempted; however, cure rate is low with surgery alone and these patients should receive adjuvant therapy. Chemoradiotherapy followed by resection is the standard of care for patients with pancoast tumors and good PS.

Neoadjuvant chemotherapy followed by surgery has been recommended in certain situations, in patients with nonbulky stage IIIA disease. There were two randomized trials that evaluated this issue. The first trial by Roth et al. (65) randomized 60 patients to receive either six cycles of perioperative chemotherapy (cyclophosphamide, etoposide, and cisplatin) and surgery, or surgery alone. For patients treated with chemotherapy and surgery, the rate of clinical major response was 35%. Patients treated with perioperative chemotherapy and surgery had an estimated median survival of 64 months compared with 11 months for patients who had surgery alone (P < .008 by log-rank test; P < .018 by Wilcoxon test). The other trial by Rosell and colleagues (66) also randomized 60 patients to chemotherapy (mitomycin, ifosfamide, and cisplatin) followed by surgery versus surgery alone. Median survival was

26 months versus 8 months ($P < .001$) and DFS was 20 months versus 5 months ($P < .001$) both in favor of the chemotherapy plus surgery arm. These trials were both planned to be larger studies, but each was stopped early due to the pronounced survival advantage of chemotherapy in interim analyses. The limitations of these trials include small sample size, use of chemotherapy regimens not in common practice today, and uncontrolled use of radiation. The Rosell trial has also been criticized for the much lower than expected survival in the surgery alone arm. A larger randomized French trial showed a survival advantage for neoadjuvant chemotherapy for N0 and N1 disease, but not for N2 disease (67).

Studies of surgery after neoadjuvant chemoradiation have not shown an overall survival benefit to the addition of surgery to standard chemoradiotherapy. The Intergroup 0139 trial (68) evaluated patients with N2 disease who were randomly assigned to two cycles of cisplatin and etoposide with 45 Gy radiation therapy followed by resection and adjuvant chemotherapy versus the nonsurgical arm in which radiation was given to 60 Gy with identical chemotherapy. The surgery arm had a significant increase in 5-year progression-free survival (PFS: 22% vs. 11%), but only a nonsignificant trend toward better overall survival (5-year survival rate: 27% vs. 20%). The lack of survival benefit in the surgical arm is attributable to more treatment-related deaths in the surgery arm compared with the chemoradiation arm (8% vs. 2%), particularly in patients undergoing pneumonectomy. Right pneumonectomy was particularly toxic in these patients with mortality in excess of 20%. EORTC 08941 (69) evaluated the role of surgery versus RT after induction chemotherapy. A total of 579 patients with biopsy-proven stage III (N2) NSCLC received three cycles of platinum-based chemotherapy, followed by randomization to surgery or thoracic RT. Median survival and 5-year overall survival rates were similar (16.4 vs. 17.5 months and 16% vs. 14% for the surgery and RT groups, respectively; HR 1.06, 95% CI 0.84–1.35).

Given these results, standard therapy for most good PS patients with stage IIIA or B NSCLC is definitive chemoradiation. Cisplatin-based therapy is preferred. The U.S. standard is etoposide and cisplatin concurrent with radiation although weekly low dose carboplatin and paclitaxel are often used. While no head-to-head comparison is available, all of the results reported with carboplatin and paclitaxel with radiation are inferior to those reported with cisplatin-etoposide. The addition of targeted agents has not yet been proven to improve outcome. Indeed, SWOG 0023 randomized patients to gefitinib or placebo after standard etoposide platinum with radiation followed by consolidation docetaxel. This trial was closed early due to a survival disadvantage in the targeted therapy arm (70). Interestingly, the control arm of this study had amongst the best survival rates ever seen in this disease. The role of consolidation chemotherapy is controversial. It is included in most trials and those trials employing consolidation have typically shown higher survival than those without. However, the Hoosier Oncology Group (HOG) conducted a study of standard cisplatin etoposide with radiation followed by docetaxel consolidation versus no consolidation and showed no benefit to the consolidation (71). This trial is criticized for lack of power as well as for an imbalance in pulmonary function in favor of the nonconsolidation arm. Despite the results of this trial, CTEP has mandated consolidation chemotherapy in several ongoing phase 3 trials.

To date, no clear advance in chemotherapy over cisplatin plus etoposide has been made for combined modality therapy. The Lilly-sponsored JMIG study is testing the newer combination of pemetrexed and cisplatin against standard etoposide and cisplatin for patients with nonsquamous stage III NSCLC in hopes of achieving better tolerance and efficacy with the newer regimen. Radiation delivery has not been optimized either. Hyperfractionated radiation has not been found superior to single daily fractionation in several trials. Ongoing studies explore radiation dosing with the RTOG now studying 60 versus 74 Gy in combination with weekly low-dose carboplatin and paclitaxel. In addition, a meta-analysis is currently being performed to evaluate the potential benefits of altered RT fractionation compared with standard daily fractionation.

Advanced NSCLC: (Stage IV) Systemic Chemotherapy

Advanced NSCLC (stage IV) is an incurable disease usually treated with palliative intent. With best supportive care (BSC) alone, the median survival of advanced NSCLC patients is approximately 3–6 months, and 1-year survival rates are less than 10% (72). It is well known that survival can be prolonged with systemic chemotherapy. Perhaps even more importantly, chemotherapy can also reduce disease-related symptoms and improve quality of life. This was established by several trials that compared BSC versus chemotherapy plus BSC. A meta-analysis of these trials conducted by the NSCLC collaborative group (11 trials of BSC vs. BSC plus chemotherapy) showed a survival benefit with cisplatin-based chemotherapy, with a 27% reduction in the risk of death, an absolute improvement in survival of 10% by 1 year and an increased median survival of about 1½ months (73).

The European Big Lung trial was conducted to confirm the survival benefit shown in the meta-analysis and also to study the impact on quality of life and cost issues (74). A total of 725 patients with advanced NSCLC were randomized to BSC alone, or BSC with cisplatin-based chemotherapy. Median survival was 8 months in the chemotherapy arm versus 5.7 months in the BSC-alone arm, (HR 0.77; 95% CI 0.66–0.89, $P = .0006$), despite an increase in treatment-related deaths of 19 (5%) in the chemotherapy arm. A total of 273 patients were included in the quality of life (QOL) substudy and although there were no significant differences in overall QOL between the two arms, a large negative effect of chemotherapy on QOL was not seen (75).

First-Line Chemotherapy

Based on the above trials, platinum-based chemotherapy was established as the standard of care for patients with advanced NSCLC and good PS. In the past, older agents such as vinca alkaloids, epipodophyllotoxins, and mitomycin were used with cisplatin (76). However, in recent years, platinum has been used in combination with other active single agents such as gemcitabine, paclitaxel, docetaxel, pemetrexed, and irinotecan with good results and better toxicity profile. For patients with poor PS, single-agent chemotherapy can be considered although trials of doublet versus single-agent chemotherapy for patients with PS 2 generally show a survival advantage to the doublet regimen (77,78).

Number of Agents

Delbaldo et al. (79) conducted a meta-analysis of 13,601 patients from 65 trials comparing a doublet regimen with a single-agent regimen or comparing a triplet regimen with a doublet regimen in patients with advanced NSCLC. The addition of a second drug increased tumor response (OR 0.42; 95% CI 0.37–0.47; $P < .0001$) and 1-year survival (OR 0.80; 95% CI 0.70–0.91; $P < .0001$). However, the addition of a third agent resulted in increased tumor response (OR 0.68; 95% CI 0.58–0.75; $P < .0001$), increased toxicity, without any impact on survival (OR 1.01; 95% CI 0.85–1.21; $P = .88$). This meta-analysis confirmed the prevailing impression that a doublet chemotherapy regimen is optimal for first-line treatment of advanced NSCLC.

Choice of Platinum Agent

There has been continued debate regarding the choice of platinum agent—cisplatin or carboplatin. Two large meta-analyses addressed this question. Ardizzoni et al. (80) included 2,968 patients from nine clinical trials. Cisplatin was associated with a higher ORR than carboplatin (30% vs. 24%, respectively; HR = 1.37; 95% CI = 1.16 to 1.61; $P < .001$). Carboplatin treatment was associated with a non-statistically significant increase in the hazard of mortality relative to treatment with cisplatin (HR = 1.07; 95% CI = 0.99 to 1.15; $P = .100$). In a subset analysis, patients with nonsquamous tumors and those treated in combination with a third-generation chemotherapy agent, carboplatin-based chemotherapy was associated with a statistically significant increase in mortality (HR = 1.12; 95% CI = 1.01–1.23 and HR = 1.11; 95% CI = 1.01–1.21, respectively). Cisplatin-based chemotherapy was associated with more severe nausea and vomiting and nephrotoxicity; however, severe thrombocytopenia was more frequent during carboplatin-based chemotherapy. Hotta et al. (81) evaluated 2,948 patients from eight trials. Cisplatin therapy was associated with higher response rates. Overall survival was not significantly different (HR = 1.050; 95% CI, 0.907–1.216; $P = .515$); however, as with Ardizzoni's analysis, subset analysis of cisplatin with a newer agent (gemcitabine, paclitaxel, or docetaxel) versus carboplatin with the same new agent revealed a statistically significant improvement in survival for cisplatin (HR = 1.106; 95% CI = 1.005 to 1.218; $P = .039$).

Overall, cisplatin has been shown to have higher response rates compared to carboplatin, and a survival benefit has been seen in several studies. Meta-analyses confirm a survival benefit to cisplatin over carboplatin when combined with the standard second agents in common use today. Although both agents are acceptable, cisplatin is preferred in a good PS patient in the absence of any contraindications.

Duration of Therapy

The optimal duration of therapy in advanced NSCLC is in flux. ASCO guidelines for treatment of patients with unresectable NSCLC (2003 update) state that first-line chemotherapy should be administered for no more than six cycles and should be stopped at four cycles in patients not responding to treatment (82). These guidelines were based on several clinical trials evaluating the duration of chemotherapy in advanced NSCLC. Smith and colleagues (83) conducted a trial in which 308 patients were randomized to three, compared with six cycles of mitomycin, vinblastine, and cisplatin (MVP). The response rate, time to disease progression, and overall survival were identical between the two arms. Fatigue was significantly decreased in the patients receiving three cycles and there was a trend toward decreased nausea and vomiting. The authors concluded that there was no benefit to continuing MVP chemotherapy beyond three cycles in patients with advanced NSCLC. A second trial by Socinski et al. (84) randomized 230 patients to four cycles of carboplatin at an area under the curve of 6 and paclitaxel 200 mg/m^2 every 21 days or continuous treatment with carboplatin/paclitaxel until progression. This study showed no overall benefit in survival, response rates, or QOL to continuing treatment with carboplatin/paclitaxel beyond four cycles in advanced NSCLC. There were no significant differences in toxicities, except neuropathy, which increased from 19.9% at cycle 4 to 43% at cycle 8. Similarly, another trial by von Plessen et al. (85) randomized 297 patients with advanced NSCLC to either three or six cycles of carboplatin plus vinorelbine. There were no response, survival, or quality-of-life differences demonstrated.

More recently, a meta-analysis of 3,027 patients from 13 trials was conducted by Soon et al. (86). This meta-analysis included trials that compared standard duration of chemotherapy (2–8 cycles) to prolonged chemotherapy that was continued until progression or unacceptable toxicity. Extending chemotherapy was associated with a clinically modest, but statistically significant improvement in overall survival with an 8% reduction in the hazard for death as compared with a standard duration of chemotherapy (HR = 0.92; 95% CI = 0.85–0.99; P = .03); PFS was substantially improved (HR = 0.75; 95% CI = 0.69–0.81; P < .00001), especially for trials extending chemotherapy with third-generation regimens rather than older regimens (HR, 0.70 interaction vs. 0.92 interaction; P = .003). Extending chemotherapy was associated with more frequent adverse effects in all trials and impaired HRQL in two of seven trials.

Maintenance Therapy

Another issue is the continuation of therapy with a single agent with known activity in advanced, refractory NSCLC following a defined duration of first-line platinum-based therapy. This is often characterized as maintenance therapy but may be better referred to as early second-line therapy. A phase 3 study by Fidias et al. (87) randomly assigned patients to either immediate or delayed docetaxel after initial treatment with gemcitabine and carboplatin. Median PFS for immediate docetaxel was significantly greater than for delayed docetaxel (5.7 vs. 2.7 months; P = .0001). Median overall survival (OS) for immediate docetaxel was greater than for delayed docetaxel, but the difference was not statistically significant (12.3 vs. 9.7 months; P = .0853). QOL results were not statistically different (P = .76) between docetaxel groups. An important confounding factor in analyzing these data is that about 37% of patients in the delayed docetaxel arm never received docetaxel therapy. OS for patients in the delayed arm who actually received docetaxel therapy was 12.5 months (95% CI, 9.6–14.6 months), which was identical to the OS observed in the immediate docetaxel arm (12.5 months; 95% CI = 10.6–15.8). These findings suggest that it may be the exposure to the active second-line agent rather than the duration or timing of therapy that confers an improvement in survival (88).

Ciuleanu et al. (89) evaluated pemetrexed and BSC versus placebo and BSC in patients with stage IIIB/IV NSCLC who had not progressed after four cycles of platinum-based chemotherapy. PFS was improved on the pemetrexed arm compared to placebo (4.3 vs. 2.6 months; HR = 0.502, 95% CI = 0.42–0.61, P < .00001) especially in patients with nonsquamous cancers. OS was 13.4 months with pemetrexed and 10.6 months with placebo (HR = 0.79, 95% CI = 0.65–0.95, P= 0.012). Toxicities were higher in the pemetrexed arm, including grade 3/4 anemia (16% vs. 4%; P < .001); fatigue (5% vs. 0.5%) and neutropenia (2.9% vs. 0%). Grade 3/4 toxicities did not increase significantly in patients who received ≥6 and ≥10 cycles of pemetrexed (4.5% vs. 1.4%). There was no survival improvement with pemetrexed in squamous cell cancers. As with the Fidias trial, there is a substantial problem in interpretetation of these data in that the majority of patients on the placebo arm did not receive pemetrexed therapy at progression. It is impossible to evaluate whether immediate versus delayed second-line pemetrexed produces a survival advantage based on these data. However, based on these results, so-called maintenance therapy with pemetrexed was approved by the FDA in 2009 for patients with advanced NSCLC who have stable disease after standard chemotherapy. Whether true maintenance with pemetrexed after initial pemetrexed-based therapy will result in a survival advantage is unknown.

Targeted therapy has also been recently evaluated as a maintenance strategy. The two trials evaluating erlotinib as maintenance in patients with nonprogressing disease after first-line platinum-based chemotherapy were the ATLAS and SATURN trials. In the ATLAS (90) trial 1,160 patients initially received four cycles of platinum-based chemotherapy with bevacizumab; following this, 768 patients with nonprogressing disease were randomized to maintenance therapy with either bevacizumab and erlotinib or bevacizumab and placebo, which was given until progression. Median PFS was 4.8 months for (B + E) versus 3.7 months for (B + P), HR = 0.722 (95% CI = 0.592–0.881), P = .0012. Overall survival data are not available.

In the SATURN trial (91), 1,949 patients with advanced NSCLC initially received four cycles of platinum-based doublet therapy; following which 889 patients with nonprogressing disease were randomized to either erlotinib or placebo. Maintenance therapy with erlotinib 150 mg/day resulted in an increase in PFS, from 40% to 53% at 12 weeks and 17% to 31% at 24 weeks, compared with placebo (HR = 0.71 [95% CI = 0.62–0.82] P < .0001). The patients were also assessed for the presence of *EGFR* mutation, and although there was some benefit even in patients with wild type *EGFR*, this was significantly higher in patients documented to have the *EGFR* mutation (HR = 0.10, 95% CI = 0.04–0.25; P < .0001). OS, which was a secondary endpoint, was also slightly but significantly improved in the erlotinib arm (12 vs. 11 months). Although erlotinib is already approved as a second-line chemotherapy agent, it is anticipated that on the basis of these results, it may be approved as a maintenance treatment in the first-line setting.

It is important to note all the above trials used agents that are approved drugs in the second-line setting (docetaxel, pemetrexed, and erlotinib). It remains unclear as to whether the survival benefit seen in these studies is due to the timing of treatment or due to actual exposure to the drug. The data from SATURN, however, are not applicable outside the setting of stage IV disease, as seen in the S0023 trial, which studied maintenance gefitinib (70). Patients included on this trial had inoperable stage III disease and were initially treated with concurrent chemoradiation therapy (cisplatin/etoposide with radiation), followed by three cycles of consolidation chemotherapy with docetaxel. Patients with nonprogressing disease were randomized to oral gefitinib 250 mg/day or placebo, until disease progression or unacceptable toxicity. With a median follow-up time of 27 months, median survival time was 23 months for gefitinib (n = 118) and 35 months for placebo (n = 125; two-sided P = 0.013).

Impact of Histology

The choice of chemotherapy can impact response rates and survival in specific histological subtypes of NSCLC. Scagliotti et al. (92) conducted a phase 3 randomized trial comparing cisplatin and gemcitabine versus cisplatin and pemetrexed for the first-line treatment of patients with advanced NSCLC. Overall survival for cisplatin/pemetrexed was noninferior to cisplatin/gemcitabine (median survival, 10.3 vs. 10.3 months, respectively; HR = 0.94; 95% CI = 0.84–1.05). In a preplanned analysis of response by histology, OS was statistically superior for cisplatin/pemetrexed versus cisplatin/gemcitabine in patients with adenocarcinoma (12.6 vs. 10.9 months, respectively) and large-cell carcinoma histology (10.4 vs. 6.7 months, respectively). In contrast, in patients with squamous cell histology, there was a significant improvement in survival with cisplatin/gemcitabine versus cisplatin/pemetrexed (10.8 vs. 9.4 months, respectively). This was the first study to show a difference in survival based on histology and has changed clinical practice for the first-line treatment of patients with metastatic NSCLC.

Targeted Agents in First-Line Setting

The epidermal growth factor receptor (*EGFR* [HER1 or c-erbB-1]) belongs to the erbB family of growth factor receptors, which also includes HER2, HER3, and HER4 proteins. EGFR is overexpressed in almost 70% of NSCLCs (93). The HER family proteins consist of an extracellular ligand-binding domain, transmembrane component and an intracellular tyrosine kinase domain. *EGFR* exists as a monomer on the cell surface, but must dimerize to activate the tyrosine kinase. *EGFR* signaling is triggered by the binding of growth factors, such as epidermal growth factor (EGF), resulting in homodimerization of *EGFR* molecules or heterodimerization with other closely related receptors, such as HER2/neu (94). Autophosphorylation and transphosphorylation of the receptors through their tyrosine kinase domains leads to recruitment of downstream effectors and activation of proliferative and cell-survival signals (95). Overexpression or mutation of *EGFR* can lead to inappropriate activation and provide a target for novel therapies.

Activating mutations of *EGFR* are seen most commonly in women, Asians, never-smokers, and patients with adenocarcinoma. Erlotinib and gefitinib are orally administered *EGFR* tyrosine kinase inhibitors that inhibit EGFR signaling by binding to the intracellular tyrosine kinase domain. *EGFR* pathway activation can be assessed by evaluation of *EGFR* mutation status by gene sequencing, *EGFR* gene copy number by FISH and *EGFR* protein expression by immunohistochemistry (IHC). The clinical use of *EGFR* active agents including TKIs and monoclonal antibodies (cetuximab) in advanced NSCLC will be briefly discussed here.

Erlotinib and gefitinib are *EGFR* TKIs and are being increasingly used in patients with advanced NSCLC. Erlotinib is approved for use in the second-line setting in the United States. Gefitinib is widely used in Asia but is no longer marketed in the United States. *EGFR* mutations were first reported in 2004 in exons 19 and 21, which correspond to the tyrosine kinase domain of *EGFR* (94,96). These mutations affect the ATP-binding cleft of the *EGFR*, which is also the *EGFR* TKI binding site. In vitro, the *EGFR* mutants appear to have prolonged and increased tyrosine kinase activity in the presence of ligand, and they display markedly enhanced susceptibility to inhibition by *EGFR* TKIs (97).

Several clinical trials are being conducted to study *EGFR* TKIs in the first-line setting. The IPASS (Iressa Pan Asia Study) (98) was an open label, randomized noninferiority trial that assessed the efficacy, safety, and tolerability of Gefitinib versus standard chemotherapy with carboplatin/paclitaxel as first-line treatment in a clinically selected population of patients from Asia. A total of 1,217 patients (never or light ex-smokers) with stage IIIB/IV adenocarcinoma were randomized to gefitinib 250 mg/day or carboplatin AUC 5 plus 6/paclitaxel 200 mg/m^2 every 3 weeks. Among all patients, PFS favored gefitinib (HR = 0.741, 95% CI = 0.651–0.845; P < .0001); although this effect was not constant over time, initially favoring the C/P arm, and then favoring the gefitinib arm. This was described as being due to the differences in PFS in patients with *EGFR* mutation positive and negative tumors. ORR was higher in the gefitinib arm and OS was similar in both arms; however, follow-up is still ongoing. When analyzed by *EGFR* mutation status, mutation positive patients (60% of this selected Asian population) had significantly longer PFS and higher ORR and mutation negative patients had significantly shorter PFS and lower ORR with G than C/P. These data emphasize the importance of assessment of *EGFR* mutation status even in patients meeting clinical criteria for enrichment in *EGFR* mutations. The detriment in survival from exposure of patients without *EGFR* mutations to first line *EGFR* TKIs is significant. The use of erlotinib as a first-line agent has been discussed under maintenance therapy and will not be repeated here.

Cetuximab is a monoclonal antibody directed against *EGFR* that has shown activity in NSCLC. The FLEX (99) trial is a phase 3 trial in which patients with *EGFR*-expressing stage wet IIIB or stage IV NSCLC were randomly assigned in a 1:1 ratio to cisplatin and vinorelbine chemotherapy plus cetuximab or chemotherapy alone. Patients on the cetuximab arm had an improved OS compared with those in the chemotherapy-alone group (median 11.3 vs. 10.1 months; HR for death = 0.871, 95% CI = 0.762–0.996; P = .044); however, toxicities including rash, diarrhea, and infusion reactions were higher in this arm.

Angiogenesis Inhibitors

Angiogenesis is the process of formation of new blood vessels and is an important step in tumor growth and metastases (100,101). Angiogenesis is primarily regulated by vascular endothelial growth factor (VEGF), which is a homodimeric glycoprotein (102). VEGF causes endothelial cell proliferation and formation of new blood vessels by binding to its tyrosine kinase receptors and inducing intracellular signaling pathways by dimerization similarly to *EGFR*. VEGF is a potentially important therapeutic target in NSCLC.

Bevacizumab is a monoclonal antibody to VEGF, which has been shown to improve survival of patients with nonsquamous lung cancer over chemotherapy alone when used in combination with carboplatin

is more likely to be adenocarcinoma or BAC, associated with *EGFR* mutations (and responsive to *EGFR-TKIs*) and carry a substantially better overall prognosis.

TNM staging in NSCLC has recently been updated with the presentation of the 7th edition by the staging committee of IASLC. The major changes are based on prognosis and therapy. Patients with early-stage (stages I and II) disease are treated with surgical resection, preferably lobectomy. All eligible patients with stage II disease and selected patients with stage IB disease should undergo adjuvant treatment with four cycles of platinum-based chemotherapy. Patients with stage III disease should optimally be managed with combined chemoradiation therapy.

Stage IV disease is treated with chemotherapy and the goal of treatment is symptom palliation and prolongation of survival. Radiotherapy is generally reserved for palliation. The optimal chemotherapy regimen depends on patient factors such as performance status, comorbidities, smoking history, and histology. Molecular factors may also be taken into account. The standard of care for first-line chemotherapy is usually a platinum-based doublet; in adenocarcinoma—pemetrexed along with a platinum agent (cisplatin preferred) is a good first choice and in squamous cell carcinoma—gemcitabine along with a platinum agent is well tolerated and effective. Elderly patients should also be treated similarly, provided they have a good performance status. In patients who cannot tolerate platinum-based doublets, single-agent chemotherapy may be given. In suitable patients, bevacizumab may be added to first-line carboplatin and paclitaxel therapy in the absence of contraindications. Treatment with platinum-based therapy beyond four to six cycles has not been associated with a survival benefit and can cause increased toxicity (126).

The issue of maintenance therapy is still unresolved; however, recent studies using pemetrexed or erlotinib as maintenance therapy have shown promise. It may be the exposure to the second-line agent more than the timing of therapy that actually provides a survival advantage. The approved agents for second-line therapy are erlotinib, docetaxel, and pemetrexed. Of these agents, pemetrexed has now been approved for use in the first-line setting in patients with adenocarcinoma. Currently bevacizumab is the only targeted agent approved for use in the first-line setting in the United States; however, it is anticipated that more drug approvals will follow in the near future.

■ SCLC

SCLC accounts for approximately 15% of all diagnosed cases of lung cancer and is more prevalent in women than in men. It is seen almost exclusively in smokers and is characterized by aggressive spread with micrometastatic disease usually present at diagnosis. The details of pathology, molecular biology, and clinical features are discussed earlier in the chapter and will not be repeated here.

Staging

The TNM staging system that is used for NSCLC is also standard for SCLC. However, the staging system most widely used for SCLC was introduced by the Veterans' Affairs Lung Study Group (VALSG). Based on this, the disease is classified as limited stage or extensive stage depending on whether the disease can be encompassed within reasonable hemithorax radiation fields.

Limited Stage: Disease confined to the ipsilateral hemithorax and regional nodes including supraclavicular nodes but excluding malignant pleural effusion.

Extensive Stage: Any metastatic disease outside the hemithorax or a malignant pleural effusion.

Treatment

Due to the aggressive behavior of SCLC and presence of micrometastatic disease at diagnosis, surgery is not appropriate treatment and systemic chemotherapy is required in almost all cases. SCLC is extremely sensitive to chemotherapy and radiation (127); treatment depends on extent of disease.

Only about one-third of all patients with SCLC present with limited-stage disease, and the remaining two-third of patients have extensive disease at the time of presentation. The standard of care for patients with limited-stage SCLC is chemotherapy with concurrent thoracic radiation. For patients with extensive-stage disease, chemotherapy alone is the standard treatment. Overall response rates with combined modality therapy in limited-stage disease exceed 90%, with complete response rates of 50% to 70%. In extensive disease, overall response rates are approximately 60% to 70% with chemotherapy alone and 20% to 30% of patients may have CR (128).

In limited-stage disease, the goal of treatment is cure. However, even with the high response rates most patients relapse. With standard etoposide/platinum and radiation, median, survival is only 18 to 24 months, with a 5-year survival rate of about 25%. Survival is extremely poor in extensive-stage SCLC, with a 2-year survival rate of less than 5% and median survival of 10 to 14 months. However, an extremely small subset of patients are cured (129). To date, no chemotherapy regimen has improved on standard cisplatin and etoposide.

Radiation Therapy

The use of thoracic radiation in limited-stage SCLC is associated with an improved local control rate and improved survival (130). Details of thoracic radiation therapy are discussed in the radiation therapy section. In general, concurrent chemoradiation is better than sequential therapy in limited-stage SCLC (131) and early radiation results in better local control and improved survival compared to late radiation. Turrisi et al. (132) conducted a randomized study in which 412 patients with limited-stage SCLC were randomized to concurrent chemoradiation using a dose of 45 Gy delivered either once daily over 5 weeks or twice daily over 3 weeks. Median survival was 23 versus 19 months and 5-year survival was 26% versus 16% in favor of the twice-daily radiation arm.

Systemic Chemotherapy

The standard chemotherapy used with concurrent radiation is cisplatin and etoposide (133). This has been shown to be superior to cyclophosphamide, doxorubicin, vincristine (CAV) in both efficacy and toxicity in limited-stage disease (134). Carboplatin is sometimes substituted for cisplatin in patients who cannot tolerate cisplatin. A small randomized Greek study comparing etoposide-cisplatin to etoposide-carboplatin showed no significant difference in median survival; however, overall response rates were slightly higher in the cisplatin group and complete response rates were substantially higher (135). Cisplatin is associated with higher incidence of emesis, neurotoxicity, and nephrotoxicity; however, carboplatin is associated with more myelosuppresion. Cisplatin should be used in the absence of contraindications especially in limited-stage disease due to the higher complete response rates and potential for cure.

Other regimens evaluated include cisplatin with irinotecan. A phase 3 Japanese trial (136) (JCOG 511) randomized 154 patients to cisplatin and irinotecan versus cisplatin and etoposide in patients with extensive-stage SCLC. The median survival was 12.8 months in the irinotecan-plus-cisplatin group and 9.4 months in the etoposide-plus-cisplatin group (P = .002). Myelosuppression was more common in the etoposide-cisplatin group. Two trials conducted in the United States attempted to confirm the Japanese data, but failed to show an improved survival with irinotecan-cisplatin. Hanna et al. (137) randomized 331 patients in a 2:1 ratio to cisplatin 30 mg/m^2 intravenously (IV) + irinotecan 65 mg/m^2 IV on days 1 and 8 every 21 days, or cisplatin 60 mg/m^2 IV on day 1, and etoposide 120 mg/m^2 IV on days 1 to 3 every 21 days for at least four cycles. There was no significant difference in response rates (48% vs. 43.6%), median time to progression (4.1 vs. 4.6 months), or overall survival (median survival time, 9.3 months vs. 10.2 months; P = 0.74). Natale et al. (138) randomized 651 patients to IP versus EP. This trial also did not show any difference in response rates, median survival, and overall survival in the two groups. The different results in the Japanese and American trials were attributed to the pharmacogenomic differences in these populations. Toxicities were similar in these trials, with more myelosuppression in the etoposide arm and more diarrhea in the irinotecan arm.

The addition of a third agent to EP has increased toxicity without improving outcome similarly to the situation for NSCLC (139). The optimal duration of treatment is four to six cycles. Prolonged duration of chemotherapy or "consolidation" chemotherapy has not been shown to provide a survival benefit. E7593 (140) was a phase 3 trial in which patients were randomized to four cycles of topotecan (1.5 mg/m^2 daily for 5 days every 3 weeks) or observation after stable or responding disease with four cycles of EP for extensive-stage SCLC. PFS was improved in the topotecan arm compared with observation (3.6 vs. 2.3 months; $P < .001$); however, there was no difference in overall survival (8.9 vs. 9.3 months; P = .43). Toxicity including myelosuppression was increased in the patients receiving topotecan.

Increased dose intensity (higher dose or more frequent cycles) of chemotherapy has been evaluated; however, no survival benefit was observed (141). Elderly patients with good performance status have a prognosis similar to younger patients and should be treated with standard platinum-based therapy in the absence of contraindications. Single-agent therapy in elderly patients has been shown to be associated with inferior survival, although toxicity is less than with combination therapy (142–144).

Salvage Therapy

Most patients with SCLC eventually relapse, and survival following relapse is generally short. Salvage chemotherapy may provide palliation in these patients. The timing of relapse plays an important role in determining response to second-line therapy. Patients who relapse within 3 months of initial therapy are usually refractory to second-line therapy with response rates <10%. For patients who relapse more than 3 months after initial therapy, response rates are approximately 25%. Patients relapsing a year or more after first-line therapy have response rates essentially the same as first line and should be treated with etoposide platinum again in the absence of contraindications. Active agents in the second-line setting include topotecan, gemcitabine, paclitaxel, and docetaxel. Topotecan is the only agent approved for use as a second-line agent in SCLC. Topotecan was compared with CAV (cyclophosphamide, doxorubicin, and vincristine) in a randomized trial of patients with relapsed SCLC (145). Response rate was 24.3% in the topotecan arm and 18.3% in the CAV arm ($P = .285$). Median times to progression were 13.3 weeks (topotecan) and 12.3 weeks (CAV) ($P = .552$). Median survival was 25 weeks for topotecan and 24.7 weeks for CAV ($P = .795$). Symptom improvement was better in the topotecan arm and toxicity including myelosuppression was lower.

Role of Surgery

Surgery has a limited role in the treatment of SCLC since most patients present with metastatic disease. Patients with T1–2, N0, M0 disease are occasionally resected largely because the diagnosis is unknown prior to surgery (146); these patients should undergo thorough staging evaluation including a mediastinoscopy to rule out occult nodal disease. After resection, all patients should receive adjuvant platinum-based chemotherapy.

Summary

SCLC is a highly aggressive malignancy that usually presents with metastatic disease or micrometastases even when apparently localized at diagnosis. It is almost exclusively a disease of smokers. Simplified staging is on the basis of whether all known gross disease can be safely encompassed within radiotherapy fields and classified as limited or extensive stage. The treatment of choice for limited-stage disease is concurrent chemoradiation therapy with cisplatin and etoposide. Twice-a-day radiation is associated with a survival advantage and is preferred in patients who can tolerate it although alternate radiation dosing and fractionation are under study. Patients with any degree of favorable response after chemoradiation should receive prophylactic cranial irradiation (PCI), which reduces brain metastases and improves survival. Extensive-stage disease is usually incurable and the treatment of choice is chemotherapy with cisplatin and etoposide for four to six cycles. PCI improves survival in these patients as well and for patients who respond completely; radiation to the primary site should be considered as it also improves survival. Patients who relapse within 3 months after first-line therapy have a poor prognosis and are considered refractory. Patients who relapse 3 months after first-line therapy may be treated with second-line therapy with topotecan.

REFERENCES

1. Brownson RC, Chang JC, Davis JR. Gender and histologic type variations in smoking-related risk of lung cancer. *Epidemiology.* 1992;3(1):61–64.
2. Horner MJ, Ries LAG, Krapcho M (eds.), et al. SEER Cancer Statistics Review, 1975–2006, National Cancer Institute. Bethesda, MD, Available at: http://seer.cancer.gov/csr/1975_2006/, based on November 2008 SEER data submission, posted to the SEER web site, 2009. Accessed July 12, 2009.
3. Alberg AJ, Samet JM. Epidemiology of Lung Cancer. *Chest.* 2003;123:21S–49S.
4. Doll, R, Hill, AB. Smoking and carcinoma of the lung; preliminary report. *Br Med J.* 1950;2:739.
5. Doll, R, Hill, AB. The mortality of doctors in relation to their smoking habits; a preliminary report. *Br Med J.* 1954;4877:1451.
6. Wynder, EL, Graham, EA. Etiologic factors in bronchiogenic carcinoma with special reference to industrial exposures; report of eight hundred fifty-seven proved cases. *A M A Arch Ind Hyg Occup Med.* 1951;4:221.
7. US Department of Health, and Human Services (USDHHS), Public Health Service, Centers for Disease

Control, and Prevention (CDC). Cigarette smoking: attributable mortality and years of potential life lost, United States, 1950–1990. *MMWR Morb Mortal Wkly Rep.* 1993;42:37–39.
8. Doll R, Peto R. Cigarette smoking and bronchial carcinoma: dose and time relationships among regular smokers and lifelong non-smokers. *J Epidemiol Community Health.*1978;32:303–313.
9. U.S. Department of Health, Education, and Welfare. *Smoking and Health: Report of the Advisory Committee to the Surgeon General of the Public Health Service.* Washington: U.S. Department of Health, Education, and Welfare, Public Health Service, Center for Disease Control; 1964. PHS Publication No. 1103.
10. US Department of Health, and Human Services (USDHHS). *The Health Benefits of Smoking Cessation: A Report of the Surgeon General.* USDHHS Publication No. 90–8416. Washington, DC: US Government Printing Office; 1990.
11. Hrubec Z, McLaughlin JK. Former cigarette smoking and mortality among US veterans: a 26-year follow-up, 1954–1980. In: Burns DM, Garfinkel L, Samet JM, eds. *Changes in Cigarette-Related Disease Risks and Their Implication for Prevention and Control.* Bethesda, MD: US Government Printing Office; 1997:501–530.
12. National Cancer Institute (NCI). *The FTC Cigarette Test Method for Determining Tar, Nicotine, and Carbon Monoxide Yields of US Cigarettes.* Monograph 7. Bethesda, MD: National Institutes of Health; 1996.
13. US Department of Health, and Human Services (USDHHS), National Cancer Institute. *Risks Associated with Smoking Cigarettes with Low Machine-Measured Yields of Tar and Nicotine.* Bethesda, MD: National Institutes of Health; 2001.
14. Newhouse ML, Berry G. Patterns of mortality in asbestos factory workers in London. *Ann N Y Acad Sci.* 1979;330:53–60.
15. Lemen RA, Dement JM, Wagoner JK. Epidemiology of asbestos-related diseases. *Environ Health Perspect.* 1980;34:1–11.
16. Economou P, Lechner JF, Samet JM. Familial and genetic factors in the pathogenesis of lung cancer. In: Samet JM, ed. Epidemiology of lung cancer. New York, NY: Marcel Dekker; 1994:353–396.
17. Nazar-Stewart V, Motulsky AG, Eaton DL, et al. The glutathione S-transferase μ polymorphism as a marker for susceptibility to lung carcinoma. *Cancer Res.* 1993;53(suppl):2313–2318.
18. Vineis P, Caporaso N. Tobacco and cancer: epidemiology and the laboratory. *Environ Health Perspect.*1995;103:156–160.
19. Alpha-Tocopheral Beta-Carotene Cancer Prevention Study Group. The effect of vitamin E and beta-carotene on the incidence of lung cancer and other cancers in male smokers.*N Engl J Med.* 1994;330:1029–1035.
20. Hennekens CH, Buring JE, Manson JE, et al. Lack of effect of long-term supplementation with beta-carotene on the incidence of malignant neoplasms and cardiovascular disease. *N Engl J Med.* 1996;334:1145–1149.
21. Omenn GS, Goodman GE, Thornquist MD, et al. Effects of a combination of beta-carotene and vitamin A on lung cancer and cardiovascular disease. *N Engl J Med.* 1996;334:1150–1155.
22. Beasley MB, Brambilla E, Travis WD. The 2004 World Health Organization Classification of Lung Tumors. *Semin Roentgenol.* 2005;40(2):90–97.
23. Hung J, Kishimoto Y, Sugio K, et al. Allele-specific chromosome 3p deletions occur at an early stage in the pathogenesis of lung carcinoma. *JAMA.* 1995;273:558–563.
24. Wenzlaff AS, Cote ML, Bock CH, et al. GSTM1, GSTT1 and GSTP1 polymorphisms, environmental tobacco smoke exposure and risk of lung cancer among never smokers: a population-based study. *Carcinogenesis.* 2005;26(2):395–401. Epub 2004 Nov 4.
25. Pasrija T, Srinivasan R, Behera D, Majumdar S. Telomerase activity in sputum and telomerase and its components in biopsies of advanced lung cancer. *Eur J Cancer.* 2007;43:476–1482.
26. Rodenhuis S, Slebos RJ. Clinical significance of ras oncogene activation in human lung cancer. *Cancer Res.* 1992;52(9)(suppl):2665s–2669s.
27. Barbacid. M. Ras genes. *Annu. Rev. Biochem.* 1987;56: 799–827.
28. Ahrendt SA, Decker PA, Alawi EA, et al. Cigarette smoking is strongly associated with mutation of the K-ras gene in patients with primary adenocarcinoma of the lung. *Cancer.* 2001;92(6):1525–1530.
29. Slebos RJ, Kibbelaar RE, Dalesio O, et al. K-ras oncogene activation as a prognostic marker in adenocarcinoma of the lung. *N Engl J Med.* 1990;323(9):561–565.
30. Tsao MS, Aviel-Ronen S, Ding K, et al. Prognostic and predictive importance of p53 and RAS for adjuvant chemotherapy in non small-cell lung cancer. *J Clin Oncol.* 2007;25(33):5240–5247.
31. Shaw AT, Costa D, Mino-Kenudson M. Clinicopathologic features of EML4-ALK mutant lung cancer. *J Clin Oncol.* 2009;27(suppl):15s (abstr 11021).
32. Brambilla E, Gazdar A. Pathogenesis of lung cancer signaling pathways: roadmap for therapies. *Eur Respir J.* 2009;33(6):1485–1497.
33. Ahrendt SA, Hu Y, Buta M, et al. p53 mutations and survival in stage I non-small-cell lung cancer: results of a prospective study. *J Natl Cancer Inst.* 2003;95(13):961–970.
34. Verri C, Roz L, Conte D, et al. Fragile histidine triad gene inactivation in lung cancer: the European Early Lung Cancer project. *Am J Respir Crit Care Med.* 2009; 179(5):396–401. Epub 2008 Dec 18.
35. Sos ML, Koker M, Weir BA, et al. PTEN loss contributes to erlotinib resistance in EGFR-mutant lung cancer by activation of Akt and EGFR. *Cancer Res.* 2009;69(8):3256–3261. Epub 2009 Apr 7.
36. Caballero OL, Cohen D, Liu Q, et al. Loss of chromosome arms 3p and 9p and inactivation of P16 ^{INK4a} in normal epithelium of patients with primary lung cancer. *Genes Chromosomes Cancer.* 2001;32(2):119–125.
37. van Tinteren H, Hoekstra OS, Smit EF, et al. Effectiveness of positron emission tomography in the preoperative

assessment of patients with suspected non-small-cell lung cancer: the PLUS multicentre randomised trial. *Lancet.* 2002;359(9315):1388–1393.
38. Fischer B, Lassen U, Mortensen J et al. Preoperative staging of lung cancer with PET-CT. *N Engl J Med.* 2009;361(1):32–39.
39. de Langen AJ , Raijmakers P , Riphagen I et al. The size of mediastinal lymph nodes and its relation with metastatic involvement: a meta-analysis. *Eur J Cardiothorac Surg.* 2006;29:26–29.
40. Goldstraw P, Crowley J, Chansky K, et al. The IASLC Lung Cancer Staging Project: Proposals for the Revision of the TNM Stage Groupings in the Forthcoming (Seventh) Edition of the TNM Classification of Malignant Tumours. *J Thorac Oncol.* 2007;2(8):706–714.
41. Deterbeck FC, Boffa DJ, Tanoue LT. The new lung cancer staging system. *Chest.* 2009;136:260–271.
42. SEER Cancer statistics review. Available at: http://seer.cancer.gov/csr/1975_2006/results_merged/sect_15_lung_bronchus.pdf. Accessed July 17, 2009.
43. Boffa DJ, Allen MS, Grab JD, et al. Data from The Society of Thoracic Surgeons General Thoracic Surgery database: the surgical management of primary lung tumors. *J Thorac Cardiovasc Surg.* 2008;135(2):247–254. Epub 2007 Dec 21.
44. Ginsberg RJ, Rubinstein LV. Randomized trial of lobectomy versus limited resection for T1 N0 non-small cell lung cancer. Lung Cancer Study Group. *Ann Thorac Surg.* 1995;60(3):615–622.
45. Koike T, Yamato Y, Yoshiya K, et al. Intentional limited pulmonary resection for peripheral T1 N0 M0 small-sized lung cancer. *J Thorac Cardiovasc Surg.* 2003;125(4): 924–928.
46. El-Sherif A, Gooding WE, Santos R et al. Outcomes of sublobar resection versus lobectomy for stage I non-small cell lung cancer: a 13-year analysis. *Ann Thorac Surg.* 2006;82(2):408–15 (discussion 415–416).
47. Kodama K, Doi O, Higashiyama M., Yokouchi H. Intentional limited resection for selected patients with T1 N0 M0 non-small-cell lung cancer: a single-institution study. *J Thorac Cardiovasc Surg.* 1997;114(3):347–353.
48. Shaw JP, Dembitzer FR, Wisnivesky JP, et al. Video-assisted thoracoscopic lobectomy: state of the art and future directions. *Ann Thorac Surg.* 2008;85(2):S705–S709.
49. Cheng D, Downey RJ, Kernstine K, et al. Video-assisted thoracic surgery in lung cancer resection: A meta-analysis and systematic review of controlled trials. *Innovations.* 2007;2(6):261–292.
50. Atkins BZ, Harpole DH Jr, Mangum JH, et al. Pulmonary segmentectomy by thoracotomy or thoracoscopy: reduced hospital length of stay with a minimally-invasive approach. *Ann Thorac Surg.* 2007;84(4):1107–1112 (discussion 1112–1113).
51. Thomas P, Doddoli C, Yena S, et al. VATS is an adequate oncological operation for stage I non-small cell lung cancer. *Eur J Cardiothorac Surg.* 2002;21(6):1094–1099.
52. Roviaro G, Varoli F, Vergani C, et al. Long-term survival after videothoracoscopic lobectomy for stage I lung cancer. *Chest.* 2004;126(3): 725–732.
53. Solaini L, Prusciano F, Bagioni P, et al. Long-term results of video assisted thoracic surgery lobectomy for stage I non-small cell lung cancer: a single-centre study of 104 cases. *Interact CardioVasc Thorac Surg.* 2004;3(1):57–62.
54. Nicastri DG, Wisnivesky JP, Litle VR, et al. Thoracoscopic lobectomy: report on safety, discharge independence, pain, and chemotherapy tolerance. *J Thorac Cardiovasc Surg.* 2008;135(3):642–647
55. Petersen RP, Pham D, Burfeind WR, et al. Thoracoscopic lobectomy facilitates the delivery of chemotherapy after resection for lung cancer. *Ann Thorac Surg.* 2007;83(4):1245–1249 (discussion 1250).
56. The International Adjuvant Lung Cancer Trial Collaborative Group. Cisplatin-based adjuvant chemotherapy in patients with completely resected non–small-cell lung cancer. *N Engl J Med.* 2004;350:351–360.
57. Pignon JP, Tribodet H, Scagliotti GV, et al. Lung Adjuvant Cisplatin Evaluation (LACE): A pooled analysis of five randomized clinical trials including 4,584 patients. *J Clin Oncol.* 2006;24:366s.
58. Douillard JY, Rosell R, De Lena M, et al. Adjuvant vinorelbine plus cisplatin versus observation in patients with completely resected stage IB-IIIA non-small-cell lung cancer (Adjuvant Navelbine International Trialist Association [ANITA]): a randomised controlled trial. *Lancet Oncol.* 2006;7(9):719–727.
59. Strauss GM, Herndon JE 2nd, Maddaus MA, Adjuvant paclitaxel plus carboplatin compared with observation in stage IB non-small-cell lung cancer: CALGB 9633 with the Cancer and Leukemia Group B, Radiation Therapy Oncology Group, and North Central Cancer Treatment Group Study Groups. *J Clin Oncol.* 2008;26(31):5043–5051. Epub 2008 Sep 22.
60. Felip E, Massuti B, Alonzo JL, et al. A Phase III randomized trial of surgery alone, or preoperative paclitaxel/carboplatin (PC) followed by surgery, or surgery followed by adjuvant PC in early stage NSCLC: NATCH follow-up data. 13th World Conference on Lung Cancer, San Francisco. August 3, 2009.
61. Dillman RO, Herndon J, Seagren SL, Eaton WL Jr, Green MR. Improved survival in stage III non-small-cell lung cancer: seven-year follow-up of cancer and leukemia group B (CALGB) 8433 trial. *J Natl Cancer Inst.*1996;88(17):1210–1215.
62. Sause W, Kolesar P, Taylor S, et al. Final results of phase III trial in regionally advanced unresectable non-small cell lung cancer: Radiation Therapy Oncology Group, Eastern Cooperative Oncology Group, and Southwest Oncology Group. *Chest.* 2000;117:358–364.
63. Furuse K, Fukuoka M, Kawahara M, et al. Phase III study of concurrent versus sequential thoracic radiotherapy in combination with mitomycin, vindesine and cisplatin in patients with unresectable stage III non-small cell lung cancer. *J Clin Oncol.* 1999;17:2692–2699.
64. Curran WJ, Scott CB, Langer CJ, Komaki R, Lee JS, Hauser S, Movsas B, Wasserman T, Sause W, Cox JD, et al. Long-term benefit is observed in a phase III comparison of sequential vs concurrent chemo-radiation for

patients with unresected state III nsclc: RTOG 9410. *Proc Am Soc Clin Oncol.* 2003;22:621 (abstr 2499).

65. Roth JA, Fossella F, Komaki R, et al. A randomized trial comparing perioperative chemotherapy and surgery with surgery alone in resectable stage IIIA non-small-cell lung cancer. *J Natl Cancer Inst.* 1994;86(9):673–680.
66. Rosell R, Gomez-Codina J, Camps C, et al. A randomized trial comparing pre-operative chemotherapy plus surgery with surgery alone in patients with non-small cell lung cancer. *N Engl J Med.* 1994;330(3):153–158.
67. Depierre A, Milleron B, Moro-Sibilot D. Preoperative chemotherapy followed by surgery compared with primary surgery in resectable stage I (except T1N0), II, and IIIa non-small-cell lung cancer. *J Clin Oncol.* 2002;20(1):247–253.
68. Albain, KS, Swann, Rs, Rusch, VR, et al. Phase III study of concurrent chemotherapy and radiotherapy (CT/RT) vs CT/RT followed by surgical resection for stage IIIA (pN2) non-small cell lung cancer (NSCLC): Outcomes update of North American Intergroup 0139 (RTOG 9309) (abstr). *J Clin Oncol.* 2005;23:624s.
69. van Meerbeeck JP, Kramer GW, Van Schil PE. Randomized controlled trial of resection versus radiotherapy after induction chemotherapy in stage IIIA-N2 non-small-cell lung cancer. *J Natl Cancer Inst.* 2007;99(6):442–450
70. Kelly K, Chansky K, Gaspar LE, et al. Phase III trial of maintenance gefitinib or placebo after concurrent chemoradiotherapy and docetaxel consolidation in inoperable stage III non-small-cell lung cancer: SWOG S0023. *J Clin Oncol.* 2008;26(15):2450–2456. Epub 2008 Mar 31.
71. Hanna NH, Neubauer M, Ansari R, et al. Phase III trial of cisplatin (P) plus etoposide (E) plus concurrent chest radiation (XRT) with or without consolidation docetaxel (D) in patients (pts) with inoperable stage III non-small cell lung cancer (NSCLC): HOG LUN 01-24/USO-023. *J Clin Oncol.* 2007;25(suppl 18S):7512.
72. Belani CP, Langer C. First line chemotherapy for NSCLC: an overview of relevant trials. *Lung Cancer.* 2002;38:S13–S19.
73. Non-small cell lung cancer collaborative group. Chemotherapy in non-small cell lung cancer: a meta-analysis using updated data on individual patients from 52 randomized clinical trials. *Br Med J.* 1995;311:899–909.
74. Spiro SG, Rudd RM, Souhami RL et al. Chemotherapy versus supportive care in advanced non-small cell lung cancer: improved survival without detriment to quality of life. *Thorax.* 2004;59(10):828–836.
75. Brown J, Thorpe H, Napp V et al. Assessment of quality of life in the supportive care setting of the big lung trial in non-small-cell lung cancer. *J Clin Oncol.* 2005;23(30):7417–7427.
76. Vokes EE, Vijayakumar S, Bitran JD et al. Role of systemic therapy in advanced non-small cell lung cancer. *Am J Med.* 1990;89:777–786.
77. Stinchcombe TE, Socinski MA. Current treatment for advanced stage non-small cell lung cancer. *Proc Am Thorac Soc.* 2009;6:233–241.
78. Socinski MA, Crowell R, Hensing TE et al. Treatment of non-small cell lung cancer, stage IV. ACCP evidence-based clinical practice guidelines. 2nd ed. *Chest.* 2007;132:277S–289S.
79. Delbaldo C, Michiels S, Syz N, Soria JC, Le Chevalier T. Pignon JP. Benefits of adding a drug to a single-agent or a 2-agent chemotherapy regimen in advanced non-small-cell lung cancer: a meta-analysis. *JAMA.* 2004;292:470–484.
80. Ardizzoni A, Boni L, Tiseo M. Cisplatin- versus carboplatin-based chemotherapy in first-line treatment of advanced non-small-cell lung cancer: an individual patient data meta-analysis. *J Natl Cancer Inst.* 2007;99(11):847–857.
81. Hotta K, Matsuo K, Ueoka H, Kiura K, Tabata M, Tanimoto M. Metaanalysis of randomized clinical trials comparing Cisplatin to Carboplatin in patients with advanced non-small-cell lung cancer. *J Clin Oncol.* 2004;22:3852–3859.
82. Pfister DG, Johnson DH, Azzoli CG, et al: American Society of Clinical Oncology treatment of unresectable of non-small cell lung cancer guideline: Update 2003. *J Clin Oncol.* 2004;22:330–353,
83. Smith IE, O'Brien ME, Talbot DC, et al. Duration of chemotherapy in advanced non-small-cell lung cancer: A randomized trial of three versus six courses of mitomycin, vinblastine, and cisplatin. *J Clin Oncol.* 2001;19:1336–1343.
84. Socinski MA, Schell MJ, Peterman A, et al: Phase III trial comparing a defined duration of therapy versus continuous therapy followed by second-line therapy in advanced-stage IIIB/IV non-small-cell lung cancer. *J Clin Oncol.* 2002;20:1335–1343.
85. von Plessen C, Bergman B, Andresen O, et al: Palliative chemotherapy beyond three courses conveys no survival or consistent quality-of-life benefits in advanced non-small-cell lung cancer. *Br J Cancer.* 2006;95:966–973.
86. Soon YY, Stockler MR, Askie LM, Boyer MJ. Duration of chemotherapy for advanced non–small-cell lung cancer: a systematic review and meta-analysis of randomized trials. *J Clin Oncol.* 2009;27:3277–3283.
87. Fidias PM, Dakhil SR, Lyss AP, et al: Phase III study of immediate compared with delayed docetaxel after front-line therapy with gemcitabine plus carboplatin in advanced non-small-cell lung cancer. *J Clin Oncol.* 2009;27:591–598.
88. Socinski MA. Re-evaluating duration of therapy in advanced non-small-cell lung cancer: is it really duration or is it more about timing and exposure? *J Clin Oncol.* 2009;27:3268–3270,
89. Ciuleanu TE, Brodowicz T, Belani CP, et al: Maintenance pemetrexed plus best supportive care (BSC) versus placebo plus BSC: A phase III study. *J Clin Oncol.* 2008;26(suppl):426s (abstr 8011).
90. Miller VA, O'Connor P, Soh C, Kabbinavar F, for the ATLAS Investigators. A randomized, double-blind, placebo-controlled, phase IIIb trial (ATLAS) comparing bevacizumab (B) therapy with or without erlotinib (E) after completion of chemotherapy with B for first-line treatment of locally advanced, recurrent, or metastatic non-small cell lung cancer (NSCLC). *J Clin Oncol.* 2009;27(suppl):18s; (abstr LBA8002).

91. Cappuzzo F, Ciuleanu T, Stelmakh L, et al. SATURN: A double-blind, randomized, phase III study of maintenance erlotinib versus placebo following nonprogression with first-line platinum-based chemotherapy in patients with advanced NSCLC. *J Clin Oncol.* 2009;27(suppl):15s (abstr 8001).
92. Scagliotti GV, Parikh P, von Pawel J, et al. Phase III study comparing cisplatin plus gemcitabine with cisplatin plus pemetrexed in chemotherapy-naive patients with advanced-stage non–small-cell lung cancer. *J Clin Oncol.* 2008;26:3543–3551.
93. Rusch VD, Klimstra E, Venkatraman P et al. Overexpression of the epidermal growth factor receptor and its ligand transforming growth factor alpha is frequent in resectable non-small cell lung cancer but does not predict tumor progression. *Clin Cancer Res.* 1997;3:515–522.
94. Lynch TJ, Bel DW, Sordella R et al. Activating mutations in the epidermal growth factor receptor underlying responsiveness of non-small cell lung cancer to gefitinib. *N Engl J Med.* 2004;350(21):2129–2139.
95. Jorissen RN, Walker F, Pouliot N, Garrett TP, Ward CW, Burgess AW. Epidermal growth factor receptor: mechanisms of activation and signaling. *Exp Cell Res.* 2003;284:31–53.
96. Paez JG et al. EGFR mutations in lung cancer: correlation with clinical response to gefitinib therapy. *Science.* 2004;304:1497–1500.
97. Dowell JE, Minna JD. EGFR mutations and molecularly targeted therapy: a new era in the treatment of lung cancer. *Nat Clin Pract Oncol.* 2006;3:170–171.
98. Mok T, Wu Y, Thongprasert S et al. Phase III, randomised, open-label, first-line study of gefitinib vs carboplatin/paclitaxel in clinically selected patients with advanced nonsmall-cell lung cancer (IPASS). 33rd ESMO Congress, 2008.
99. Von Pawel J, Park K, Pereira JR, et al. A. Phase III study comparing cisplatin/vinorelbine plus cetuximab versus cisplatin/vinorelbine as first-line treatment for patients with epidermal growth factor (EGFR)-expressing advanced non-small cell lung cancer (NSCLC) (FLEX). *J Clin Oncol ASCO Ann Meeting Proc.* 2006;24(18)(pt I.)(suppl):7109.
100. Folkman J. Tumor angiogenesis: therapeutic implications. *N Engl J Med.* 1971;285:1182–1186.
101. Hanahan D, Folkman J. Patterns and emerging mechanisms of the angiogenic switch during tumorigenesis. *Cell.* 1996;86:353–364.
102. Schiller JH. ASCOSEP: Medical Oncology Self-Evaluation Program. 4th ed. Alexandria, VA: American Society of Clinical Oncology; 2007:126.
103. Sandler A, Gray R, Perry MC, et al. Paclitaxel–carboplatin alone or with bevacizumab for non–small-cell lung cancer. *N Eng J Med.* 2006;355:2542–2550.
104. Manegold C, et al (AVAIL): A Phase III Randomised Study of First-Line Bevacizumab Combined with Cisplatin/Gemcitabine in Patients with Advanced or Recurrent non-squamous, Non-Small-Cell-Lung Cancer. ESMO Meeting 2008.
105. Bunn, PA Jr, Lilenbaum, R. Chemotherapy for elderly patients with advanced non-small-cell lungcancer. *J Natl Cancer Inst.* 2003;95(5):341.
106. Effects of vinorelbine on quality of life and survival of elderly patients with advanced non-small-cell lung cancer. The Elderly Lung Cancer Vinorelbine Italian Study Group. *J Natl Cancer Inst.*1999;91(1):66–72.
107. Gridelli C, Perrone F, Gallo C, et al. Chemotherapy for elderly patients with advanced non-small cell lung cancer: the Multicenter Italian Lung Cancer in the Elderly Study (MILES) phase III randomized study. *J Natl Cancer Inst.* 2003;95:362–372.
108. Frasci G, Lorusso V, Panza N, Comella P, Nicolella G, Bianco A, et al. Gemcitabine plus vinorelbine versus vinorelbine alone in elderly patients with advanced non-small-cell lung cancer. *J Clin Oncol.* 2000;18:2529–2536.
109. Langer CJ, Manola J, Bernardo P, et al. Cisplatin-based therapy for elderly patients with advanced non-small-cell lung cancer: implications of Eastern Cooperative Oncology Group 5592, a randomized trial. *J Natl Cancer Inst.* 2002;94(3):173–181.
110. Lilenbaum RC, Herndon JE 2nd, List MA, et al. Single-agent versus combination chemotherapy in advanced non-small-cell lung cancer: the cancer and leukemia group B (study 9730). *J Clin Oncol.* 2005;23(1):190–196.
111. Shepherd FA, Dancey J, Ramlau R, et al. Prospective randomized trial of docetaxel versus best supportive care in patients with non-small-cell lung cancer previously treated with platinum-based chemotherapy. *J Clin Oncol.* 2000;18:2095–2103.
112. Fossella FV, DeVore R, Kerr RN, et al. Randomized phase III trial of docetaxel versus vinorelbine or ifosfamide in patients with advanced non-small-cell lung cancer previously treated with platinum-containing chemotherapy regimens. The TAX 320 Non-Small Cell Lung Cancer Study Group. *J Clin Oncol.* 2000;18:2354–2362.
113. Chen YM, Shih JF, Perng RP, et al. A randomized trial of different docetaxel schedules in non-small cell lung cancer patients who failed previous platinum-based chemotherapy. *Chest.* 2006;129:1031–1038.
114. Camps C, Massuti B, Jimenez A, et al. Randomized phase III study of 3-weekly versus weekly docetaxel in pretreated advanced non-small-cell lung cancer: a Spanish Lung Cancer Group trial. *Ann Oncol.* 2006;17:467–472
115. Hanna N, Shepherd FA, Fossella FV, et al. Randomized phase III trial of pemetrexed versus docetaxel in patients with non-small-cell lung cancer previously treated with chemotherapy. *J Clin Oncol.* 2004;22:1589–1597.
116. Shepherd FA, Pereira JR, Ciuleanu T, et al. Erlotinib in previously treated non–small-cell lung cancer. *N Eng J Med.* 2005;353:123–132.
117. Zheng Z, Chen T, Li X, Haura E, Sharma A, Bepler G. DNA synthesis and repair genes *RRM1* and *ERCC1* in lung cancer. *N Engl J Med.* 2007;356(8):800–808.
118. Ceppi P, Volante M, Novello S, et al. *ERCC1* and *RRM1* gene expressions but not EGFR are predictive of

shorter survival in advanced non-small-cell lung cancer treated with cisplatin and gemcitabine. *Ann Oncol.* 2006;17(12):1818–1825.
119. Olaussen KA, Dunant A, Fouret P et al. DNA repair by ERCC1 in non-small-cell lung cancer and cisplatin-based adjuvant chemotherapy. *N Engl J Med.* 2006;355(10):983–991.
120. Taron M, Rosell R, Felip E, et al. BRCA1 mRNA expression levels as an indicator of chemoresistance in lung cancer. Hum. Mol. Genet. 2004;13(20):2443–2449.
121. Monzó M, Rosell R, Sánchez JJ, et al. Paclitaxel resistance in non-small-cell lung cancer associated with beta-tubulin gene mutations. *J Clin Oncol.* 1999;17(6):1786–1793.
122. Danenberg PV. Thymidylate synthetase—a target enzyme in cancer chemotherapy. *Biochim Biophys Acta.* 1977;473:73–92.
123. Sigmond J, Backus HHJ, Wouters D et al. Induction of resistance to the multitargeted antifolate Pemetrexed (ALIMTA) in WiDr human colon cancer cells is associated with thymidylate synthase overexpression. *Biochem Pharmacol.* 2003;66(3):431–438.
124. Giovannetti E, Mey V, Nannizzi S et al. Cellular and pharmacogenetics foundation of synergistic interaction of pemetrexed and gemcitabine in human non–small-cell lung cancer cells. *Mol Pharmacol.* 2005;68:110–118.
125. Ceppi P et al. *Cancer.* 2006;107:1589.
126. Socinski MA, Stinchcombe TE: Duration of first-line chemotherapy in advanced non small-cell lung cancer: Less is more in the era of effective subsequent therapies. *J Clin Oncol.* 2007;25:5155–5157.
127. Simon G, Ginsberg RJ, Ruckdeschel JC. Small cell lung cancer. *Chest Surg Clin N Am.* 2001;11:165–188.
128. Simon M, Argiris A, Murren JR. Progress in the therapy of small cell lung cancer. *Crit Rev Oncol Hematol.* 2004;49:119–133.
129. Chute JP, Chen T, Feigal E et al. Twenty years of phase III trials for patients with extensive-stage small cell lung cancer: A Hoosier Oncology Group Study. *J Clin Oncol.* 1995;13:2594–2599.
130. Warde P, Payne D. Does thoracic irradiation improve survival and local control in limited-stage small-cell carcinoma of the lung? A meta-analysis. *J Clin Oncol.* 1992;10(6):890–895.
131. Takada M, Fukuoka M, Kawahara M. Phase III study of concurrent vs. sequential radiation therapy in combination with cisplatin and etoposide for limited-stage small cell lung cancer: Results of the Japan Clinical Oncology Group study 9104. *J Clin Oncol.* 2002;20:3054–3060.
132. Turrisi AT 3rd, Kim K, Blum R, et al. Twice-daily compared with once-daily thoracic radiotherapy in limited small-cell lung cancer treated concurrently with cisplatin and etoposide. *N Engl J Med.* 1999;340(4): 265–271.
133. Evans WK, Shepherd FA, Feld R, et al. VP-16 and cisplatin as first line therapy for small cell lung cancer. *J Clin Oncol.* 1985;3(11):1471–1477.
134. Sundstrom S, Bremnes RM, Kaasa S, et al. Cisplatin and etoposide regimen is superior to cyclophosphamide, epirubicin, and vincristine regimen in small-cell lung cancer: results from a randomized phase III trial with 5 years' follow-up. *J Clin Oncol.* 2002;20(24):4665–4672.
135. Skarlos DV, Samantas E, Kosmidis P, et al. Randomized comparison of etoposide-cisplatin vs. etoposide-carboplatin and irradiation in small-cell lung cancer. A Hellenic Co-operative Oncology Group study. *Ann Oncol.* 1994;5(7):601–607.
136. Noda K, Nishiwaki Y, Kawahara M. Irinotecan plus cisplatin compared with etoposide plus cisplatin for extensive small-cell lung cancer. *N Engl J Med.* 2002;346(2):85–91.
137. Hanna N, Bunn PA Jr, Langer C, et al. Randomized phase III trial comparing irinotecan/cisplatin with etoposide/cisplatin in patients with previously untreated extensive-stage disease small-cell lung cancer. *J Clin Oncol.* 2006;24(13):2038–2043.
138. Lara PN Jr, Natale R, Crowley J, et al. Phase III trial of irinotecan/cisplatin compared with etoposide/cisplatin in extensive-stage small-cell lung cancer: clinical and pharmacogenomic results from SWOG S0124. *J Clin Oncol.* 2009;27(15):2530–2535. Epub 2009 Apr 6.
139. Niell HB, Herndon JE 2nd, Miller AA, et al. Randomized phase III intergroup trial of etoposide and cisplatin with or without paclitaxel and granulocyte colony-stimulating factor in patients with extensive-stage small-cell lung cancer: Cancer and Leukemia Group B Trial 9732. *J Clin Oncol.* 2005;23(16):3752–3759.
140. Schiller JH, Adak S, Cella D, DeVore RF 3rd, Johnson DH. Topotecan versus observation after cisplatin plus etoposide in extensive-stage small-cell lung cancer: E7593—a phase III trial of the Eastern Cooperative Oncology Group. *J Clin Oncol.* 2001;19(8):2114–2122.
141. Klasa R, Murray N, Coldman A. Dose intensity meta-analysis of chemotherapy regimens in small cell carcinoma of the lung. *J Clin Oncol.* 1991;9(3):499–5098.
142. Shepherd FA, Amdemichael E, Evans WK, Chalvardjian P, Hogg-Johnson S Coates R. Paul K Treatment of small cell lung cancer in the elderly. *J Am Geriatr Soc.* 1994;42(1):64–70.
143. Girling DJ. Comparison of oral etoposide and standard intravenous multidrug chemotherapy for small-cell lung cancer: a stopped multicentre randomised trial. Medical Research Council Lung Cancer Working Party. *Lancet.* 1996;348(9027): 563–566.
144. Souhami RL, Spiro SG, Rudd RM, et al. Five-day oral etoposide treatment for advanced small-cell lung cancer: randomized comparison with intravenous chemotherapy. *J Natl Cancer Inst.*1997;89(8):577–580.
145. von Pawel J, Schiller J, Shepherd F, et al. Topotecan versus CAV for the treatment of recurrent small cell lung cancer. *J Clin Oncol.* 1999;17(2):658–667.
146. Inoue M, Miyoshi S, Yasumitsu T et al. Surgical results for small cell lung cancer based on the new TNM staging system. Thoracic surgery study group of Osaka University, Osaka, Japan. *Ann Thorac Surg.* 2000;70:1615–1619.

TABLE 1 Prospective randomized clinical trials involving chemoradiotherapy in the management of esophageal cancer

Study	Study Interval	Patient Number	Histology	Treatment Arms	Radiation Dose	Chemotherapy Agents	Median Survival[a]	Overall Survival	*P*
Definitive radiotherapy vs. definitive chemoradiotherapy									
Herskovic et al. (3)	1986–	123	SCC (88%)	RT	64 Gy/32 fx	PF	9.3	0% (5 yr)	<.0001
(RTOG 8501)	1990		ACA (12%)	CRT → C	50 Gy/25 fx		14.1	27% (5 yr)	
Definitive chemoradiotherapy vs. surgery									
Chui et al. (32)	2000–	80	SCC	S	50–60 Gy	PF		54.5% (2 yr)	.45
(Hong Kong)	2004			CRT				58.3	
Preoperative chemoradiotherapy vs. surgery alone									
Nygaard et al. (21)	1983–	186	SCC	S	35 Gy/20 fx	PB		9 %(3-yr)	.009
(Scandinavia)	1988			C → S	35 Gy/20 fx	PB		3%	(no RT
				RT → S				21%	vs. RT
				CRT → S				17%	arms)
Le Prise et al. (38)	1988–	86	SCC	S	20 Gy/10 fx	PF		14% (3-yr)	.56
(Rennes, France)	1991			CRT → S				19%	
Apinop et al. (39)	1986–	69	SCC	S	40 Gy/20 fx	PF	7.4	10% (5-yr)	.4
(Thailand)	1992			CRT → S			9.7	24%	
Urba et al. (13)	1989–	100	ACA (75%)	S	45 Gy/20 fx	PFV	17.6	16% (3-yr)	.15
(Univ. of Michigan)	1994		SCC (25%)	CRT → S			16.9	30%	
Bosset et al. (14)	1989–	282	SCC	S	37 Gy/20 fx	P	18.6	~26% (5 yr)	.78
(EORTC)	1995			CRT → S			18.6	~26%	
Walsh et al. (6)	1990–	113	ACA	S	40 Gy/15 fx	PF	11	6% (3 yr)	.01
(Dublin, Ireland)	1995			CRT → S			16	32%	
Tepper et al. (4)	1997–	56	ACA (75%)	S	50.4 Gy/28 fx	PF	21	16% (5 yr)	.002
(CALGB 9781)	2000		SCC (25%)	CRT → S			54	39%	
Burmeister et al.(37)	1994–	256	ACA (62%)	S	35 Gy/15 fx	PF	19.3	~25% (5 yr)	.57
(TROG/AGITG)	2000		SCC (38%)	CRT → S			22.2	~25%	
Lee et al. (15)	1999–	101	SCC	S	45.6 Gy/38 fx	PF	27.3	57% (2 yr)	.69
(Seoul, Korea)	2002			CRT → S			28.2	55%	
Preoperative chemoradiotherapy with surgery vs. definitive chemoradiotherapy									
Bedenne et al. (33)	1993–	259	SCC	CRT → S	46 Gy/23 fx	PF	17.7	33.6% (2 yr)	.44
(FFCD 9102)	2000			CRT	66 Gy/33 fx	PF	19.3	39.8%	
Stahl et al. (25)	1992–	172	SCC	C→ CRT→ S	40 Gy/20 fx	PE	16.4	31.3% (2 yr)	NS
(Germany)	2002			C→ CRT	60–65 Gy	PE	14.9	24.4%	
Preoperative chemotherapy vs. preoperative chemoradiotherapy									
Stahl et al. (5)	2000–	119	ACA	C → S	30 Gy/15 fx	PFL	21.1	27.7% (3 yr)	.07
(Germany)	2005			CRT → S			33.1	47.4%	

ACA, adenocarinoma; B, bleomycin; C, chemotherapy; CRT, chemoradiotherapy; E, etoposide; F, 5-fluorouricil; Fx, fractions; L, leucovorin; P, cisplatin; NS, not significant; RT, radiotherapy; SCC, squamous cell carcinoma; S, surgery; V, vinblastine.

[a]months.

improved from 41% to 64% ($P = .003$) with surgery. An important finding from the French trial, FFCD (Federation Francophone de Cancerologie Digestive) 9102, is that on subsequent analysis (33,34) of the 192 patients who did not clinically respond to neoadjuvant CRT (and were thus not randomized), patients who subsequently underwent surgery had equivalent outcome to patients who had clinically responded and were randomized on the trial.

The results of neither of these trials preclude the role of surgical resection among all patients with esophageal cancer who undergo neoadjuvant CRT. But among patients with SCC who clinically respond favorably, observation without resection is reasonable. Such a decision should be made based on multiple factors including age and medical fitness of the patient, thoroughness of clinical restaging after CRT, and dose of radiotherapy delivered. It is noted that in both of these trials, patients randomized to CRT alone received a total radiation dose of 60 to 65 Gy.

Neoadjuvant Chemoradiotherapy

Table 1 provides a detailed review of prospective randomized trials evaluating CRT in the management of locally advanced esophageal cancer. Such trials are dominated primarily by studies comparing neoadjuvant chemoradiotherapy followed by surgery to surgical resection alone. The primary rationale for the use of preoperative therapy is the high local recurrence rates documented among patients undergoing resection alone for advanced disease, particularly among patients for whom tumor-free microscopic margins (R0) cannot be achieved.

The reported rates of local or regional recurrence among resected esophageal cancer patients probably underestimate the true rate of recurrence for a variety of factors. Many clinical trials report data regarding first failure only. In addition, local recurrence is often initially underdetected due to the limitations of CT in discovery of recurrences in the thorax, especially prior to the advent of positron emission tomography (PET). Nevertheless, prospective randomized trials with treatment arms that exclude radiotherapy report locoregional recurrence rates of 17% to 75% (35,36), with most trials rates exceeding 30% to 40% (5,13,31,37). The inclusion of CRT in the preoperative management of esophageal cancer has been associated with a reduction in locoregional recurrence. The results of four randomized trials of neoadjuvant CRT have demonstrated a 40% to 54% relative reduction in the locoregional recurrence rates (5,13,14,37).

An update of RTOG 8911/INT 113, a randomized trial of surgical resection alone or with neoadjuvant chemotherapy (no radiotherapy), reported a strong relationship between completeness of surgical resection and patient overall survival (30). Patients who underwent a complete resection of the tumor had a 3-year overall survival rate of 39%, while patients with microscopic involved margins (R1) or gross-residual disease after surgery (R2) had survival rates of 12% and 4%, respectively ($P < .0001$). Table 2 lists the various changes in resectability rates among patients who underwent neoadjuvant therapy (chemotherapy or chemoradiotherapy) for esophageal cancer. Though inconsistently reported, at least four randomized trials of preoperative CRT show an advantage in resectability compared with initial surgery alone.

Though multiple randomized trials demonstrate improvement in locoregional control and resectability with preoperative CRT, some but not all trials reported improved patient overall survival with neoadjuvant therapy. Limitations of the trials are noted. Though all nine trials listed in Table 1 included concurrent cisplatin-based chemotherapy during radiation, many of the trials employed radiotherapy regimens considered subtherapeutic by current standards (14,21,37,38). In addition, there is disparity between proportion of tumor histologies (SCC vs. ACA) in the trials, statistical limitations due to the study size of the trials (13,21,38,39), and some trials even closed prematurely (4,5,15). Furthermore, the efficacy of therapy may be less identifiable in studies conducted in the 1980s and early 1990s due to less-modern radiotherapy techniques and initial understaging of patients with distant metastases due to imaging limitations compared with today's standards.

Nevertheless, four of these trials support the use of preoperative CRT for patients with esophageal cancer. The CALBG (Cancer and Leukemia Group B) 9781 trial (4) may be the most relevant to current practice as the dose of radiotherapy (50.4 Gy), and the described technique is most consistent with current standards. Also, the majority of patients had ACA, which is common to most oncology practices in the United States currently. Despite premature closure of the study to enrolment (56 out of planned 475 planned), with long-term follow-up there was a

TABLE 2 Pathologic complete response rate and resectability rates in prospective randomized trials of neoadjuvant therapy

Study	Patient number	Histology	Treatment arms	Regimen	Change in resectability	pCR %
Le Prise et al. (38) (Rennes, France)	86	SCC	S CRT → S	20 Gy + PF	15% increase in "easy" tumor removal	13
Urba et al. (13) (Univ. Michigan)	100	ACA (75%) SCC (25%)	S CRT → S	45 Gy + PFV		28
Bosset et al. (14) (EORTC)	282	SCC	S CRT → S	37 Gy + P	12% increase in "curative" resections (*P* = .017)	26
Walsh et al. (6) (Dublin, Ireland)	113	ACA	S CRT → S	40 Gy + PF		25
Tepper et al. (4) (CALGB 9781)	56	ACA (75%) SCC (25%)	S CRT → S	50.4 Gy + PF		40
Burmeister et al.(37) (TROG/AGITG)	256	ACA (62%) SCC (38%)	S CRT → S	35 Gy + PF	21% increase in R0 resections (*P* = .0002)	16
Lee et al. (15) (Seoul, Korea)	101	SCC	S CRT → S	45.6 Gy + PF	12% increase in R0 resections	43
Bedenne et al. (33) (FFCD 9102)	444	SCC	CRT → S CRT	46 Gy + PF 66 Gy + PF		23
Stahl et al. (25) (Germany)	172	SCC	C → CRT→ S C → CRT	40 Gy + PE 60 Gy + PE		35
Stahl et al. (5) (Germany)	119	ACA (EG junction)	C → S CRT → S	30 Gy PLF	No difference in "complete resections"	2 16[a]
Kelsen et al. (31) (INT 113)	440	ACA (55%) SCC (45%)	S C → S	PF	11% reduction in R1 resections (*P* = .001)	3
Boige et al. (11) (FFCD 9703)	224	ACA (esophagus/ stomach)	S C → S	PF	Increase R0 resections (*P* = .04)	
Ancona et al. (36) (Padova, Italy)	94	SCC	S C→	PF	No change in resectability	13
Law et al. (59) (Hong Kong)	147	SCC	S C→ S	PF	32% increase "curative" resections (*P* = .0003)	7
Medical Research Council (35)	802	ACA (66%) SCC (31%)	S C → S	PF	No difference in R0 resections	4

ACA, adenocarinoma; C, chemotherapy; CRT, chemoradiotherapy; F, 5-fluorouricil; L, leucovorin; P, cisplatin; pCR, pathologic complete response; R0, resection with tumor-fee margins; R1, resection with microscopically-involved margins; RT, radiotherapy; S, surgery; SCC, squamous cell carcinoma; V, vinblastine.

[a]*P* = .03.

significant improvement in the 5-year overall survival rate from 16% to 39% (*P* = .002) and an improvement in median survival from 1.8 to 4.5 years.

Walsh et al. (6) reported a similar improvement in overall survival with preoperative CRT in a randomized trial from Ireland. Although the poor results of the surgical-alone arm (3-year survival of 6%) have led some to be uncertain about the conclusions of the study, the 3-year survival rate of the trimodality arm (32%) is consistent with other trials. The initial results of a German trial (5) randomizing patients to neoadjuvant chemotherapy versus CRT showed a strong trend toward improved 3-yr survival with the combined treatment arm (27.7% vs. 47.4%, *P* = .07) in addition to improvement in other endpoints. Finally, the randomized trial of neoadjuvant CRT versus surgery alone from the University of Michigan lends support to the benefit of neoadjuvant CRT (13). Treatment was associated with nearly doubling the 3-year overall survival (16% vs. 30%,

P = .15). Though only a statistical trend in improvement, the study had been designed to detect a rather large improvement in median survival, which it may have had insufficient patients to do.

Acknowledging the individual limitations of many of these trials of neoadjuvant CRT, collective analyses of patient outcome has provided further support for the benefit of this treatment strategy. The largest meta-analysis to date was reported in 2007 from Gebski et al. (7), evaluating the outcome of over 1,200 patients from 10 randomized trial of neoadjuvant CRT. Preoperative CRT was associated with 13% absolute improvement in overall survival at 2 years and a hazard ratio for mortality of 0.81 (P = .002). Significant benefit was found in both SCC and ACA histologies. Two other meta-analyses of neoadjuvant CRT demonstrate a reduction in the 3-year mortality rate with therapy, reporting similar odds ratios of 0.43 (P = .001) (40) and 0.45 (P = .005) (41).

Thus despite disparity in the results and conclusions of individual trials, as a whole the trials support benefit from neoadjuvant CRT among patients who are sufficiently fit to undergo trimodality therapy.

Evaluation of Response

Compared to CT and endoscopic evaluation, the development of CT-PET imaging has dramatically improved not only the initial staging of esophageal cancer but also the assessment of clinical response to therapy. Among patients who undergo neoadjuvant therapy, clinical restaging is primarily important to identify patients who develop early distant metastatic disease and should be excluded from surgery. The gold standard of evaluation of primary tumor response to preoperative therapy is pathologic evaluation of the surgical specimen. Thus, it is unclear to what degree clinical decision making or patient prognosis is influenced by evaluation of response of the primary tumor (by endoscopy, endoscopic ultrasound [EUS], or imaging) prior to resection. Among patients who undergo definitive CRT or for whom completeness of response to initial CRT will influence decisions regarding surgery or observation (e.g., SCC), accurate evaluation of response is crucial.

Among patients who undergo repeat endoscopy with biopsy after neoadjuvant CRT, only between 36% and 45% of patients with negative biopsies are subsequently confirmed to have pathologic complete response (pCR) in the esophagectomy specimen (37,38,42). The accuracy of EUS is only between 29% and 59% in identifying residual tumor in the esophagus, mainly due to challenges in distinguishing residual tumor from necrosis and inflammatory tissue (43).

It should be noted that after neoadjuvant CRT, biopsy and esophagectomy pathologic rates of complete tumor eradication likely *underestimate* the true eradication rate of disease. Most patients undergo clinical restaging and esophagectomy after neoadjuvant CRT within 4 to 8 weeks after treatment completion. Such timing on the whole is premature in assessing completeness of response to therapy as minor amounts detectable residual disease at that time point may not prove viable in time among some patients. The clinical experience with SCC of the anal canal has demonstrated that tumor regression can take months in patients with eventual complete resolution of disease (44,45). Similarly, ACA of the rectum treated with neoadjuvant CRT may continue to respond over an extended period of time (46) and improved tumor downstaging and pathologic complete response rates are associated with longer interval to surgery (47). Computed tomography (CT) has also not proven to be very useful in identifying responders to neoadjuvant therapy, with reported sensitivity and specificity rates of 33% to 55% and 5% to 70%, respectively (48).

Generally, PET or CT-PET has proven more successful in identifying response to neoadjuvant therapy than other imaging techniques (see example in Figure 9.1). Reported sensitivity and specificity rates of PET in identifying major responders range from 47% to 100% and 52% to 100%, respectively (48–52). The broad range of sensitivity and specificity to some degree is related to the strictness in defining a major response to therapy. The best detection rates are with series that define response as <10% viable neoplasm (50,52), while lower rates apply when strictly predicting the complete eradication of disease (pCR) (49).

Not only is PET useful in determining response after completion of neoadjuvant CRT, but also in predicting responders as early as 14 days into treatment (50,53,54). Such early reimaging has not yet found role in routine clinical practice. In addition to predicting tumor response, the relative reduction in tracer uptake at the primary tumor from after neoadjuvant therapy has been shown to strongly correlate with prognosis. Relative reduction in tumor SUV (specific uptake value) from a range of 52% to 80% after neoadjuvant therapy has been shown to correlate with improved patient survival (51,52,55).

who are not eligible for curative attempt due to distant metastasis or who are medically unfit to endure aggressive therapy. Dysphagia is certainly the most common indication, but pain and bleeding are also appropriately palliated with RT.

Palliative radiotherapy alone is associated with lasting improvement in dysphagia in about two-thirds of patients (60). Results of randomized trials of full-dose external beam radiotherapy (50–64 Gy), with or without concurrent chemotherapy have documented improvement in swallowing among 58% to 78% of patients, with little difference in symptom response rate with our without concurrent chemotherapy (3,61).

More moderate doses of RT can also provide long-term palliation of swallowing. A simple regimen of 35 Gy in 14 fractions with concurrent 5-FU achieved a 78% improvement in swallowing grade among 106 patients with esophageal cancer (62). Furthermore, 98% were able to complete the course of therapy and 51% maintained their improved swallowing function until death.

There has been one prospective randomized trial of radiotherapy and esophageal stents in the management of malignant dysphagia (63). A total of 209 patients were randomized to either endoscopic placement of a stent or a single 12 Gy dose of high dose-rate brachytherapy. Stenting provided more instantaneous relief of dysphagia, but the single dose of radiation provided greater long-term relief with fewer complications, particularly late hemorrhage.

■ RADIOTHERAPY TECHNIQUES

It should be emphasized that radiotherapy treatment techniques have significantly improved since the eras in which many of the above trials were conducted. CT-based treatment planning is now standard practice for target and normal tissue localization. Normal organ tolerances to radiotherapy continue to be better defined. Advances in diagnostic imaging, particularly CT-PET, have improved tumor identification. Esophageal tumor movement due to respiration has been both acknowledged and defined. More sophisticated computerized treatment planning allows improved dose delivery and reduction in exposure to normal tissues. Though the benefits of these radiotherapy treatment tools have not been systemically studied, it is anticipated that their employment will lead to improved patient outcomes.

Simulation

To maximize setup reproducibility during treatment, patients are preferably immobilized and simulated in the supine position. Though prone positioning has been reported to displace the esophageal lumen at an average of 1.7 cm anterior from the vertebral column, allowing more distance from the spinal cord (64), periesophageal soft tissue posterior to the esophagus remains fixed to the spine and is part of the clinical target volume (CTV) and thus remains unchanged. Therefore, in the era of three-dimensional (3D) treatment planning, there does not seem to be advantage to prone positioning.

In order to allow for lateral or oblique fields, the arms must be simulated over the head using a wing board or other device to ensure setup reproducibility. When the target volumes will include a portion of the stomach, such as for GEJ tumors, consideration should be given to simulating and treating the patient with an empty stomach to minimize variation in gastric distension.

CT-based simulation and treatment planning is mandatory for accurate tumor identification and calculation of dose to lung, heart, spinal cord, and possibly liver and kidneys. Despite tumor location and extent, the entire thorax must be imaged to allow dose-volume histogram analysis of the entire lungs. Similarly, for lower esophageal tumors, treatment volumes often include upper abdominal lymph nodes as far as the celiac nodes, necessitating the imaging of the entire liver and kidneys. Fluoroscopic simulation may aid in identification of suture lines and staples as well as possibly mucosal extent of disease with use of oral contrast, but in no way should this alone be considered adequate simulation in the absence of CT. Relying on conventional RT treatment planning alone based on two-dimensional (2D) plain films, the appropriate field size can be easily underestimated and has been associated with poor patient outcome compared to CT-based techniques (65).

Both the esophagus and regional lymph nodes can move significantly during respiration, especially distal tumors located near the diaphragm. Fluoroscopic simulation may provide assessment of approximate movement of the esophagus during free breathing. Four-dimensional (4D) CT-simulation, however, provides complete information regarding not only esophageal movement of but nodal tissues as well that are not visible by fluoroscopy. In addition, imaging data sets from 4D simulation can be used in the construction of an internal target volume (ITV).

Target Volumes

Early trials of radiotherapy-specified treatment fields that encompassed the entire esophagus for at least a majority of the treatment course (3,21). Subsequent studies have almost uniformly followed the convention of treating a minimum 5 cm mucosal or crandiocaudad margin and 2 to 3 cm radial margin from the primary tumor to the block edge (4,6,13,14,37,66). More recent studies have described radiotherapy treatment using 3D target volume nomenclature (5,25). Though the use of 3D target volumes (GTV, CTV, ITV, and PTV) is preferred, it should be emphasized that conversion from previous conventions of tumor expansion to block edge is not directly convertible to CTV or PTV delineation. The CTV expansion from the GTV is often asymmetric in the axial plane depending on individual distribution of periesophageal tissue. Furthermore, previous definitions of tumor margin to block edge incorporated beam penumbra that may vary from 5 to 12 mm beyond the PTV depending on beam orientation. The discussion below describes 3D treatment volumes that will at least create similar irradiated volumes compared with the techniques of past trials.

Among patients who have not undergone surgery, the GTV includes the maximal extent of all gross disease, esophageal and nodal, identified by upper gastrointestinal radiography, endoscopy, EUS, CT, MRI, and/or CT-PET. Barium esophagram is of little benefit in planning for most patients as it underestimates the radial and often longitudinal tumor extent. For some patients with early disease, however, mucosal irregularity on esophagram combined with CT may improve confidence in GTV determination. It is crucial that the radiation oncologist review endoscopic and EUS reports while determining the GTV, as the mucosal extent of tumor may be described beyond what is appreciated on any imaging. In addition, the described location of tumor in relationship to incisors can be used to verify there is concordance between imaging and endoscopy. Useful anatomic landmarks for correlation of CT anatomy and endoscopic distance from the incisors include the thoracic inlet at 18 cm, carina at 24 cm, and GEJ at 40 to 42 cm (12). For smaller tumors that are not readily visible with CT, coordination with the endoscopist can facilitate accurate identification of the tumor by placing radio-opaque clips on the tumor.

Whenever possible, CT-PET imaging should be used not only in staging but also in contouring the GTV as well. Relying on CT alone may actually lead to larger target volumes in some patients compared with PET (67). But given the limitations of any imaging modality, the GTV should be defined based on the reasonable maximal extent of disease from combined consideration of all modalities (68). If patients have undergone neoadjuvant chemotherapy with response prior to simulation, the GTV should encompass the full extent of pretreatment disease.

For patients who have not undergone surgery, the CTV includes all areas at risk of harboring microscopic disease. This includes possible direct extension of the primary tumor in to periesophageal tissue and spread to lymph nodes. Radial expansion of the CTV beyond the GTV generally includes the 0.5 to 2 cm of periesophageal soft tissue. Often such tissue is distributed asymmetrically in the posterior mediastinum. It includes but does not extend beyond all the tissue bounded by the anterior spine, aorta, parietal pleura, trachea, and posterior pericardium.

Of special note is the propensity of esophageal carcinomas to spread along submucosal lymphatics. Autopsy series have described skip lesions from 2 to 10 cm from the primary tumor in 13% of patients (69). Thus, greater longitudinal (mucosal) margins compared with radial margins are required in esophageal cancer. When taking into consideration beam penumbra and an approximately 1 cm PTV for patient movement and set error, previous conventions of 5 cm longitudinal margins from the tumor are probably analogous to 3 to 3.5 cm longitudinal expansion beyond the GTV to create the CTV.

The regional lymphatics within the CTV mainly include not only the periesophageal nodes, but also the upper abdominal nodes in lowers esophageal lesions, and the supraclavicular nodes in patient with upper tumors. As the periesophageal nodes lie chiefly within the posterior mediastinum, in the fatty tissue around the esophagus, they are naturally included in the CTV as above described above when contouring periesophageal soft tissue. In the mid-esophagus this will include the subcarinal nodes and in the upper esophagus the paratracheal nodes. Hilar and anterior mediastinal nodes are not generally included. Patients with tumors of the lower esophagus and GEJ are at particular risk of nodal spread to the upper abdomen. In such patients, the CTV should include pericardial nodes and the nodes along the lesser gastric curvature and gastrohepatic ligament. Depending on patient stage and field size, consideration can also be given to extending the CTV to retroperitoneal nodes all the way to the celiac nodes, given the common involvement in this location. Among patients with GEJ cancer who have significant gastric involvement, nodal treatment volumes should include nodes along the greater gastric curvature, suprapancreatic nodes, and splenic hilar nodes.

For patients treated postoperatively, similar principles apply with some caveats. Preoperative staging in addition to operative findings and pathology need all be reviewed for proper definition of the CTV that must include the tumor bed. There may be some inclination to exclude the anastomosis from treatment, as it does lead to extended treatment fields, especially among patients with anastomosis in the neck. Such exclusion should be avoided, as omitting the anastomosis from treatment has been associated with a 29% recurrence rate compared with 0% in one series (70).

Among patients who undergo 4DCT-simulation, an ITV can be constructed to account for target movement in all phases of free respiration. A PTV of 10 mm is appropriate in most patients for whom respiratory movement has been taken into consideration. A smaller margin of 5 to 7 mm may be appropriate for patients undergoing daily image guidance and may particularly reduce lung exposure. Among patients who have not undergone assessment of tumor motion, asymmetric expansion of the PTV should be considered to account for such, especially among patients with lower esophageal and GEJ cancers. Cumulative data from respiratory motion of esophageal tumors has led to the recommendation of incorporating at least 1.5 cm longitudinal and 0.75 cm radial margin within the PTV for patients that have not undergone 4D imaging (71,72). Respiratory movement of upper abdominal lymph nodes can also be substantial and should be taken in to consideration (72).

Dose

As shown in Table 1, a wide range of total doses and fraction size have been used on trials of neoadjuvant CRT. Given concerns regarding late toxicity with fraction sizes greater than 2.0 Gy and possible inferior efficacy of doses less than 40 to 45 Gy, most of the listed RT regimens are not commonly used in the United States. The CALGB 9781 trial (4) probably best reflects a current dose standard among patients undergoing preoperative CRT, 50.4 Gy in 28 fractions. An appropriate dose schedule in most patients is 45 Gy in 1.8 Gy fractions delivered to the CTV, followed by a 5.4 Gy boost in three fractions to the GTV without planned treatment break. Although dose escalation may be possible with modern treatment planning, it is not clear that increased dose would be of benefit or be wise among such patients if subsequent resection is planned.

Among patients who are treated with definitive CRT, there is still lack of consensus regarding optimal dose. RTOG 9405/INT 123 evaluated dose escalation to 64 Gy with a standard dose of 50.4 Gy, both treatment arms with concurrent chemotherapy (66). There was no apparent improvement in local control or survival with increased dose. However, many still question how 50 Gy could be optimal radiotherapy dose to extinguish gross disease, even with concurrent chemotherapy. Subsequent retrospective series have detected improved disease control with doses above 51 Gy (73). In addition, recent prospective randomized trials of definitive CRT in the management of SCC of the esophagus have used doses of 60 to 66 Gy in treatment arms that did not include subsequent surgical resection (25,33). Therefore, in the absence of clinical trial enrolment, total dose of 50 to 60 Gy seems appropriate in the definitive setting when exposure of normal thoracic structures can be kept within acceptable tolerance.

Normal Tissue Constraints

For more detailed discussion regarding the normal tissue constraints with thoracic radiotherapy in general see Chapter 13, "Normal Tissue Toxicity." Below are some selected points of emphasis specific to esophageal cancer.

Particular attention needs to be made to lung exposure from radiation especially among patients who are to undergo subsequent surgery. Large volumes of lung exposure, even to low doses of radiation in the preoperative setting, may increase the risk of postoperative lung complications such as pneumonia and ARDS (adult respiratory distress syndrome). Although V20 (volume of lung receiving 20 Gy or more) had been a traditional benchmark and should be kept to less than 25% to 30 % when possible, excessive V5, V10, and mean lung dose have been shown to be more predictive of lung complication in the postoperative period (74). Reliance on V20 alone with excessive low-dose exposure to the large lung volumes has led to disastrous pulmonary complications in other thoracic malignancies (75). In general, it is advisable to reduce the V5 to less than 50% to 60% when possible, acknowledging there is no absolute level at which exposure is without risk.

Heart exposure is difficult to avoid for tumors of the lower esophagus and GEJ. With modern treatment planning it is generally possible to limit the whole heart to 30 Gy or less and restrict one half of the heart to less than 40 Gy. The left ventricle should be preferentially spared when possible. Spinal cord tolerance should be closely respected, with caution given when exceeding 45 Gy.

Among patients whose fields include the upper abdomen, doses to liver and kidney cannot be overlooked but rarely should be a challenge to restrain exposures within organ tolerances. Mean dose to liver can usually be kept below 20 to 25 Gy and certainly doses should not exceed 30 Gy to greater than 60% of the liver. Traditional limits for kidney exposure are the sparing of two-thirds of one whole kidney or the conglomerate of one entire kidney from doses in excess of 18 Gy. Rarely would such dose limits be challenged even in the treatment of GEJ tumors. In settings where the large majority of one kidney (usually the left) may be exposed beyond kidney tolerance, it is prudent to obtain renal scan to ensure the contralateral kidney has adequate function.

Treatment Planning

In esophageal cancer, 3D treatment planning is crucial given the complexity of treatment targets, the proximity of thoracic and upper abdominal organs, and potential for serious treatment toxicity without proper RT delivery. AP-PA fields expose the least amount of lung to radiation, but often include a significant amount of heart and are limited by spinal cord tolerance when treatment doses exceed 40 to 45 Gy. Oblique fields may avoid spinal cord and reduce cardiac exposure in some orientations but increase lung exposure.

A common field arrangement includes a four-field technique with the majority of dose being delivered from AP and PA fields, using lateral fields to reduce dose to the spinal cord and heart (see Figure 2). Care must be taken to minimize lateral field contribution so that lung tolerances as discussed above are not exceeded. Another common beam orientation is a three-field technique with an AP and two posterior oblique fields with at least one field excluding the spinal cord. Noncoplanar beams such as an anterior-inferior beam for lower lesions may produce dosimetric gain by reducing dose to the heart while sparing lung.

There are a few dosimetric and clinical reports of using intensity-modulated radiotherapy (IMRT) in the treatment of esophageal cancer. In the upper and cervical esophagus, the employment of IMRT is logical given the similarities to head and neck cancer and need for sparing structures such as the spinal cord and salivary glands (76,77). Within the thorax, IMRT must be used cautiously in treating esophageal cancer because of the risk of pneumonitis associated with low-dose exposure to large volumes of the lungs (75). However, with careful treatment planning IMRT may actually reduce meaningful lung exposure. A dosimetric comparison between IMRT and 3D conformal RT at the M.D. Anderson Cancer Center described a 10% median reduction in V10, 5% reduction in V20, and 2.5 Gy reduction in mean lung dose with IMRT (78). Other dosimetric reports have shown improvements in lung and heart parameters with IMRT (79,80). The only large clinical experience of the use of IMRT in the treatment of esophageal cancer is reported from Hsu et al. (81) describing 52 patients treated preoperatively for esophageal cancer. No dosimetric factors were found to correlate with postoperative complications, and no conclusions were made regarding toxicity and efficacy of IMRT.

Side Effects and Complications

Given the extensive disease presentation and impaired nutritional and performance status of many patients, invasiveness of esophagectomy, and rigors of cisplatin-based chemotherapy and thoracic radiotherapy, it is not surprising that combined-modality therapy in this disease is associated with significant toxicity and risk of mortality. Such treatment justifies a multidisciplinary team committed to aggressive supportive care during treatment and experience in patient selection for combined therapy.

Common treatment-related side effects during a course of CRT include severe esophagitis and or

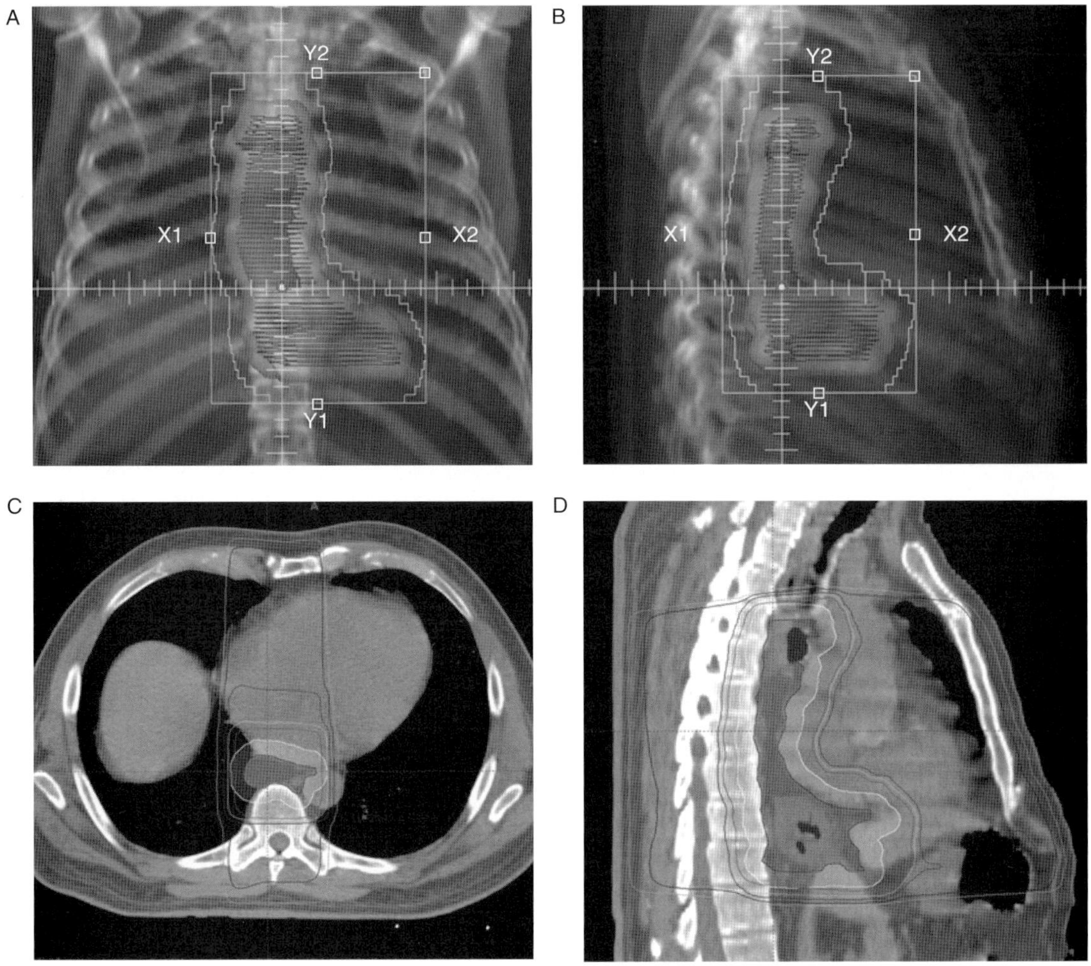

FIGURE 2 Radiation fields and dosimetry of a patient with a cT3N1 ACA of the distal esophagus treated with a four-field technique (AP:PA and laterals). A. AP field. B. Right lateral field. C. Axial dosimetry. D. Sagittal dosimetry.

spasm, gastritis, nausea and vomiting, anorexia, dermatitis, weight loss, and hematological compromise. Patients with moderate to severe nutritional compromise prior to CRT often benefit from placement of a feeding tube prior to initiating therapy. A jejunostomy tube is generally preferred over gastrostomy if surgery with gastric pull-up is anticipated.

Most of the randomized trials of neoadjuvant CRT have assessed whether or not treatment increases postoperative morbidity, hospital stay, or perioperative mortality. The majority of these studies have found no difference in these endpoints (4–6,13,15,37–39). However, the EORTC trial did observe an 8% increase in postoperative deaths (P = .012) with neoadjuvant CRT mainly due to respiratory failure and infection (14). In addition, one meta-analysis reported an increased risk of postoperative death among patients who received preoperative CRT (OR of 2.1, P = .01) (40).

There is little data regarding late toxicity from RT in esophageal cancer mainly because of the limited survival of most patients. The EORTC trial did report no difference in late pulmonary, esophageal, or cardiac toxicity at 2 years among those treated with CRT versus surgery alone (14). However, the lack of data does not imply that such late effects do not exist. Certainly given the aggressiveness of combined modality therapy, residual effects upon survivors would be expected although not yet well described.

■ CONTROVERSIES

Perhaps the greatest controversy in the treatment of advanced esophageal cancer is not the administration of neoadjuvant therapy, rather whether such preoperative treatment should entail chemoradiotherapy or chemotherapy alone. Though RTOG 8911/INT 113 (30,31) and randomized trials from Italy (36) and Hong Kong (59) showed no evidence of benefit of to neoadjuvant cisplatin and 5-FU when compared with surgery alone, three trials from Europe have reported a survival advantage to neoadjuvant chemotherapy followed by resection for esophageal or gastroesophageal cancers. A randomized trial conducted by the Medical Research Council of over 800 patients with esophageal cancer found 5-year overall survival rate improved from 17% to 23% (*P* = .03) with two cycles of neoadjuvant cisplatin and 5-FU compared with surgery alone (35,82). Benefit was seen among patients with both SCC and ACA. Furthermore, two other randomized trials of neoadjuvant therapy for gastric cancer that included GEJ tumors (10) or lower esophageal ACA (11) showed significant improvement in patient overall survival with induction chemotherapy. On the basis of the favorable results of these trials of neoadjuvant chemotherapy, this approach is an accepted treatment strategy (especially among patients with ACA of the distal esophagus and GEJ) as a competing alternative to neoadjuvant chemoradiotherapy (26).

One randomized trial, among patients with GEJ tumors, has been completed comparing neoadjuvant chemotherapy followed by surgery compared to a shorter course of the same chemotherapy, followed by preoperative CRT, and surgery (5) (see Table 1). Though the study was closed prematurely due to slow accrual, the 3-year survival rate favored CRT (27.7% vs. 47.4, *P* = .07). In addition, with neoadjuvant CRT there was a significant increase in pCR rate (15.6% vs. 2.0%, *P* = .03) and tumor-free lymph nodes (64.4% vs. 36.7%, *P* = .01) compared with chemotherapy alone. These differences in patient outcome were observed despite only 30 Gy of radiotherapy delivered on the study (40% less dose than CALGB 9781).

In addition to changes in resectability with neoadjuvant therapy, Table 2 lists the pCR rates from randomized trials of preoperative CRT or preoperative chemotherapy. Note the pCR rates from neoadjuvant CRT trials range from 13% to 43% and are consistently higher than the pCR rates found on neoadjuvant chemotherapy trials where pCR rates are generally less than 10%.

Finally, meta-analyses of neoadjuvant therapies for esophageal cancer favor neoadjuvant CRT over chemotherapy alone. Three-year odds ratios of survival with neoadjuvant CRT have been reported to 0.43 (*P* = .001) (40) and 0.45 (*P* = .005) (41), while trials with neoadjuvant chemotherapy alone have been associated with only a 4% increase in 5-year survival (HR 0.87, *P* = .003) (83). There has been one meta-analysis that evaluated both neoadjuvant chemotherapy (5 trials) and chemoradiotherapy trials (10 trials) (7). Preoperative CRT was associated with a 13% absolute improvement in 2-year survival (HR 0.81, *P* = .002) compared with a 7% survival benefit (HR 0.90, *P* = .05) with chemotherapy alone.

■ ALGORITHM

A simplified algorithm for esophageal cancer is shown in Figure 3. There may be institutional difference in preference regarding the use of neoadjuvant CRT versus chemotherapy alone among patients with advanced disease.

■ FUTURE RESEARCH AND THERAPIES

Given the rich history of clinical trials in esophageal cancer, it is anticipated that the oncology community can look forward to many more efforts to continue to improve outcome in this disease. Active clinical trials continue to define the benefit of neoadjuvant CRT such as FFCD 9901 or the CROSS trial (84). Alternative chemotherapy regimens, particularly those that are taxane based, are being evaluated in hopes of improved patient outcome and tolerance. Biologic agents such as cetuximab are being assessed in conjunction with CRT. In addition, some trials are incorporating the strategy of both neoadjuvant chemotherapy and CRT followed by surgery (5).

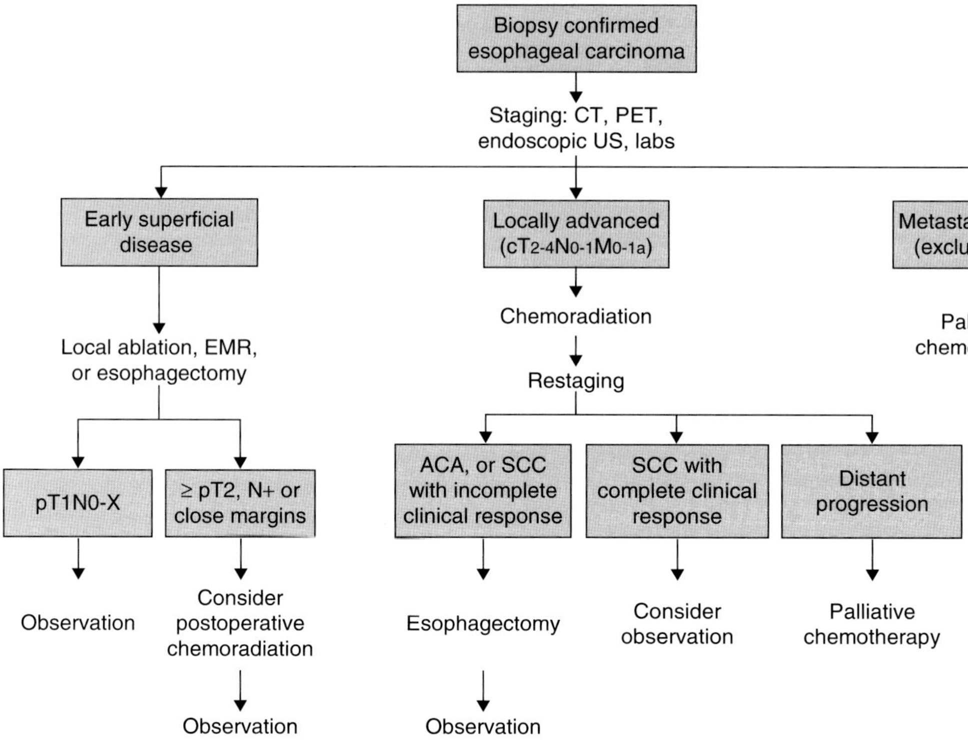

FIGURE 3 Treatment algorithm for esophageal cancer. ACA, adenocarcinoma. SCC, squamous cell carcinoma. EMR, endoscopic mucosal resection.

Further investigation needs to focus on improved methods for detection of complete response to CRT and improved selection of patient for subsequent esophagectomy. Advances in radiotherapy planning and delivery need further study to determine how such tools can improve patient outcome, particularly to reduce morbidity from therapy and possibly to dose escalate.

SUMMARY

Esophageal cancer represents a therapeutic challenge to the radiation and medical oncologist as well as surgeon. The outcome is not universally dismal and has improved with multimodality therapy. The results of multiple randomized trials, as reviewed, have defined the benefit of radiotherapy particularly as definitive or neoadjuvant therapy when combined with concurrent chemotherapy. Multidisciplinary evaluation and cooperation is crucial in the proper selection of patients for aggressive multimodality strategies with curative intent. Further investigation, particularly prospective clinical trials, is imperative to improve the outcome of patients suffering from this disease.

REFERENCES

1. Jemal A, Siegel R, Ward E, et al. Cancer statistics, 2009. *CA Cancer J Clin.* 2009;59(4):225–249.
2. Devesa SS, Blot WJ, Fraumeni JF, Jr. Changing patterns in the incidence of esophageal and gastric carcinoma in the United States. *Cancer.* 1998;83(10):2049–53.
3. Herskovic A, Martz K, al-Sarraf M, et al. Combined chemotherapy and radiotherapy compared with radiotherapy alone in patients with cancer of the esophagus. *N Engl J Med.* 1992;326(24):1593–1598.
4. Tepper J, Krasna MJ, Niedzwiecki D, et al. Phase III trial of trimodality therapy with cisplatin, fluorouracil, radiotherapy, and surgery compared with surgery alone for esophageal cancer: CALGB 9781. *J Clin Oncol.* 2008;26(7):1086–1092.
5. Stahl M, Walz MK, Stuschke M, et al. Phase III comparison of preoperative chemotherapy compared with chemoradiotherapy in patients with locally advanced

adenocarcinoma of the esophagogastric junction. *J Clin Oncol.* 2009;27(6):851–856.

6. Walsh TN, Noonan N, Hollywood D, et al. A comparison of multimodal therapy and surgery for esophageal adenocarcinoma. *N Engl J Med.* 1996;335(7):462–467.
7. Gebski V, Burmeister B, Smithers BM, et al. Survival benefits from neoadjuvant chemoradiotherapy or chemotherapy in oesophageal carcinoma: a meta-analysis. *Lancet Oncol.* 2007;8(3):226–234.
8. Kamangar F, Dores GM, and Anderson WF. Patterns of cancer incidence, mortality, and prevalence across five continents: defining priorities to reduce cancer disparities in different geographic regions of the world. *J Clin Oncol.* 2006;24(14):2137–2150.
9. Blot WJ, Devesa SS, Kneller RW, et al. Rising incidence of adenocarcinoma of the esophagus and gastric cardia. *JAMA.* 1991;265(10):1287–1289.
10. Cunningham D, Allum WH, Stenning SP, et al. Perioperative chemotherapy versus surgery alone for resectable gastroesophageal cancer. *N Engl J Med.* 2006;355(1):11–20.
11. Boige V, Pignon J, Saint-Aubert B, et al. Final results of a randomized trial comparing preoperative 5-fluorouracil (F)/cisplatin (P) to surgery alone in adenocarcinoma of stomach and lower esophagus (ASLE): FNLCC ACCORD07-FFCD 9703 trial. *J Clin Oncol.* 2007;25:4510.
12. *Esophagus.* In: F.L. Green, et al., ed. *AJCC Cancer Staging Handbook.* Philadelphia: Lippincott Raven Publishers;2005:101–109.
13. Urba SG, Orringer MB, Turrisi A, et al. Randomized trial of preoperative chemoradiation versus surgery alone in patients with locoregional esophageal carcinoma. *J Clin Oncol.* 2001;19(2):305–313.
14. Bosset JF, Gignoux M, Triboulet JP, et al. Chemoradiotherapy followed by surgery compared with surgery alone in squamous-cell cancer of the esophagus. *N Engl J Med.* 1997;337(3):161–167.
15. Lee JL, Park SI, Kim SB, et al. A single institutional phase III trial of preoperative chemotherapy with hyperfractionation radiotherapy plus surgery versus surgery alone for resectable esophageal squamous cell carcinoma. *Ann Oncol.* 2004;15(6):947–954.
16. Burmeister B, Smithers B, Fitzgerald L, et al. A randomized phase III trial of preoperative chemoradiation followed by surgery (CR-S) versus surgery alone (S) for localized resectable cancer of the esophagus, #518 in ASCO;2002.
17. Lee PC, Port JL, Paul S, et al. Predictors of long-term survival after resection of esophageal carcinoma with nonregional nodal metastases. *Ann Thorac Surg.* 2009;88(1):186–192 (discussion 192–193).
18. Hofstetter W, Correa AM, Bekele N, et al. Proposed modification of nodal status in AJCC esophageal cancer staging system. *Ann Thorac Surg.* 2007;84(2):365–373 (discussion 374–375).
19. Wang M, Gu XZ, Yin WB, et al. Randomized clinical trial on the combination of preoperative irradiation and surgery in the treatment of esophageal carcinoma: report on 206 patients. *Int J Radiat Oncol Biol Phys.* 1989;16(2);325–327.
20. Gignoux M, Roussel A, Paillot B, et al. The value of preoperative radiotherapy in esophageal cancer: results of a study by the EORTC. *Recent Results Cancer Res.* 1988;110:1–13.
21. Nygaard K, Hagen S, Hansen HS, et al. Pre-operative radiotherapy prolongs survival in operable esophageal carcinoma: a randomized, multicenter study of preoperative radiotherapy and chemotherapy. The second Scandinavian trial in esophageal cancer. *World J Surg.* 1992;16(6):1104–1109 (discussion 1110).
22. Teniere P, Hay JM, Fingerhut A, et al. Postoperative radiation therapy does not increase survival after curative resection for squamous cell carcinoma of the middle and lower esophagus as shown by a multicenter controlled trial. French University Association for Surgical Research. *Surg Gynecol Obstet.* 1991;173(2):123–130.
23. Fok M, Sham JS, Choy D, et al. Postoperative radiotherapy for carcinoma of the esophagus: a prospective, randomized controlled study. *Surgery.* 1993;113(2):138–147.
24. Zieren HU, Muller JM, Jacobi CA, et al. Adjuvant postoperative radiation therapy after curative resection of squamous cell carcinoma of the thoracic esophagus: a prospective randomized study. *World J Surg.* 1995;19(3):444–449.
25. Stahl M, Stuschke M, Lehmann N, et al. Chemoradiation with and without surgery in patients with locally advanced squamous cell carcinoma of the esophagus. *J Clin Oncol.* 2005;23(10):2310–2317.
26. *The NCCN Clinical Practice Guidelines in Oncology. Esophageal Cancer (V.I.2009). National Comprehensive Cancer Network, Inc.* 2009. To view the most recent and complete version of the NCCN Guidelines, go online to NCCN.org. Accessed August 27, 2009.
27. Okawa T, Tanaka M, Kita-Okawa M, et al. Superficial esophageal cancer: multicenter analysis of results of definitive radiation therapy in Japan. *Radiology.* 1995;196(1):271–274.
28. Yamada K, Murakami M, Okamoto Y, et al. Treatment results of chemoradiotherapy for clinical stage I (T1N0M0) esophageal carcinoma. *Int J Radiat Oncol Biol Phys.* 2006;64(4):1106–1111.
29. al-Sarraf M, Martz K, Herskovic A, et al. Progress report of combined chemoradiotherapy versus radiotherapy alone in patients with esophageal cancer: an intergroup study. *J Clin Oncol.* 1997;15(1):277–284.
30. Kelsen DP, Winter KA, Gunderson LL, et al. Long-term results of RTOG trial 8911 (USA Intergroup 113): a random assignment trial comparison of chemotherapy followed by surgery compared with surgery alone for esophageal cancer. *J Clin Oncol.* 2007;25(24):3719–3725.
31. Kelsen DP, Ginsberg R, Pajak TF, et al. Chemotherapy followed by surgery compared with surgery alone for localized esophageal cancer. *N Engl J Med.* 1998; 339(27):1979–1984.

32. Chiu PW, Chan AC, Leung SF, et al. Multicenter prospective randomized trial comparing standard esophagectomy with chemoradiotherapy for treatment of squamous esophageal cancer: early results from the Chinese University Research Group for Esophageal Cancer (CURE). *J Gastrointest Surg.* 2005;9(6):794–802.
33. Bedenne L, Michel P, Bouche O, et al. Chemoradiation followed by surgery compared with chemoradiation alone in squamous cancer of the esophagus: FFCD 9102. *J Clin Oncol.* 2007;25(10):1160–1168.
34. Jouve J, Michel P, Mariette C, et al. Outcome of the nonrandomized patients in the FFCD 9102 trial: Chemoradiation followed by surgery compared with chemoradiation alone in squamous cancer of the esopahgus. *J Clin Oncol.* 2008;26(supp) (abstr 4555).
35. Surgical resection with or without preoperative chemotherapy in oesophageal cancer: a randomised controlled trial. *Lancet.* 2002;359(9319):1727–1733.
36. Ancona E, Ruol A, Santi S, et al. Only pathologic complete response to neoadjuvant chemotherapy improves significantly the long term survival of patients with resectable esophageal squamous cell carcinoma: final report of a randomized, controlled trial of preoperative chemotherapy versus surgery alone. *Cancer.* 2001;91(11):2165–2174.
37. Burmeister BH, Smithers BM, Gebski V, et al. Surgery alone versus chemoradiotherapy followed by surgery for resectable cancer of the oesophagus: a randomised controlled phase III trial. *Lancet Oncol.* 2005;6(9):659–668.
38. Le Prise E, Etienne PL, Meunier B, et al. A randomized study of chemotherapy, radiation therapy, and surgery versus surgery for localized squamous cell carcinoma of the esophagus. *Cancer.* 1994;73(7):1779–1784.
39. Apinop C, Puttisak P, Preecha N. A prospective study of combined therapy in esophageal cancer. *Hepatogastroenterology.* 1994;41(4):391–393.
40. Fiorica F, Di Bona D, Schepis F, et al. Preoperative chemoradiotherapy for oesophageal cancer: a systematic review and meta-analysis. *Gut.* 2004;53(7):925–930.
41. Urschel JD and Vasan H. A meta-analysis of randomized controlled trials that compared neoadjuvant chemoradiation and surgery to surgery alone for resectable esophageal cancer. *Am J Surg.* 2003;185(6):538–543.
42. Bates BA, Detterbeck FC, Bernard SA, et al. Concurrent radiation therapy and chemotherapy followed by esophagectomy for localized esophageal carcinoma. *J Clin Oncol.* 1996;14(1):156–163.
43. Das A, Chak A. Reassessment of patients with esophageal cancer after neoadjuvant therapy. *Endoscopy.* 2006;38(suppl 1), S13–S!7.
44. Cummings BJ, Keane TJ, O'Sullivan B, et al. Epidermoid anal cancer: treatment by radiation alone or by radiation and 5-fluorouracil with and without mitomycin C. *Int J Radiat Oncol Biol Phys.* 1991;21(5):1115–1125.
45. Nigro ND. An evaluation of combined therapy for squamous cell cancer of the anal canal. *Dis Colon Rectum.* 1984;27(12):763–766.
46. Habr-Gama A, de Souza PM, Ribeiro U, Jr., et al. Low rectal cancer: impact of radiation and chemotherapy on surgical treatment. *Dis Colon Rectum.* 1998;41(9):1087–1096.
47. Moore HG, Gittleman AE, Minsky BD, et al. Rate of pathologic complete response with increased interval between preoperative combined modality therapy and rectal cancer resection. *Dis Colon Rectum.* 2004;47(3): 279–286.
48. Westerterp M, van Westreenen HL, Reitsma JB, et al. Esophageal cancer: CT, endoscopic US, and FDG PET for assessment of response to neoadjuvant therapy—systematic review. *Radiology.* 2005;236(3):841–851.
49. Erasmus JJ, Munden RF, Truong MT, et al. Preoperative chemo-radiation-induced ulceration in patients with esophageal cancer: a confounding factor in tumor response assessment in integrated computed tomographic-positron emission tomographic imaging. *J Thorac Oncol.* 2006;1(5):478–486.
50. Kroep JR, Van Groeningen CJ, Cuesta MA, et al. Positron emission tomography using 2-deoxy-2-[18F]-fluoro-D-glucose for response monitoring in locally advanced gastroesophageal cancer; a comparison of different analytical methods. *Mol Imaging Biol.* 2003;5(5):337–346.
51. Flamen P, Van Cutsem E, Lerut A, et al. Positron emission tomography for assessment of the response to induction radiochemotherapy in locally advanced oesophageal cancer. *Ann Oncol.* 2002;13(3):361–368.
52. Brucher BL, Weber W, Bauer M, et al. Neoadjuvant therapy of esophageal squamous cell carcinoma: response evaluation by positron emission tomography. *Ann Surg.* 2001;233(3):300–309.
53. Weber WA, Ott K, Becker K, et al. Prediction of response to preoperative chemotherapy in adenocarcinomas of the esophagogastric junction by metabolic imaging. *J Clin Oncol.* 2001;19(12):3058–3065.
54. Wieder HA, Brucher BL, Zimmermann F, et al. Time course of tumor metabolic activity during chemoradiotherapy of esophageal squamous cell carcinoma and response to treatment. *J Clin Oncol.* 2004;22(5):900–908.
55. Downey RJ, Akhurst T, Ilson D, et al. Whole body 18FDG-PET and the response of esophageal cancer to induction therapy: results of a prospective trial. *J Clin Oncol.* 2003;21(3):428–432.
56. Swisher SG, Maish M, Erasmus JJ, et al. Utility of PET, CT, and EUS to identify pathologic responders in esophageal cancer. *Ann Thorac Surg.* 2004;78(4):1152–1160 (discussion 1152–60).
57. Rice TW, Adelstein DJ, Chidel MA, et al. Benefit of postoperative adjuvant chemoradiotherapy in locoregionally advanced esophageal carcinoma. *J Thorac Cardiovasc Surg.* 2003;126(5):1590–1596.
58. Macdonald JS, Smalley SR, Benedetti J, et al. Chemoradiotherapy after surgery compared with surgery alone for adenocarcinoma of the stomach or gastroesophageal junction. *N Engl J Med.* 2001;345(10):725–730.
59. Law S, Fok M, Chow S, et al. Preoperative chemotherapy versus surgical therapy alone for squamous cell carcinoma of the esophagus: a prospective randomized trial. *J Thorac Cardiovasc Surg.* 1997;114(2):210–217.
60. Wara WM, Mauch PM, Thomas AN, et al. Palliation for carcinoma of the esophagus. *Radiology.* 1976;121(3) (pt.1):717–720.

61. Roussel A, Bleiberg H, Dalesio O, et al. Palliative therapy of inoperable oesophageal carcinoma with radiotherapy and methotrexate: final results of a controlled clinical trial. *Int J Radiat Oncol Biol Phys.* 1989; 16(1):67–72.
62. Harvey JA, Bessell JR, Beller E, et al. Chemoradiation therapy is effective for the palliative treatment of malignant dysphagia. *Dis Esophagus.* 2004;17(3):260–265.
63. Homs MY, Steyerberg EW, Eijkenboom WM, et al. Single-dose brachytherapy versus metal stent placement for the palliation of dysphagia from oesophageal cancer: multicentre randomised trial. *Lancet.* 2004; 364(9444):1497–1504.
64. Corn BW, Coia LR, Chu JC, et al. Significance of prone positioning in planning treatment for esophageal cancer. *Int J Radiat Oncol Biol Phys.* 1991;21(5):1303–1309.
65. Sykes AJ, Burt PA, Slevin NJ, et al. Radical radiotherapy for carcinoma of the oesophagus: an effective alternative to surgery. *Radiother Oncol.* 1998;48(1):15–21.
66. Minsky BD, Pajak TF, Ginsberg RJ, et al. INT 0123 (Radiation Therapy Oncology Group 94–05) phase III trial of combined-modality therapy for esophageal cancer: high-dose versus standard-dose radiation therapy. *J Clin Oncol.* 2002;20(5):1167–1174.
67. Konski A, Doss M, Milestone B, et al. The integration of 18-fluoro-deoxy-glucose positron emission tomography and endoscopic ultrasound in the treatment-planning process for esophageal carcinoma. *Int J Radiat Oncol Biol Phys.* 2005;61(4):1123–1128.
68. Vrieze O, Haustermans K, De Wever W, et al. Is there a role for FGD-PET in radiotherapy planning in esophageal carcinoma? *Radiother Oncol.* 2004;73(3):269–275.
69. Mandard AM, Chasle J, Marnay J, et al. Autopsy findings in 111 cases of esophageal cancer. *Cancer.* 1981; 48(2):329–335.
70. Yu E, Dar R, Rodrigues GB, et al. Is extended volume external beam radiation therapy covering the anastomotic site beneficial in post-esophagectomy high risk patients? *Radiother Oncol.* 2004;73(2):141–148.
71. Yaremko BP, Guerrero TM, McAleer MF, et al. Determination of respiratory motion for distal esophagus cancer using four-dimensional computed tomography. *Int J Radiat Oncol Biol Phys.* 2008;70(1):145–153.
72. Patel AA, Wolfgang JA, Niemierko A, et al. Implications of respiratory motion as measured by four-dimensional computed tomography for radiation treatment planning of esophageal cancer. *Int J Radiat Oncol Biol Phys.* 2009;74(1):290–296.
73. Zhang Z, Liao Z, Jin J, et al. Dose-response relationship in locoregional control for patients with stage II–III esophageal cancer treated with concurrent chemotherapy and radiotherapy. *Int J Radiat Oncol Biol Phys.* 2005;61(3):656–664.
74. Wang SL, Liao Z, Vaporciyan AA, et al. Investigation of clinical and dosimetric factors associated with postoperative pulmonary complications in esophageal cancer patients treated with concurrent chemoradiotherapy followed by surgery. *Int J Radiat Oncol Biol Phys.* 2006; 64(3):692–699.
75. Allen AM, Czerminska M, Janne PA, et al. Fatal pneumonitis associated with intensity-modulated radiation therapy for mesothelioma. *Int J Radiat Oncol Biol Phys.* 2006;65(3):640–645.
76. Fenkell L, Kaminsky I, Breen S, et al. Dosimetric comparison of IMRT vs. 3D conformal radiotherapy in the treatment of cancer of the cervical esophagus. *Radiother Oncol.* 2008;89(3):287–291.
77. Wang SL, Liao Z, Liu H, et al. Intensity-modulated radiation therapy with concurrent chemotherapy for locally advanced cervical and upper thoracic esophageal cancer. *World J Gastroenterol.* 2006;12(34):5501–5508.
78. Chandra A, Guerrero TM, Liu HH, et al. Feasibility of using intensity-modulated radiotherapy to improve lung sparing in treatment planning for distal esophageal cancer. *Radiother Oncol.* 2005;77(3):247–253.
79. Mayo CS, Urie MM, Fitzgerald TJ, et al. Hybrid IMRT for treatment of cancers of the lung and esophagus. *Int J Radiat Oncol Biol Phys.* 2008;71(5):1408–1418.
80. Chen YJ, Liu A, Han C, et al. Helical tomotherapy for radiotherapy in esophageal cancer: a preferred plan with better conformal target coverage and more homogeneous dose distribution. *Med Dosim.* 2007;32(3):166–171.
81. Hsu FM, Lee YC, Lee JM, et al. Association of clinical and dosimetric factors with postoperative pulmonary complications in esophageal cancer patients receiving intensity-modulated radiation therapy and concurrent chemotherapy followed by thoracic esophagectomy. *Ann Surg Oncol.* 2009;16(6):1669–1677.
82. Allum WH, Fogarty PJ, Stenning SP, et al., *Long Term Results of the MRC OEO2 Randomized Trial of Surgery with or Without Preoperative Chemotherapy in Resectable Esophageal Cancer*, in *Gastrointestinal Cancers Symposium*. Orlando: American Society of Clinical Oncology; 2008:74.
83. Thirion PG, Michiels S, Le Maitre A, et al. Individual patient data-based meta-analysis assessing pre-operative chemotherapy in resectable oesophageal carcinoma. *J Clin Oncol.* 2007;25(suppl 1) (abstract 4512).
84. van Heijl M, van Lanschot JJ, Koppert LB, et al. Neoadjuvant chemoradiation followed by surgery versus surgery alone for patients with adenocarcinoma or squamous cell carcinoma of the esophagus (CROSS). *BMC Surg.* 2008;8, 21.

demos MEDICAL

RADIATION MEDICINE ROUNDS

Surgery for Esophageal Cancer

Dawn E. Jaroszewski and JoDee Winter*
Mayo Clinic, Scottsdale, AZ

ABSTRACT

Esophageal Cancer is a highly lethal malignancy that continues to rise in incidence. More than 16,000 new cases are diagnosed each year. Treatment options include chemotherapy as well as radiation and surgical resection. Minimally invasive esophagectomy is rapidly emerging as a surgical alternative to open resections. This approach offers a lower incidence of postoperative pain and pulmonary complications without compromise to pathological or oncologic outcome. Patients may have a shorter length of stay and a quicker return to activity. Esophagectomy continues to play the critical role in the treatment of esophageal cancer. The procedures are well tolerated with low complications at centers with high volume and experience. Long-term function and quality of life for survivors should be equivalent to that of the normal population.

BACKGROUND AND PATHOLOGY

Cancer of the esophagus is a highly lethal malignancy with a rising incidence. There are approximately 16,000 new diagnoses each year (12,900 men 3,500 women). The two most common types are squamous cell carcinoma and adenocarcinoma. The incidence of adenocarcinoma has been increasing steadily with the fastest growth rate of all cancers; while squamous cell has declined overall (1).

Risk factors for squamous cell esophageal cancer have been clearly linked to the African American race as well as tobacco and alcohol use. Squamous cell cancer accounts for more cases worldwide, with a high incidence in China, and the southern republics of the former Soviet Union. Adenocarcinoma is more common in patients who have recurrent reflux resulting in Barrett's esophagus. Other risk factors are obesity, male gender, and Caucasian race (2,3).

Due to the general lack of screening for esophageal cancer, most cases are not discovered until the cancer has progressed to cause symptoms and is locally advanced. Treatment options include chemotherapy, radiation, and surgical resection (4). The standard of care at most large-volume cancer centers includes neoadjuvant chemotherapy and radiation for all cancers with a depth greater than T2 or any evidence of lymph node involvement (5–10).

Evaluation and staging of suspected esophageal cancer includes endoscopic ultrasound (EUS) with fine needle aspiration (FNA), positron emission tomography (PET) scan, computerized tomography (CT), as well as final pathological staging with surgical resection of the primary tumor and lymph node examination (11).

*Corresponding author, Division of Thoracic Surgery, Mayo Clinic, 13400 Shea Blvd., Scottsdale, AZ 85259
E-mail address: winter.jodee@mayo.edu

Radiation Medicine Rounds 1 (2010) 161–172.

DOI: 10.5003/2151-4208.1.1.161

■ PATIENT SELECTION FOR ESOPHAGECTOMY

Surgery remains the mainstay of potentially curative treatment. The definition of patients considered "resectable" can vary from center to center, but generally the definition includes those medically stable for surgery, with the disease confined to the area of the esophagus and local lymph nodes. Locally advanced T4 tumors and stage IV tumors that have shown localized regression of disease or complete PET resolution of distant disease after neoadjuvant therapy can be considered for surgical resection in selected cases. Use of intraoperative radiation and en-bloc resections are occasionally performed in high-volume centers in an effort to salvage these patients.

Advances in perioperative and postoperative care have improved survival following esophageal resections. Perioperative mortality and morbidity have declined from 29% in 1979 (Earlam) to less than 5% in large-volume centers. (3,12–17). Critical to maintaining standards of low morbidity and mortality remains high experience and volume. Multiple studies have shown that centers performing <10 cases per year have prohibitively high morbidity and mortality. In countries such as the Netherlands, facilities performing <10 esophagectomies per year are now prohibited from doing so (18).

Factors independently associated with postoperative complications include induction therapy, diabetes, increased age, and intraoperative blood transfusions (19,20). Pulmonary complications were among the most frequent causes of morbidity among all patients. Postoperative epidural analgesia for better pain control improve pulmonary mechanics and postoperative lung activity (21,22).

Patients often present with a multitude of comorbidites including obesity, significant weight loss, diabetes, coronary and peripheral arterial disease, and many others (12,23). Neoadjuvant therapy may add additional morbidity to an already sick patient population. A thorough preoperative workup is necessary including assessment of pulmonary functions, electrocardiogram, and cardiac stress testing if indicated. Cessation of any tobacco products and stabilized weight with a preoperative serum pre-albumin that is above 10–15 mg/dl (24) is critical. The morbidly obese patient is technically difficult for the surgeon and at increased risk of postoperative complications. However, obesity alone should not be a contraindication to surgery. The majority of patients can safely undergo resection in a high-volume institution specializing in esophageal treatment.

Two contraindications we maintain before proceeding with surgery include active tobacco abuse and significant total body weight loss. Two of the more frequent complications following esophagectomy are pneumonia and pulmonary failure. These complications are associated with significant mortality (16). Respiratory complications account for nearly two-thirds of postesophagectomy mortality (16,25). Patients who develop pneumonia after esophagectomy face a 20% risk of death (16).

Active smoking increases the perioperative risk and can contribute to distal small vessel constriction. This increases the risk of anastomotic leaks and strictures (16,25). Anti-tobacco counseling and aids can be provided. However, if the patient refuses to cease smoking, surgery is not performed. The patient who has lost greater than 10% of his or her usual body weight in 3 to 6 months or >5% in 1 month or has a preoperative serum pre-albumin less than 10 mg/dl (24,26–27) has a documented increased risk of postoperative complications. Laparoscopic jejunal feeding tube placement is performed in the majority of patients with significant dysphagia and weight loss before surgery and often prior to neoadjuvant treatment in order to prevent this wasting syndrome (28–31). Placement of a jejunostomy tube avoids potential injury to the stomach. Catastrophic anastomotic complications and high morbidity/mortality can be avoided with this tactic of regaining patient's nutritional status prior to operating (26,32–35).

The elderly patient is always a concern for undergoing a large operative procedure. Controversy exists concerning the effect of advanced age on outcome of esophagectomy (21,36–38). Memorial Sloan Kettering reviewed their octogenarian esophageal cancer patient population (39). Postoperative death, length of stay, and survival, were significantly worse in this patient population. In a logistic regression model controlling for comorbidites, age older than 80 years was significantly associated with increased perioperative mortality. Because of this risk, the octogenarian patients did not have the same survival benefit from esophagectomy as the younger patients, despite similar rates of tumor stage, postoperative complications, choice of operation, and completeness of resection (38). Other investigators have reported similar outcomes for both elderly and younger patients (21,37). With current advances in surgical management and perioperative care, age should not be a limiting factor as esophagectomy can be safely performed. However, some measure of caution should be used especially in patients 80 years of age and those with significant comorbidities.

■ THE BASICS OF ESOPHAGECTOMY

What to Use for Conduit to Replace the Resected Esophagus?

A viable and functional esophageal conduit is one of the most important factors affecting postoperative outcome and quality of life. Esophageal conduit options are the stomach, colon, and jejunum. Option for replacement use may be limited by previous surgeries and coexisting diseases, especially previous gastric surgery.

Stomach

The stomach is by far the most commonly used conduit to replace the resected esophagus (Figure 1). The submucosal blood supply is based solely on the right gastroepiploic artery after mobilization and rarely has anatomic variants. The stomach is easily mobilized to reach as high as the upper neck and only requires a single anastomosis (Figure 2). Graft necrosis rates are low and the stomach retains its shape and function over time (40–42).

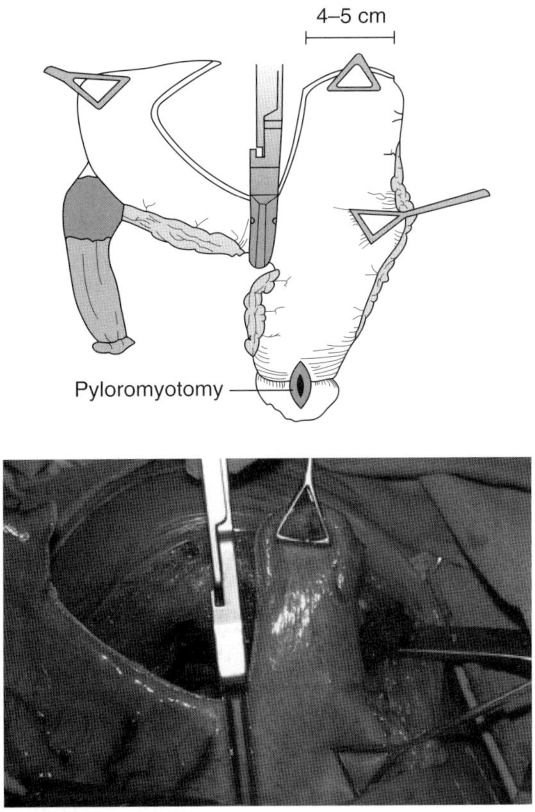

FIGURE 1 The stomach is most commonly used because of its excellent submucosal blood supply and low rate of postoperative complications. An endostapler is used to divide and shape the stomach into a tube.

Colon

When the stomach has a compromised blood supply or has undergone previous resection for ulcer treatment or other causes, jejunum or colon must be used for conduit (Figure 3). The colon can safely replace the esophagus. However, the morbidity and mortality resulting from the use of this type of conduit is relatively high. This includes anastomotic stricture, reflux and a 4% to 10% mortality rate (40,43). Prior to use of the colon for the conduit, a very thorough examination must be made to ensure that there are no unsuspected lesions and the colonic blood supply is adequate. The marginal artery is highly variable and many surgeons will have a CT angiogram prior to completely evaluate the blood supply before surgery. Nutritional status is crucial in this patient population. Both the left and right colon can be used. However, most surgeons prefer the left colon due to the better blood supply, smaller lumen, and easier positioning (40,43).

Jejunum

The Jejunum may also be used as a conduit and is mobilized and used as a Roux-en-Y limb. In contrast to using the colon the jejunum does not require preoperative bowel prep, is easily mobilized, size is comparable to the esophagus and it contains large mesenteric blood vessels. Jejunal graft necrosis rates of 5% to 15% have been reported (40). The location of the blood vessels away from the bowel wall within the mesentary makes long-segment bowel grafting

TABLE 1 Advantages and disadvantages of the intrathoracic anastomosis

Advantages
Mediastinal lymph node dissection
Wide resection of paraesophageal mediastinal tissues
Minimal risk to recurrent laryngeal nerve
Less graft ischemia
Lower leak rate
Less strictures
(45, 46) (12,17,19,21–23,41,43,47–50)
Disadvantages
Thoracic pain. Post operative pulmonary complications
Leaks have higher morbidity
Margins of resection less for proximal esophagus (15,19,23,25,35,37,43,48,51–53)

TABLE 2 Advantages and disadvantages of the cervical anastomosis

Advantages
More complete proximal resection of esophageal tissue
Easier to control and minimize morbidities of leaks
No thoracic pain? Better postoperative pulmonary function
Some also do cervical lymph node dissection
Disadvantages
Damage to recurrent laryngeal nerve
Increased dysphagia and aspiration post operative
Significantly higher leak rates
Most do not do intrathoracic lymph node dissection
Higher rates of anastomotic strictures (14,21,22,49,50,54,55)

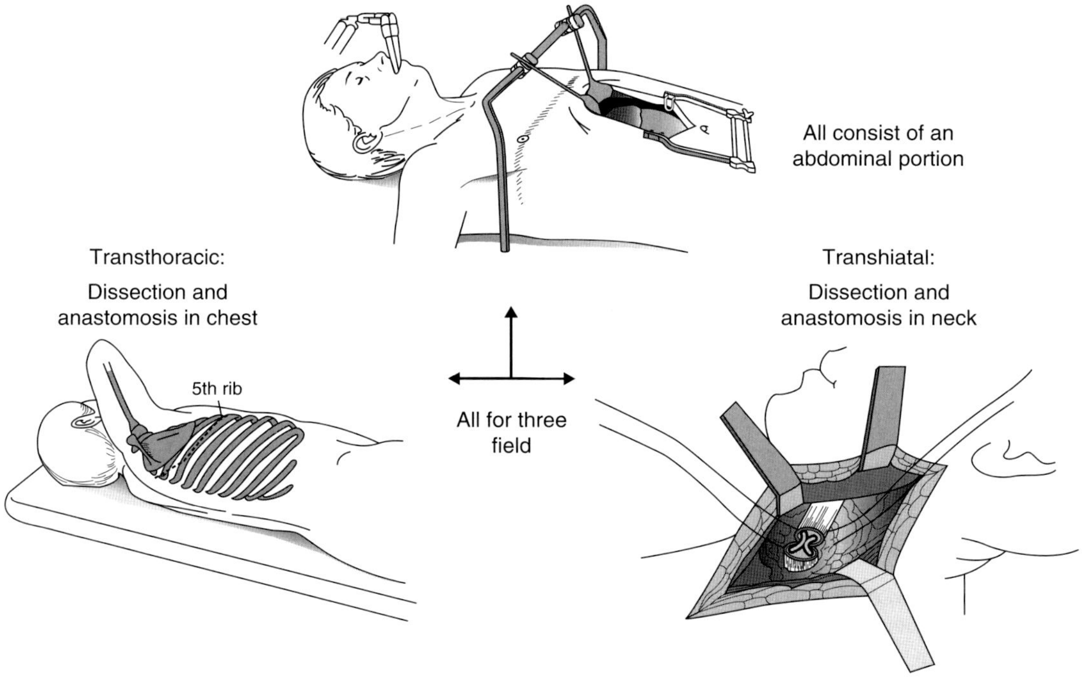

FIGURE 4 The three main types of esophagectomies, transhiatal, transthoracic and three field.

end-to-end, circular stapling and side-to-side linear stapling (Figure 8).

Minimally Invasive Esophagectomy (MIE)

Minimally invasive esophagectomy is rapidly emerging as a surgical alternative to open resections. Over the past decade, MIE has emerged as effective treatment without compromise to pathologic or oncologic outcome (45,51,55–58). MIE offers several potential benefits for patients including a lower incidence of postoperative pain and pulmonary complications, shorter length of stay, and quicker return to activity (4,19,22,45,51,54–63). The learning curve required to perform MIE is steep. High-volume centers with extensive experience in the care of these patients, rather than any specific technique are

A Step 1: Abdominal procedure to assess metastases and create stomach conduit. Can be done either open or with laparoscopy

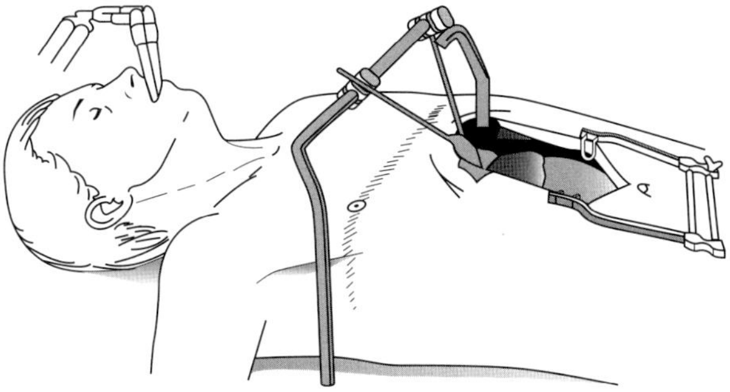

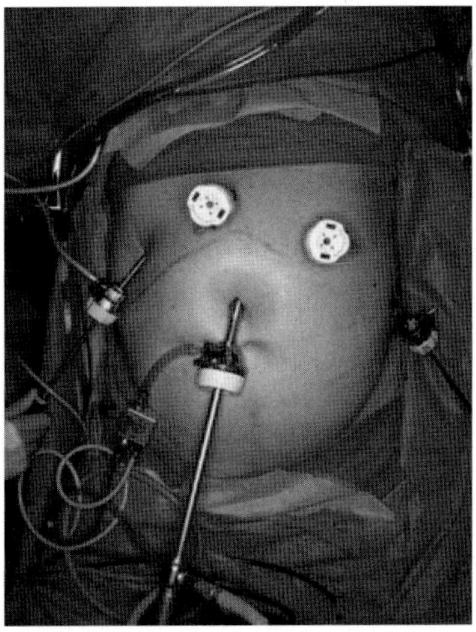

B Step 2: The esophagus is freed through a cervical incision and from below the diaphragm and the specimen brought out through the neck incision.

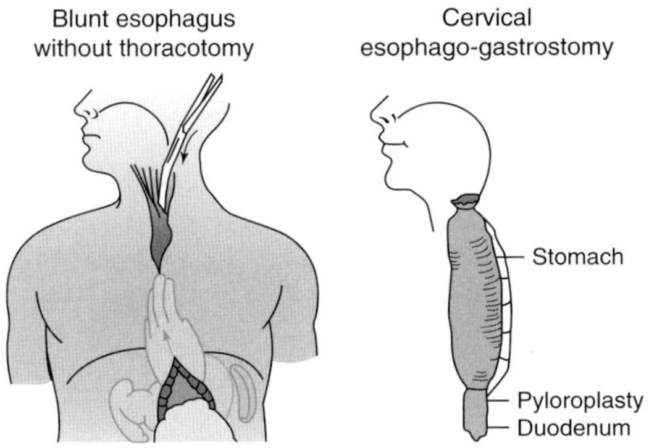

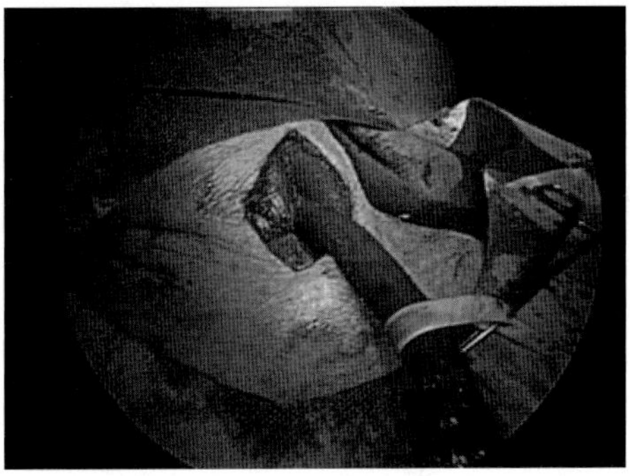

C Step 3: The conduit is anastomosed to the proximal esophagus in the neck. This can be performed hand sewn or with stapling devices

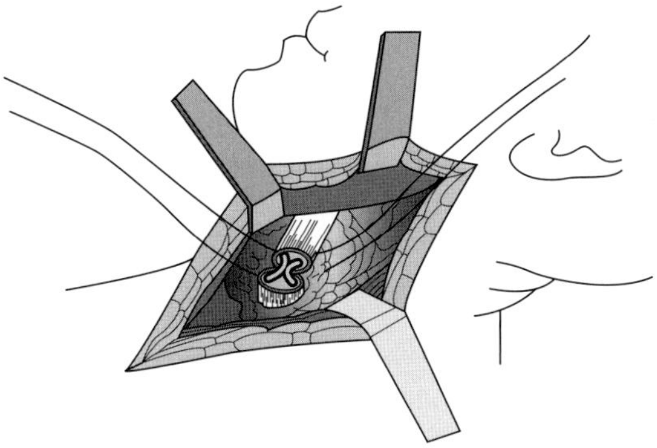

FIGURE 5 Transhiatal Esophagectomy: Steps 1, 2, and 3.

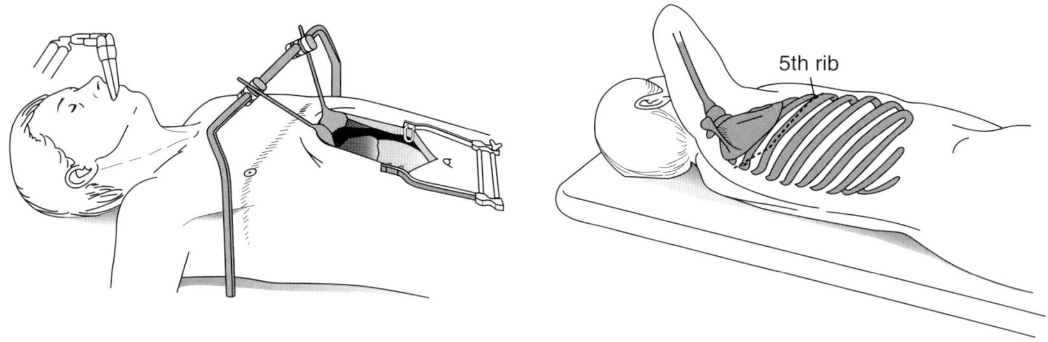

FIGURE 6 Transthoracic Ivor Lewis–open procedure steps 1 and 2.

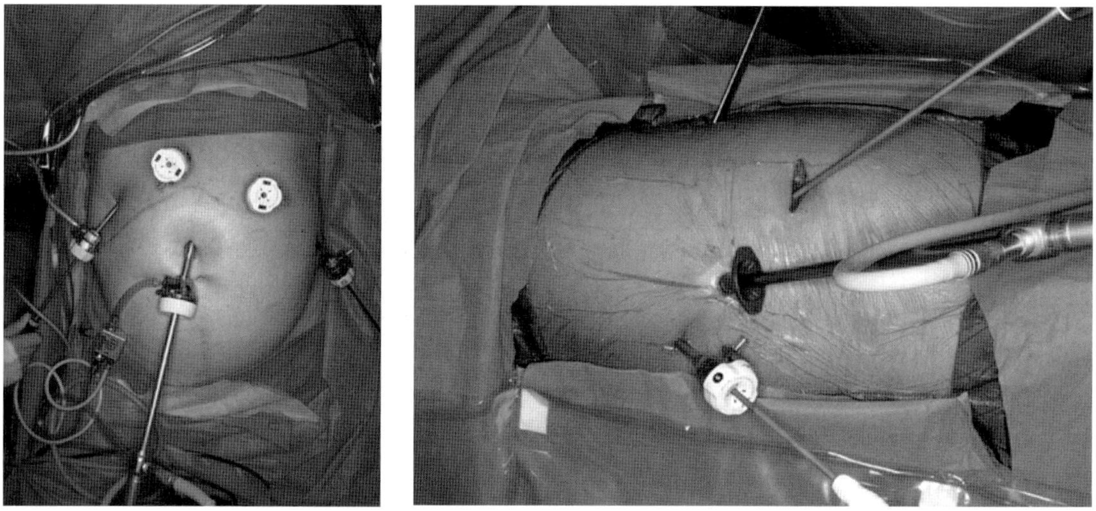

FIGURE 7 Transthoracic Ivor Lewis–minimally invasive steps 1 and 2.

associated with decreased morbidity and mortality. A multi-institution trial is underway to determine the potential advantages of MEI. This trial is being performed by the Eastern Cooperative Oncology Group (ECOG 2202).

The future includes increased options for robotically assisted esophagectomy (Figure 9). Robotically assisted esophagectomy provides a higher accuracy, finer tissue technique, and a wider range of motion than even the laproscopic/thoracoscopic technique. Successful series with excellent results have been published (64,65).

Extent of Lymph Node Dissection

The extent of lymph node dissection occurring at the time of surgery has remained controversial (17,48,51,53,56,66,67). Several published reports have stated that use of three-field lymph node dissection significantly increases long-term survival rates (48,53,66,68). There has been limited acceptance

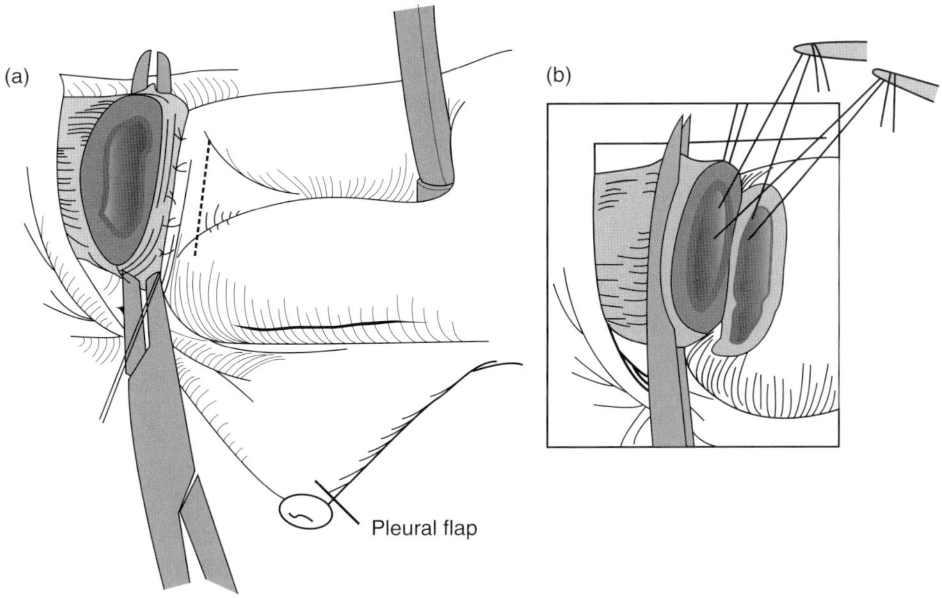

FIGURE 8 Anastomosis of the proximal esophageal stump and the gastric conduit is shown.

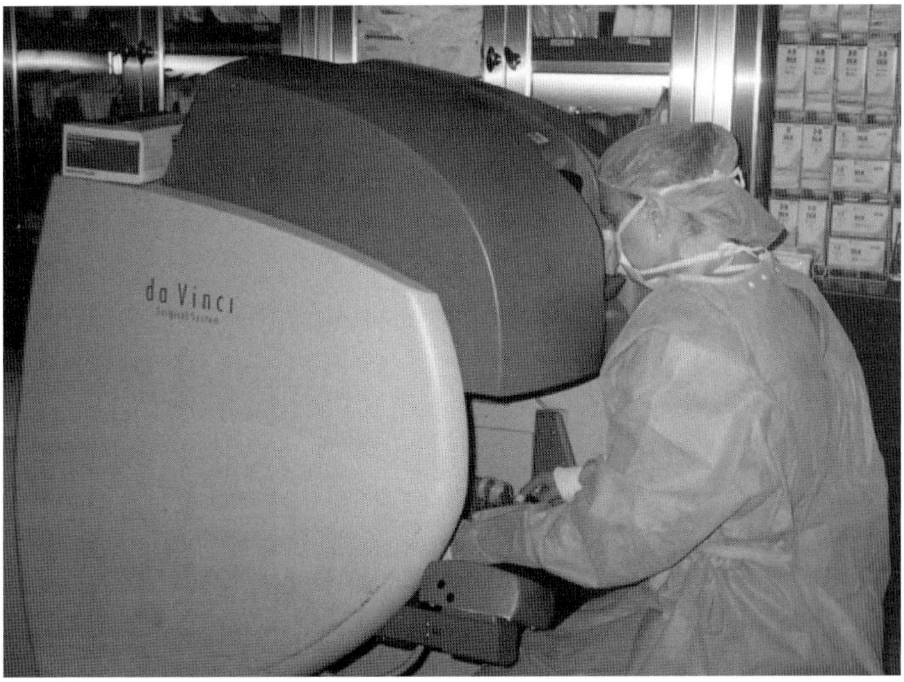

FIGURE 9 The future of esophagectomy includes robotic minimally invasive surgery.

among U.S. oncologic centers that advocate extended en block lymphadenectomy in certain patients (66,69).

RESULTS OF ESOPHAGECTOMY

The optimal approach to esophagectomy remains controversial, however morbidity and mortality continues to improve as experience accrues. Results are clearly superior in hospitals with surgeons performing >15 esophagectomies per year (4,12–14,16,18,20, 21,23,34,36,46,67,70). Pneumonia, atrial fibrillation, anastomoic leaks, and strictures continue to be the most common complications (4,12–14,16,18,20,21, 23,34,36,46,52,67,70).

Quality of life is always the primary concern of patients and physicians alike. Interestingly, dysphagia and overall quality of life are excellent with patient's Standardized Form 36 scores comparable to the U.S. norms following esophagectomy (50,52,56,71–73) (Figure 10).

CONCLUSION

Esophagectomy continues to play a critical role in the treatment of esophageal cancer. The procedures are well tolerated with low complications at centers with high experience and long-term function, and quality of life for the survivors is equivalent to that of the normal population.

REFERENCES

1. Fisichella PM, Patti MG. *Esophageal Cancer.* 2009, Available at: eMedicine Oncology. Accessed July 2009.
2. Livstone EM. *Esophageal Cancer.* 2007, Available at: Merck.com. Accessed July 2009.
3. Chak AFG, Grady WM, et al. Assessment of familiality, obesity and other risk factors for early age of cancer diagnosis in adenocarcinomas of the esophagus and gastoesophageal junction. *Am J Gastro.* 2009;104(8):1913–1921.
4. Collins G, Johnson E, Kroshus T, et al. Experience with minimally invasive esophagectomy. *Surg Endosc.* 2006;20:298–301.
5. Medical Research Council Oesophageal Cancer Working Group. Surgical resection with or without preoperative chemotherapy in oesophageal cancer: a randomised controlled trial. *Lancet.* 2002;359:1727–1733.
6. Burmeister BH, Smithers BM, Gebski V, et al. Surgery alone versus chemoradiotherapy followed by surgery for resectable cancer of the oesophagus: A randomised controlled phase III trial. *Lancer Oncol.* 2005;6:659–668.
7. Greer SE, GP, Sutton JE, et al. Neoadjuvant chemoradiotherapy for esophageal carcinoma: a meta-analysis. *Surgery.* 2005;137:172–177.

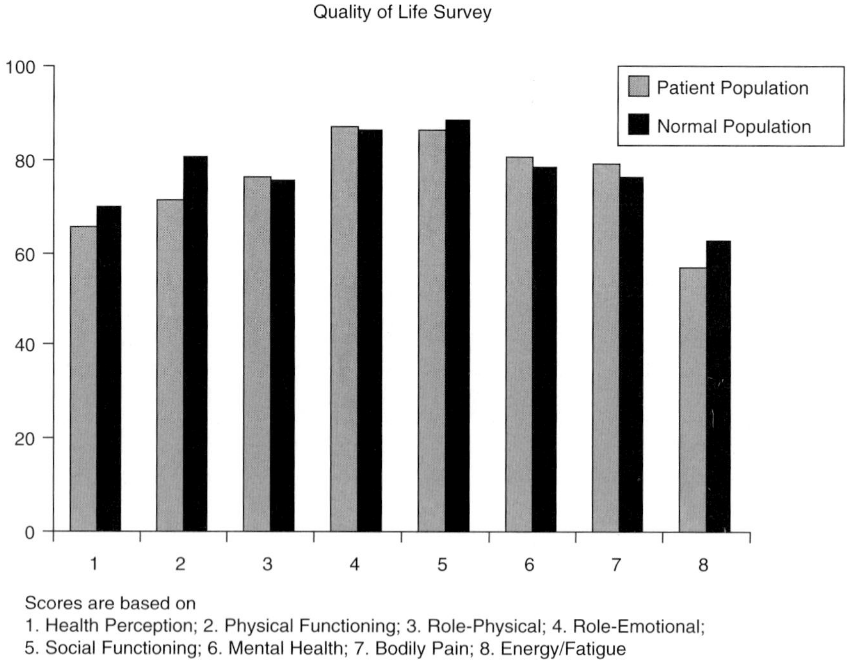

FIGURE 10 Quality of life survey. (From Ref. 73).

8. Graham AJ, Shrive FM, Ghali WA, et al. Defining the optimal treatment of locally advanced esophageal cancer: a systematic review and decision analysis. *Ann Thorac Surg.* 2007;83:1257–1264.
9. Gebski V, Burmeister B, Smithers BM, et al. Survival benefits from neoadjuvant chemoradiotherapy or chemotherapy in oesophageal carcinoma: a meta-analysis. *Lancet Oncol.* 2007;8:226–234.
10. Tepper J, Krasha M, Niedzwiecki D, et al. Phase III trial of trimodality therapy with cisplatin, fluorouracil, radiotherapy, and surgery compared with surgery alone for esophageal cancer: CALGB 9781. *J Clin Oncol.* 2008;26(7):1086–1092.
11. Botet J, Lightdale C, Zarber A, et al. Preoperative staging of esophageal cancer: comparison of endoscopic US and dynamic CT. *Radiology.* 1991;181:419–425.
12. Steyerberg EW, Neville BA, Koppert KW, et al. Surgical mortality in patients with esophageal cancer: development and validation off a simple risk score. *J Clin Oncol.* 2006;24:4277–4284.
13. Swisher SG, Deford L, Merriman KW, et al. Effect of operative volume on morbidity, mortality, and hospital use after esophagectomy for cancer. *J Thorac Cardiovasc Surg.* 2000;119:1126–1132.
14. Whooley BP, Law S, Murthy SC, et al. Analysis of reduced death and complication rates after esophageal resection. *Ann Surg.* 2001;233:338–44.
15. Chu KM, Law SY, Fok M, Wong J. A prospective randomized comparison of transhiatal and transthoracic resection for lower-third esophageal carcinoma, *Am J Surg.* 1997;174:320–324.
16. Atkins BZ, Shah AS, Hutcheson KA, et al. Reducing hospital morbidity and mortality following esophagectomy. *Ann Thorac Surg.* 2004;78:1170–1176.
17. Low DE, Kunz S, Schembre D, et al. Esophagectomy—it's not just about mortality anymore: standardized perioperative clinical pathway improve outcomes in patients with esophageal cancer. *J Gastrointest Surg.* 2007;11:1395–1402.
18. Wouters MW, Krijnen P, LeCessie S, et al. Volume- or outcome-based referral to improve quality of care for esophageal cancer surgery in the Netherlands. *J Surg Oncol.* 2009;99:481–487.
19. Ferguson MK, Reeder LB, Olak J. Mortality after esophagectomy: risk factor analysis. *World J Surg.* 1997;21:599–604.
20. Bailey SH, Bull DA, Harpole DH, et al. Outcomes after esophagectomy: a ten-yearr prospective cohort. *Ann Thorac Surg.* 2003;75:217–222.
21. Ruol A, Portale G, Zaninotto G, et al. Results of esophagectomy for esophageal cancer in elderly patients: Age has little influence on outcome and survival. *J Thorac Cardiovasc Surg.* 2007;133(5):1186–1192.
22. Shulman M, Sandler AN, Bradley JW, Young PS, Brelomer. Post-thoracotomy pain and pulmonary function following epidural and systemic morphine. *Anesthesiology.* 1984;61:569–575.
23. Ra J, Paulson EC, Kucharczuk J, et al. Postoperative mortality after esophagectomy for cancer: development of a preoperative risk prediction model. *Ann Surg Oncol.* 2008;15(6):1577–1584.
24. Gibbs J, Cull W, Henderson W, et. al. Preoperative serum albumin level as a predictor of operative mortality and morbidity. *Arch of Surg.* 1999;134(1):36–42.
25. Dumont P, Wihlm JM, Hentz JG, et al. Respiratory complications after surgical treatment of esophageal cancer: a study of 309 patients according to the type of resection. *Eur J Cardiothorac Surg.* 1995;9:539–543.
26. Bower M, Jones W, Vessesl B. Nutritional management during neoadjuvant therapy for esophageal cancer. *J Surg Oncol.* 2009;100:82–87.
27. Knight CE. Nutrition considerations in esophagectomy patients. *Nutr Clinic Prac.* 2008;23(5):521–528.
28. Han-Geurts IJM, Lim A, Stijnen T, Bonjer HJ, Laparoscopic feeding jejunostomy. *Surg Endosc.* 2005; 19:951–957.
29. Scolapio JS, DeArment J, Hurley DL Roamno M. Prophylactic placement orf gastrostomy feeding tubes before radiotherapy in patients with head and neck cancer: is it worthwhile? *J Clin Gastro.* 2001;33(3): 215–217.
30. Jenkinson AD, Lim J, Agrawal N, Menzies D. Laparoscopic feeding jejunostomy inesophagogastric cancer. *Surg Endosc.* 2007;21:299–302.
31. Schattner M. Enteral nutritional support of the patient with cancer. *J Clin Gastroenterol.* 2003;36(4):297–302.
32. Pedersen H, Hansen HS, Cederqvist C. The prognostic significance of weight loss and its integration in stage grouping of esophageal cancer. *Acta Chir Scand.* 1982;148: 363–366.
33. Bozzetti F, Cozzaglio L, Gavazzi C, et al. Nutritional support in patients with cancer of the esophagus: impact on nutritional status, patient compliance to therapy and survival. *Tumori.* 1998;84:681–686.
34. Conti S, West JP, Fitzpatrick HF. Mortality and morbidity after esophago-gastrectomy for cancerr of the esophagus and cardia. *Am Surg.* 1977;43:92–96.
35. Zheng Y, Li F, Qi B, et al. Application of perioperative immunonutrition for gastrointestinal surgery: a meta-analysis of randomized controlled trials. *Asia Pac J Cliln Nutr.* 2007;16(suppl I):253–257.
36. Internullo E, Moons J, Nafteux P, et al. Outcome after esophagectomy for cancer of the esophagus and GEJ in patients aged over 75 years. *Eur J Cardiothorac Surg.* 2008;33(6):1096–1104.
37. Rice TW, Rusch VW, Apperson-Hansen C, et al. Worldwide esophageal cancer collaboration. *Dis Esophagus.* 2008;22:1–8.
38. Moskovitz AM, Rizk NP, Venkatraman E, et al. Mortality Increases for Octogenarians Undergoing Esophagogastrectomy for Esophageal Cancer. *Ann Thorac Surg.* 2006;82:2031–2036.
39. Moskovitz AM, Rizk NP, Venkatraman E, et al. Mortality increases for octogenarians undergoing esophagogastrectomy for esophageal cancer. *Ann Thorac Surg.* 2006;82:2031–2036.
40. Wormuth JM, Heitmiller RF. Esophageal conduit necrosis. *Thorac Surg Clin.* 2006;16:11–22.

41. Nguyen NTM, Longoria M, Sabio A, et al. Preoperative laparoscopic ligation of the left gastric vessels in preparation for esophagectomy. *Ann Thorac Surg.* 2006;81: 2318–2320.
42. Mitchell JD. Anastomotic leak after esophagectomy. *Thorac Surg Clin.* 2006;16:1–9.
43. Cerfolio RM, Allen MS, Deschamps CD, et al. Esophageal replacement by colon interposition. *Ann Thorac Surg.* 1995;59:1382–1384.
44. Blewett CJ, Miller JD, Young JE, et al. Anastomotic leaks after esophagectomy for esophageal cancer: a comparison of thoracic and cervical anastomoses. *Ann Thorac Cardiovasc Surg.* 2001;7(2):75–78.
45. Braghetto I, Csendes A, Cardemil G, et al. Open transthoracic or transhiatal esophagectomy versus minimally invasive esophagectomy in terms of morbidity, mortality and survival. *Surg Endosc.* 2006;20:1681–1686.
46. Briel JW, Tamhankar AP, Hagan JA, et al. Prevalence and risk factors for ischemia, lead, and stricture of esophageal anastomosis: gastric pull-up versus colong interposition. *J Am Coll Surg.* 2004;198(4):536–541.
47. Heitmiller RF, Jones B. Transient diminished airway protection after transhiatal esophagectomy. *Am J Surg.* 1991;162:442–446.
48. Lerut T, Nafteux P, Moons J, et al. Three-field lymphadenectomy for carcinoma of the esophagus and gastroesophageal junction in 174 R0 resections: impact on staging, disease-free survival and outcome. *Ann Surg.* 2004;240: 962–974.
49. Rentz J, Bull D, Harpole D, et al. Transthoracic versus transhiatal esophagectomy: a prospective study of 945 patients. *J Thorac Cardiovasc Surg.* 2003;125:1114–1120.
50. Moraca RJ, Low DE. Outcomes and health-related quality of life after esophagectomy for high-grade dysplasia and intramucosal cancer. *Arch Surg,* 2006;141:545–551.
51. Bussieres JS. Open or minimally invasive esophagectomy: are the outcomes different? *Curr Opin Anaesthesiol.* 2009; 22:55–60.
52. deBoer AG, van Lanschot JJ, van Sandick JW, et al. Quality of life after transhiatal compared with extended thrasthoracic resection for adenocarcinoma of the esophagus. *J Clin Oncol.* 2004;22:4202–4208.
53. Shimada H, Okazumi S, Shiratori T, et al. Mode of lymphadenectomy and surgical outcome of upper thoracic esophageal squamous cell carcinoma. *J Gastrointest Surg.* 2009;13:619–625.
54. Sanders G, Borie F, Husson E, et al. Minimally invasive transhiatal esophagectomy: lessons learned. *Surg Endosc.* 2007;21:1190–1193.
55. Dapri G, Himpens J, Cadiere GB. Minimally invasive esophagectomy for cancer: laparoscopic transhiatal procedure or thoracoscopy in prone position followed by laparoscopy? *Surg Endosc.* 2008;22:1060–1069.
56. Luketich JD, Alvelo-Rivera M, Buenaventura PO, et al. Minimally invasive esophagectomy: outcomes in 222 patients. *Ann Surg.* 2003;238(4):486–496.
57. Kent MS, Schuchert M, Fernando H, Luketich JD. Minimally invasive esophagectomy: state of the art. *Dis Esophagus.* 2006;19:137–145.
58. Avital S, Zundel N, Szomstein S, Rosenthal R. Laparoscopic transhiatal esophagectomy for esophageal cancer. *Am J Surg.* 2005;190:69–74.
59. Maloney JD, Weigel TL. Minimally invasive esophagectomy for malignant and premalignant diseases of the esopohagus. *Surg Clin N Am.* 2008;88:979–990.
60. Nguyen NTM, Roberts P, Follette DM, et al. Thorascopic and laproscopic esophagectomy for benign and malignant disease: lessons learned from 46 consecutive procedures. *J Am Coll Surg.* 2003;197(6):902–913.
61. Senkowski C, Adams MT, Beck AN, Brower ST. Minimally invasive esophagectomy: early experience and outcomes. *Am Surg.* 2006;72(8):677–683.
62. Bizekis C, Kent MS, Luketich JD, et al. Initial experience with minimally invasive Ivor Lewis Esophagectomy. *Ann Thorac Surg.* 2006;82:402–407.
63. Law SM. Minimally invasive techniques for oesophageal cancer surgery. *Baillieres Best Pract Res Clin Gastroenterol.* 2006;20(5):925–940.
64. Galvani C, Gorodner MV, Moser F, et al. Robotically assisted laproscopic transhiatal esophagectomy. *Surg Endosc.* 2008;22:188–195.
65. Kernstine K. The first series of completely robotic esophagectomies with three-field lymphadenectomy: initial experience. *Surg Endosc.* 2008;22(9):2102.
66. Hagen JA, DeMeester SR, Peters JH, Chandrasoma P, DeMeester TR. Curative resection for esopageal adenocarcinoma: analysis of 100 en bloc esophagectomies. *Ann Surg.* 2001;234:520–530.
67. Chen YJ, Schultheiss TE, Wong JY, Kernstine KH. Impact on the number of resected and involved lymph nodes on esophageal cancer survival. *J Surg Oncol.* 2009;100(2):127–132.
68. Hulsched JB, van Sandick JW, De Boer AG, et al. Extended thransthoracic resection compared with limited transhiateal resection for adenocarcinoma of the esophagus. *N Engl J Med.* 2002;347:1662–1669.
69. Swanson SJ, B.H., Bueno R, et al. Transthoracic esophagectomy with radical mediastinal and abdominal lymph node dissection and cervical esophagogastrostomy for esophageal carcinoma. *Ann Thorac Surg.* 2001;72:1918–24.
70. Blazeby JM, F.J., Donovan J, et al. A prospective longitudinal study examining the quality of life of patients with esophageal carcinoma. *Cancer.* 2000;88:1781–1787.
71. Headrick JR, N.F., Miller DL, et al. High-grade esophageal dysplasia: long-terrm survival and quality of life after esophagectomy. *Ann Thorac Surg.* 2002;73(6): 1697–1702.
72. McLarty AJ, Deschamps C, Trastek VF, et al. Esophageal resection for cancer of the esophagus: long-term function and quality of life. *Ann Thorac Surg.* 1997;63:1568–1572.
73. Martin JT, Federico JA, McKelvey AA, et al. Prevention of delayed gastric emptying after esophagectomy:a single center's experience with botulinum toxin. *Ann Thorac Surg.* 2009;87(6):1713–1714.

demos MEDICAL

RADIATION MEDICINE ROUNDS

Systemic Therapy for Esophageal Cancer

Kelly K. Curtis* and Helen J. Ross
Mayo Clinic, Scottsdale, AZ

■ ABSTRACT

Pathology and Natural History: Until recently in the United States, a cancer of squamous cell histology was most often seen after years of tobacco and alcohol use. However, adenocarcinomas of the distal esophagus and gastroesophageal junction are increasing in incidence especially among caucasians.

The mucosal layer of the esophagus contains abundant lymphatics, allowing esophageal malignancies easy access to lymph channels for local and distant spread. Thus, most patients with esophageal cancer present with locally advanced or metastatic disease. Due to its proclivity for lymphatic spread, a majority of patients have occult micrometastatic disease at presentation. Squamous cell carcinomas of the esophagus invade lymphatics in the lamina propria early in their development, spreading to cervical and superior mediastinal lymph nodes (if in the upper third of the esophagus), or paratracheal/hilar/subcarinal, periesophageal, and pericardial lymph nodes (if in the middle third). Celiac node metastases can represent regional disease for lower esophageal and gastroesophageal junction tumors. Distant sites of spread commonly include lung, liver, and bone.

The histology of esophageal cancer appears to affect patterns of recurrence, with squamous cell carcinomas more likely to recur locally and adenocarcinomas more likely to recur distantly. Combined modality treatment strategies employing surgery, chemotherapy, and radiation may reduce local recurrence rates, but may result in increased rates of distant relapse as patients live long enough for systemic micrometastases to develop into measurable disease.

Therapy: Multiple combination chemotherapy regimens show activity against metastatic esophageal cancer. Few trials have compared combination regimens and no regimen is clearly superior to another. In general, combination chemotherapy regimens produce response rates of 30% to 40%, and median overall survivals of 8 to 12 months. Most regimens incorporate a fluoropyrimidine, such as 5-fluorouracil, with a platinum, such as cisplatin. Newer regimens and ongoing clinical trials incorporate targeted agents against the epidermal growth factor receptor and vascular endothelial growth factor, and third-generation chemotherapy agent such as taxanes. Second-line therapy options for patients with metastatic esophageal cancer are few, with low-response rates.

Patients with unresectable esophageal cancer may be treated with definitive chemoradiotherapy. Cisplatin is given on day 1 and day 29 and 5-fluorouracil via 96-hour continuous IV infusion given on days 1 to 4 and days 29 to 33 with radiation (50.4 Gy in 2 Gy per day fractions), followed by two cycles of the same drugs every 3 weeks

*Corresponding author, Division of Hematology and Oncology, Mayo Clinic, 13400 E. Shea Blvd., Scottsdale, AZ 85259
E-mail address: curtis.kelly1@mayo.edu

Radiation Medicine Rounds 1 (2010) 173–210.

DOI:10.5003/2151–4208.1.1.173

demosmedpub.com/rmr

after radiation. This regimen has become one standard of care for this patient population, on the basis of results from the Radiation Therapy Oncology Group 85–01 trial. No recent trials of definitive chemotherapy are available demonstrating superiority for this regimen.

Trimodality therapy with chemotherapy and radiation prior to surgery (neoadjuvant therapy) is currently the most recommended treatment approach for patients with locally advanced, resectable esophageal cancer. Two meta-analyses of trials of neoadjuvant chemoradiotherapy and surgery versus surgery alone found a significant improvement in long-term survival with neoadjuvant chemoradiotherapy followed by surgery. Cisplatin and 5-fluorouracil are the most studied drugs with radiation.

Several studies have investigated induction chemotherapy prior to chemoradiotherapy and surgery, but in the absence of trials comparing induction chemotherapy plus neoadjuvant chemoradiotherapy followed by surgery to neoadjuvant chemoradiotherapy followed by surgery (without induction chemotherapy), this strategy remains investigational, and probably should be employed only in the context of a clinical trial. Published trials of induction chemotherapy show results comparable to, but no better than, conventional neoadjuvant chemoradiotherapy followed by surgery.

Gastroesophageal (GE) junction adenocarcinoma managemet is controversial with some authors suggesting it be treated as esophageal cancer or others as gastric cancer. For patients with locally advanced adenocarcinoma of the distal esophagus and stomach, induction chemotherapy prior to surgery is an acceptable treatment approach based on results from the United Kingdom Medical Research Council Adjuvant Gastric Infusional Chemotherapy (MAGIC) trial that included both gastric and gastroesophageal junction cancers, and in which induction chemotherapy with epirubicin, cisplatin and infusional 5-fluorouracil significantly improved 5-year survival compared with surgery alone.

Algorithm: An algorithm for esophageal cancer treatment is presented in Chapter 9, "Radiotherapy for Esophageal Cancer."

■ INTRODUCTION

There has been an alarming increase in the number of new esophageal cancer cases. Once a condition seen mainly in men with exposure to tobacco and alcohol and typically of squamous cell histology, esophageal adenocarcinoma is increasingly common among caucasians. Indeed, esophageal adenocarcinoma increased at the greatest rate of any malignancy in the United States over the past 25 years (1).The reasons for this dramatic increase are not well understood. The reasons for this shift remain unclear, but may relate to increasing obesity resulting in more GI reflux which predisposes to Barrett's esophagus, a precursor lesion.

This chapter will provide an overview of systemic therapy for locally advanced and metastatic esophageal cancer. A review of esophageal cancer epidemiology, natural history, and pathology will be provided.

■ EPIDEMIOLOGY

The annual incidence of esophageal cancer in the United States has increased from an estimated 12,300 cases in 2000 to 16,470 in 2008 (2,3). This diagnosis is a death sentence for the majority of patients, resulting in an estimated 14,280 deaths in the United States in 2008 (3). Five-year survival rates have improved over the last 50 years from 4% in 1950–1954 to 17.5% from 1996 to 2003, but more than 80% of patients will still die within 5 years of diagnosis (4). Esophageal cancer is now the sixth most common cause of cancer-related death in the world (5).

The major histologic subtypes of esophageal cancer are squamous cell carcinoma and adenocarcinoma which account for 93% of esophageal cancer cases. Although squamous cell carcinoma of the esophagus continues to occur, adenocarcinomas are now more commonly diagnosed in the Western world (6,7). This shift likely occurred sometime in the 1990s, with esophageal adenocarcinoma comprising approximately half of all esophageal cancer cases by 1990 (7,8). The overall incidence of squamous cell carcinoma of the esophagus has decreased by 50% since the 1970s (9). However, a trend of increasing esophageal adenocarcinoma cases among caucasians has been observed.

Along with the change in histology, a change has been noted in the most common anatomic location at which esophageal cancer arises. Unlike squamous cell carcinoma of the esophagus, which arises in the midesophagus in 75% of cases, 94% of esophageal adenocarcinomas affect the distal esophagus, including the gastroesophageal junction, now making esophageal carcinoma primarily a disease of the distal esophagus and gastroesophageal (GE) junction (6,10,11).

Racial disparities in incidence, histology, and survival of esophageal cancer have been well documented. For example, in 2002, African American males living in the District of Columbia in the United States had the fifth highest incidence of esophageal cancer in the world (149 cases per 100,000 population). African American females in Connecticut had the 14th highest incidence of esophageal cancer in the world (36 cases per 100,000 population) (6). The age-adjusted incidence of esophageal cancer is approximately twofold higher for African Americans compared with whites with age-adjusted mortality rate also twice that of whites (12). Squamous cell carcinoma remains the most common esophageal cancer histology in African Americans, with adenocarcinoma incidence in African Americans 30% the rate of whites (10,12,13). African Americans also appear to have a lower 5-year survival rate stage-for-stage compared to whites, with a 20% 5-year survival for localized lesions (compared with 36% for whites), and 11% 5-year survival for locally advanced cancers (compared with 18% for whites) (6). African Americans with metastatic disease appear to have comparable survival to whites (6).

As with disparities in race, sex also appears to impact incidence and histology of esophageal cancer. The discrepancies in sex, as it relates to esophageal cancer, are illustrated by the incidence of esophageal adenocarcinoma of the gastroesophageal junction in men, which outnumbered that in women 5:1 in a study of patients in Connecticut over a 20-year study period ending in 1989 (10). Furthermore, females still are more likely to be diagnosed with squamous cell carcinoma of the esophagus than men, although the incidence of esophageal adenocarcinoma in women is increasing, as noted previously (9,12). While the incidence of esophageal cancer in white men has increased, the incidence of esophageal cancer in women held steady (9). This constant rate is due mainly to the decrease in squamous cell carcinoma of the esophagus that was replaced by the increase in esophageal adenocarcinoma in women (9). Although 5-year survival does not appear to differ between men and women (6% vs. 7% for African American males and females, respectively and 11% vs. 12% for white males and females, respectively), mortality rates are higher for men than women (12).

In summary, esophageal cancer is a disease in evolution. The overall incidence of esophageal cancer is increasing, and survival has improved only slightly over the past 50 years. Adenocarcinoma of the esophagus is now more common than squamous cell carcinoma. Squamous cell carcinoma of the esophagus continues to affect predominantly African Americans and women, whereas esophageal adenocarcinoma (especially of the gastroesophageal junction) has become increasingly common in caucasians. African Americans have lower survival rates from esophageal cancer than whites. The reasons for these patterns are not fully understood.

■ ANATOMY, PATHOLOGY, AND NATURAL HISTORY

The esophagus is a 25 to 30 cm-long portion of the alimentary canal. It extends from the cricopharyngeus muscle at the level of the sixth cervical vertebra through the esophageal hiatus at the level of the tenth thoracic vertebra to the gastroesophageal junction. It is typically divided into thirds for descriptive purposes—the upper third comprising the portion of the esophagus extending from the thoracic inlet to the level of the carina, the middle third extending from the carina to the inferior pulmonary veins, and the distal third comprising the remainder of the organ to the gastroesophageal junction (14). It is comprised of a mucosal layer lined by nonkeratinized squamous epithelium, overlaid by lamina propria containing lymphatics and the muscularis mucosa, submucosa, muscularis externa, and adventitia. As mentioned previously, squamous cell carcinoma is found typically in the upper two-thirds of the esophagus (60% in the middle third, 30% in the upper third, and 10% in the distal third) (15,16), and adenocarcinoma arises predominantly in the distal third (17,18).

Esophageal squamous cell carcinoma invades lymphatics in the lamina propria early, spreading to cervical and superior mediastinal lymph nodes (if in the upper third of the esophagus), or paratracheal/hilar/subcarinal, periesophageal, and pericardial lymph nodes (if in the middle third) (14). Fistula formation may result from invasion of local structures, such as a tracheoesophageal fistula, or erosion into the aorta with massive hemorrhage. Distant sites of spread include lung, liver, and bone.

TABLE 2 Tumor suppressor genes associated with esophageal adenocarcinoma

Tumor Suppressor Gene	Chromosome Location	Event	Function
FHIT	3p14	Gene deletion	Unknown, but frequently found deleted in many carcinogen-related cancers
VHL	3p25-26	Loss of heterozygosity	Targets HIF1a for degradation, thereby decreasing angiogenesis.
PPARγ	3p25-26	Loss of heterozygosity	Unknown in esophageal cancer; may regulate cell growth and differentiation.
APC	5q21	Loss of heterozygosity and/or promoter hypermethylation	Targets beta catenin for degradation, thereby decreasing transcription of cell proliferation genes.
P16	9p21	Loss of heterozygosity and/or gene deletion	Inhibits cyclin dependent kinases 4 and 6, preventing cells from progressing from G1 to S phases.
Rb	13q14	Gene deletion	Inhibits E2F family transcription factors necessary for cells to progress from G1 to S phases; may regulate apoptotic pathways.
P53	17p	Loss of heterozygosity	Arrests cells prior to S phase; induces apoptosis of cells with irreparable DNA damage.
SMAD4 and *DCC*	18q	Loss of heterozygosity	Arrest cell proliferation and migration.

APC, Adenomatosis Polyposis Coli; DCC, deleted in colorectal carcinoma; FHIT, Fragile Histidine Triad; HIF1a, hypoxia inducible factor; PPARγ, peroxisome proliferator-activator receptor; Rb, Retinoblastoma; VHL, von Hippel Lindau.

The list of genes and proteins involved in esophageal adenocarcinoma development and progression can be duplicated for squamous cell carcinoma (14,92,93). Among proto-oncogenes, *EGFR*, *c-erbB2*, *myc*, and *ras*-family oncogenes are known to be associated with development of squamous cell carcinoma of the esophagus (94–99). *p53*, *p16*, *Rb*, *PPARγ*, *APC* and the tylosis esophageal cancer (TOC) gene are tumor suppressor genes known to be mutated and/or inactivated in esophageal squamous cell carcinoma (100–111). Fas-receptor, survivin, and bcl-2 family proteins involved in apoptosis are known to be dysregulated in this form of esophageal cancer (112–116). Cyclin D1 amplification has been found in many studies of esophageal squamous cell carcinoma tumor samples (93,105,117–119). Thus, it appears that adenocarcinomas and squamous cell carcinomas both arise because of similar disruptions in the cellular machinery. These similarities may have important implications as new therapies are developed. If each form of esophageal cancer has the same or similarly aberrant pathways, drugs targeting these pathways might successfully treat either.

■ RISK FACTORS

There are several well-established risk factors for esophageal cancer. Some are common to both squamous cell carcinoma and adenocarcinoma; others are unique to one particular form (Table 3).

Tobacco and Alcohol

Tobacco and alcohol use are known to increase esophageal cancer risk. Each agent increases risk independently of the other; used together and in heavy amounts, risk is multiplied (120). The proportion of squamous cell carcinoma of the esophagus attributable to ever-smoking (population attributable risk) is estimated at 56.9%, and for those consuming 30 or more alcoholic beverages per week, 44.9% (121). Smoking 20 or more cigarettes per day for 35 or more years appears to increase risk of esophageal squamous cell carcinoma at least 10-fold (122). This amount of smoking, in combination with more than 70 g of alcohol or 5 drinks of 1½ ounces of hard alcohol each week, appears to increase the risk of esophageal squamous

TABLE 3 Risk factors associated with adenocarcinoma and squamous cell carcinoma of the esophagus development

Adenocarcinoma	Squamous Cell Carcinoma
Barrett's esophagus	Achalasia
Bisphosphonates	Alcohol
Demographics (race, sex, geography, socioeconomics)	Bisphosphonates?
Diet?	Caustic injury
Gastroesophageal reflux disease	Demographics (race, sex, geography, socioeconomics)
Helicobacter pylori infection (↓ risk)?	Diet?
Medications decreasing lower esophageal sphincter pressure	Human papilloma virus infection?
Obesity	Prior upper aerodigestive tract malignancy
Tobacco	Tobacco
	Tylosis

cell carcinoma at least 23-fold (122). The proportion of esophageal adenocarcinoma in the population attributed to ever-smoking is 39.7% (121). Combined with heavy alcohol use (more than 70 g of alcohol per week), smoking increases esophageal adenocarcinoma risk at least twofold (122). Smoking cessation lowers squamous cell carcinoma of the esophagus risk by up to 50%, with less risk over time since exposure to tobacco was stopped (123,124). Esophageal adenocarcinoma risk appears to persist despite smoking cessation (123,124). Consumption of one or more alcoholic beverage per day alone is a risk factor found in 80% of squamous cell carcinoma of the esophagus (125). A dose-response relationship to alcohol consumption and risk of squamous cell carcinoma of the esophagus may exist, and cessation of alcohol use appears to reduce risk over time (126). The risk of adenocarcinoma of the esophagus from alcohol consumption is less well established, with some studies showing no increased risk with beer or hard liquor intake (121,124).

Diet

The role of diet in development of esophageal cancer is less clear. Case-control studies have attempted to show links, but evidence is far from definitive. Diets high in antioxidants (vitamin C, β-carotene, vitamin E), and fruits and vegetables had significantly lower odds of Barrett's esophagus in one case-control study (127). Another case-control study, in which cases and controls were interviewed with regard to dietary habits, showed diets high in fiber, β-carotene, folate, and vitamins B6 and C lowered odds of esophageal adenocarcinoma and squamous cell carcinoma, whereas diets high in animal protein, cholesterol, and vitamin B12 increased the risk (128). Diets high in folate were shown to decrease the relative risk of esophageal squamous cell carcinoma and adenocarcinoma in one meta-analysis (129). Dietary intake of N-nitrosamines has been linked to an increased risk of squamous cell carcinoma of the esophagus in China, and vitamin C intake has been found to reduce N-nitrosamine levels in gastric juice, suggesting a possible protective effect from vitamin C (130,131). Chronic ingestion of hot beverages (greater than 65°C), diets low in selenium, and low tissue levels of zinc have also been reported as risk factors for squamous cell carcinoma of the esophagus (132–134).

Demographics

As discussed previously, race and sex appear to impact esophageal cancer incidence, histology and survival. Additionally, socioeconomics impact esophageal cancer risk, with higher-income, higher-educated individuals having lower odds of esophageal adenocarcinoma and squamous cell carcinoma than the lowest quintile (those with less than $15,000 per year income and less than 12 years of education completed) (124).

Tylosis

Tylosis, an autosomal dominant condition caused by mutations in or deletions of the tylosis esophageal cancer (TOC) gene on chromosome 17, is associated with a high risk of squamous cell carcinoma of the esophagus (110,111). The condition results in hyperkeratosis of the palms and soles, with a high number of esophageal papillomas. Abnormal maturation of squamous cells and inflammation are noted on histopathological examination (135).

Infection

Human papilloma virus (HPV) serotypes 16 and 18 have been shown to inactivate *p53* and *Rb* tumor suppressor genes (136). Associations between HPV and squamous cell carcinoma of the esophagus have been established in high-incidence regions, with HPV detected in as few as 8.5% and as many as 65% of esophageal squamous cell carcinoma cases in Eastern countries (137,138). In contrast, the association of HPV and squamous cell carcinoma of the esophagus in low-incidence regions of the West is less clear, with no HPV detected in studies of tumor specimens in Slovenia, Italy, and the United States, and no association between HPV and squamous cell carcinoma of the esophagus in a case-control study in Sweden (139–142). Thus, it is unclear whether HPV causes squamous cell carcinoma of the esophagus, and the association between high-risk sexual behaviors, HPV transmission, and squamous cell carcinoma of the esophagus are not well understood.

In contrast to HPV infection, which possibly increases the risk of squamous cell carcinoma, *Helicobacter pylori* infection may decrease the risk of adenocarcinoma of the esophagus. One review of the literature concluded that *Helicobacter pylori* infection may be associated with a lower risk of reflux esophagitis, due to achlorhydria induced by atrophic gastritis, which is caused by *Helicobacter pylori* infection (143). One might speculate, then, that as the risk of reflux esophagitis is reduced with *Helicobacter pylori* infection, the risk of esophageal adenocarcinoma is reduced, as was suggested by one meta-analysis (144). Other studies have found that high levels of antibodies to the cagA+ strain of *Helicobacter pylori* may lower risk of esophageal adenocarcinoma (145,146). The data are conflicting, however, with some studies showing *Helicobacter pylori* infection not related to Barrett's esophagus risk (147,148). Thus, the role of *Helicobacter pylori* in the development of Barrett's esophagus, reflux esophagitis, and esophageal adenocarcinoma remains speculative. It does not appear that *Helicobacter pylori* infection is linked to squamous cell carcinoma of the esophagus (144).

Prior Malignancies

Patients with a history of aerodigestive tract cancers (e.g., head and neck, lung) are at increased risk for developing a second aerodigestive tract cancer. One study of head and neck cancer patients identified an annual incidence of second aerodigestive tract cancers of 4%, with esophageal cancer arising in 9% of such patients (149). Similarly, esophageal cancer may be found eventually in up to 10% of patients with a history of lung cancer (150). Synchronous esophageal squamous cell carcinoma has been found in up to 14% of newly diagnosed patients with squamous cell carcinoma of the head and neck (151). These findings are likely due to a "field defect" created by tobacco and alcohol use, which increases the risk of cancer at multiple aerodigestive sites (151).

Esophageal Disorders

Disorders and injuries of the esophagus, such as achalasia or caustic injury from lye ingestion, are recognized risk factors for squamous cell carcinoma of the esophagus (152,153). Plummer-Vinson syndrome has also been associated with an increased risk of squamous cell carcinoma of the esophagus (154). In the case of achalasia and Plummer-Vinson syndrome, cancer may develop as a result of chronic irritation of the esophagus from retained food particles (14,154).

Medications

Certain medications, including those that decrease pressure of the lower esophageal sphincter, have been linked to an increased risk of esophageal cancer, although evidence is weak. A case-control study of newly diagnosed esophageal adenocarcinoma patients in Sweden identified an almost fourfold higher odds ratio of this cancer in patients using medications that relax the lower esophageal sphincter (such as aminophyllines, nitroglycerin, anticholinergics, beta-agonists, and benzodiazepines) compared with controls (155). However, another case-control study found an increased risk of esophageal adenocarcinoma only with use of beta-agonists and theophylline, and not with nitrates (156). Yet another case-control study found an increased risk of Barrett's esophagus with use of beta-agonists and theophylline in patients less that 70 years of age. When the results were adjusted for presence of asthma symptoms, the association was much less, suggesting that gastroesophageal reflux may be triggering asthma and Barrett's esophagus, instead of the asthma medications causing Barrett's esophagus (157). Finally, diagnoses of esophageal squamous cell carcinoma and adenocarcinoma have been made in patients on long-term bisphosphonate therapy. The U.S. Food and Drug Administration recommends that patients with known Barrett's esophagus not take bisphosphonates orally (158).

Obesity and Gastroesophageal Reflux Disease

It is believed that the increased incidence of esophageal adenocarcinoma seen over the past two decades is, in part, due to the increased prevalence of obesity in Western society (159). Whether this increased incidence of adenocarcinoma is solely because obesity increases gastroesophageal acid reflux, or if it is because of other factors, is not certain. Studies have shown that obesity increases the risk of gastroesophageal reflux disease (160,161). Gastroesophageal reflux disease, in turn, has been found to increase the risk of esophageal adenocarcinoma, with frequent, severe, long-lasting reflux increasing the odds by the greatest amount (162,163). However, obesity is known to be an independent risk factor for esophageal adenocarcinoma, regardless of gastroesophageal reflux disease symptoms (159,161). Furthermore, approximately 40% of patients with adenocarcinoma of the esophagus have no history of reflux (26,162). Therefore, it does not appear that a stepwise progression of weight gain, leading to symptomatic gastroesophageal reflux, leading to Barrett's esophagus, leading to adenocarcinoma, necessarily occurs. Obese patients, with or without symptomatic gastroesophageal reflux, have an increased risk of esophageal adenocarcinoma, just as normal-weight patients with gastroesophageal reflux appear to be at an increased risk.

Barrett's Esophagus

As noted, Barrett's esophagus is the single most important risk factor for developing esophageal adenocarcinoma (19,20). Patients found to have Barrett's esophagus have a 40 to 125-fold higher risk of developing esophageal adenocarcinoma, with an absolute risk of 1 in 200 in a given year (19,20,164–166). Central adiposity increases the risk of Barrett's esophagus (167,168). In addition, Barrett's esophagus can be identified in up to 15% of patients with antecedent histories of gastroesophageal reflux, and is the most common medical complication of long-standing gastroesophageal reflux disease (169,170). Despite this known association between obesity, gastroesophageal reflux, Barrett's esophagus, and adenocarcinoma, less than 5% of patients undergoing surgery for esophageal adenocarcinoma had documented Barrett's esophagus prior to presenting with symptomatic cancer, and 40% of patients with adenocarcinoma of the esophagus have no history of reflux (26,162). This suggests that screening obese patients or those patients with a history of gastroesophageal reflux disease for Barrett's esophagus is unlikely to impact esophageal adenocarcinoma outcomes, and even surveillance endoscopy for patients with established Barrett's esophagus is the subject of controversy (171). A review of screening for Barrett's esophagus in patients with a history of gastroesophageal reflux disease, surveillance, and treatment of established Barrett's esophagus, and treatment of esophageal dysplasia, is beyond the scope of this chapter.

■ EVALUATION AND STAGING

The evaluation and staging of esophageal cancer is covered in Chapter 10, "Surgery for Esophageal Cancer." Detailed descriptions of the TNM system for staging of esophageal cancer, preoperative evaluation with imaging (including the role of EUS and PET, and the role of diagnostic laparoscopy and bronchoscopy in the initial evaluation of esophageal cancer) are provided.

■ SYSTEMIC THERAPY FOR ESOPHAGEAL CANCER IN NONSURGICAL CANDIDATES

Systemic Therapy for Metastatic Esophageal Cancer

Many drugs have activity against both esophageal squamous cell carcinoma and adenocarcinoma. Early trials of systemic therapy for esophageal cancer were conducted at a time when squamous cell histology predominated, and investigated mostly agents active in squamous cell carcinomas of the head and neck. Drugs such as bleomycin, 5-fluorouracil, cisplatin, doxorubicin, etoposide, methotrexate, and mitomycin-C, which have activity in head and neck cancer, also have been shown to produce responses in patients with metastatic squamous cell carcinoma of the esophagus. However, responses are rarely complete and generally short-lived (172–181). As esophageal adenocarcinoma has become the more common histology, esophageal cancer trials have investigated drugs known to be active in gastric adenocarcinoma. Furthermore, most trials conducted over the past two decades have included patients with both squamous cell carcinoma and adenocarcinoma of the esophagus, as well as adenocarcinoma of the gastroesophageal junction and gastric cardia, with the regimens investigated considered active in each type of cancer. Therefore, this discussion of systemic therapy for metastatic esophageal cancer will not delineate between esophageal adenocarcinoma and squamous cell carcinoma, nor between cancers of the proximal esophagus, gastroesophageal junction, or gastric cardia. Survival and response rates that are observed with particular combinations of drugs will be presented for "esophageal cancer" as a whole, incorporating all of these forms, since this is the approach of most of the clinical trials whose data are presented.

In modern clinical practice, single-agent chemotherapy for metastatic esophageal cancer is rarely used.Only a few trials have compared combination chemotherapy to single-agent treatment. These trials showed improved response rates with combination therapy, but no differences in overall survival (178,182–184). However, a meta-analysis demonstrated improved survival with combination chemotherapy compared to use of single agents (185). These data, plus a consensus among most oncologists that combination chemotherapy is more effective, means that most patients now being treated for esophageal cancer in the metastatic setting are receiving multidrug regimens. Indeed, guidelines from the National Comprehensive Cancer Network do not list single-agent therapy as a consideration for treatment of metastatic esophageal cancer. Only combination regimens are recommended (186). Thus, a detailed overview of response rates and survival with single-agent chemotherapy for metastatic esophageal cancer is of historical interest, and will not be presented in detail.

Combination chemotherapy regimes for treatment of metastatic esophageal cancer are many and varied. Table 4 summarizes combinations recommended by the National Comprehensive Cancer Network for metastatic esophageal cancer or locally advanced esophageal cancer for which chemoradiation is not feasible (186).

Epirubicin-Based Therapy

Among these combinations, epirubicin given with cisplatin and infusional 5-fluorouracil (ECF) has shown promising results. One trial of ECF found a 71% response rate with 12% of study patients having complete responses. Overall median survival was 8.2 months, with a 30% and 10% survival rate at 1 and 2 years, respectively. Significant leukopenia was observed in 21% of patients, and grade 3 or 4 emesis in 13% (187). Another trial of ECF versus 5-fluorouracil, doxorubicin and methotrexate (FAMTX) showed an overall response rate of 45% with ECF versus 21% with FAMTX, and significantly improved median overall survival with ECF (8.9 months) versus FAMTX (5.7 months). Alopecia and emesis were more common with ECF, compared to infection and bone marrow suppression with FAMTX (188). A meta-analysis of randomized phase 2 and 3 trials of first-line therapy in advanced gastric cancer found that combination therapy with 5-fluorouracil, an anthracycline and cisplatin improved overall survival (185), so that ECF is now considered a reference standard for treatment of advanced upper gastric (i.e., gastroesophageal junction and gastric cardia) adenocarcinoma.

Modifications of ECF are probably also effective. A noninferiority trial substituted oxaliplatin for cisplatin, and capecitabine for infusional 5-flurorouracil, to create the regimens of epirubicin plus cisplatin and capecitabine (ECX), epirubicin plus oxaliplatin and infusional 5-fluorouracil (EOF), and epirubicin plus oxaliplatin and capecitabine (EOX). These combinations, along with ECF, were compared in a two-by-two randomization. Noninferiority of ECX compared to ECF, and of EOX to EOF, was demonstrated, suggesting that oxaliplatin and capecitabine may be substituted for cisplatin and infusional 5-fluorouracil. A secondary analysis also found significantly longer overall survival for EOX compared to ECF (11.2 vs. 9.9 months). Use of oxaliplatin resulted in less neutropenia and renal toxicity compared to cisplatin, while infusional 5-fluorouracil and capecitabine treated patients experienced similar toxicities (189).

Fluoropyrimidine-Based Therapy

Infusional 5-fluorouracil, combined with cisplatin, has been used for treatment of localized esophageal cancer prior to surgical resection. When investigated in 44 patients with advanced esophageal cancer, a 35% response rate was observed, compared with a 19% response rate in 44 patients given cisplatin alone. Median overall survival was 8 months. Gastrointestinal and hematological toxicities were

TABLE 4 Combination chemotherapy regimens for treatment of metastatic esophageal cancer

Drugs	Dosage	Response Rate	Median Overall Survival	Reference
Epirubicin + Cisplatin + Infusional 5FU	Epirubicin 50mg/m² IV every 21 days Cisplatin 60 mg/m² IV every 21 days 5FU 200 mg/m²/day via continuous IV infusion for 21 days	41%–71%	8.9 mos	187, 188, 189
Epirubicin + Oxaliplatin + Capecitabine	Epirubicin 50 mg/m² IV day 1 Oxaliplatin 130 mg/m² IV day 1 Capecitabine 625 mg/m² po twice daily days 1 to 14 Repeated every 21 days	48%	11.2 mos	189
Epirubicin + Cisplatin + Capecitabine	Epirubicin 50mg/m² IV day 1 Cisplatin 60 mg/m² IV day 1 Capecitabine 625 mg/m² po twice daily days 1 to 14 Repeated every 21 days	46%	9.9 mos	189
Epirubicin + Oxaliplatin + Infusional 5FU	Epirubicin 50 mg/m² IV day 1 every 21 days Oxaliplatin 130 mg/m² IV day 1 every 21 days 5FU 200 mg/m²/day via continuous IV infusion for 21 days	42%	9.3 mos	189
Cisplatin + Infusional 5FU	Cisplatin 100 mg/m² IV day 1 5FU 1000 mg/m²/day via continuous IV infusion days 1–5 Repeated every 3 weeks	35%	8 mos	178
Docetaxel+ Cisplatin + Infusional 5FU	Docetaxel 75 mg/m² IV day 1 Cisplatin 75 mg/m² IV day 1 5FU 750 mg/m²/day via continuous IV infusion days 1–5 Repeated every 21 days	37%	9.2 mos	201
Docetaxel + Capecitabine	Docetaxel 75 mg/m² IV day 1 Capecitabine 825 mg/m² po twice daily days 1–14 Repeated every 21 days Docetaxel 75 mg/m² IV day 1 Capecitabine 1000 mg/m² po twice daily days 1–14 Repeated every 21 days Docetaxel 36 mg/m² IV days 1 and 8 Capecitabine 1000 mg/m² po twice daily days 1–14 Repeated every 21 days	39%–46%	8–12 mos	204–206
Irinotecan + Cisplatin	Irinotecan 65 mg/m² IV with Cisplatin 30 mg/m² IV days 1 and 8 every 21 days Irinotecan 65 mg/m² with Cisplatin 30 mg/m² IV weekly for 4 weeks followed by 2 weeks rest Irinotecan 70 mg/m² IV days 1 and 15 Cisplatin 80 mg/m² IV day 1 Repeated every 28 days	30%–58%	9–14 mos	211–213
Irinotecan + Infusional 5FU	Irinotecan 80 mg/m² IV day 1 Folinic acid 500 mg/m² IV day 1 5FU 2000 mg/m² via 22-hour continuous IV infusion Weekly for 6 out of 7 weeks	31.8	9 mos	216
Irinotecan + Capecitabine	Irinotecan 130 mg/m² IV days 1 and 15 Capecitabine 3500 mg/m² po BID days 1–6 and 16–22 Repeated every 28 days	43.6%	11 mos	217

Continued

TABLE 4 Combination chemotherapy regimens for treatment of metastatic esophageal cancer (*Continued*)

Drugs	Dosage	Response Rate	Median Overall Survival	Reference
Paclitaxel + Cisplatin	Paclitaxel 180 mg/m² IV day 1 Cisplatin 60 mg/m² IV day 1 Repeated every 2 weeks Paclitaxel 175 mg/m² IV Cisplatin 75 mg/m² IV day 1 Repeated every 3 weeks	43%–49%	9–13 mos	193, 194
Paclitaxel + Carboplatin	Paclitaxel 200 mg/m² IV day 1 Carboplatin AUC 5 mg/h/ml IV day 1 Repeated every 21 days	43%	9 mos	197
Cisplatin + Paclitaxel + Etoposide	Paclitaxel 50 mg/m² IV twice weekly for 3 weeks Cisplatin 15 mg/m² IV twice weekly for 3 weeks Etoposide 40 mg/m² IV twice weekly for 3 weeks Repeated every 28 days	70%–100%	12–13 mos	198, 199
Oxaliplatin + Infusional 5FU	Oxaliplatin 100 mg/m² IV day 1 Folinic acid 400 mg/m² IV day 1 5FU 400 mg/m² IV bolus 5FU 3000 mg/m² via 46-hour continuous IV infusion Repeated every 14 days Oxaliplatin 50 mg/m² IV day 1, 8, 15, 22 Folinic acid 500 mg/m² IV day 1, 8, 15, 22 5FU 2000 mg/m² via 24-hour continuous IV infusion day 1, 8, 15, 22 Repeated every 5 weeks Oxaliplatin 85 mg/m² IV day 1 5FU 2.6 g/m² via 24-hour continuous IV infusion Folinic acid 500 mg/m² IV day 1 Repeated every 2 weeks	43%–54%	8–11 mos	207, 299, 300
Oxaliplatin + Capecitabine	Oxaliplatin 130 mg/m² IV day 1 Capecitabine 1000 mg/m² po twice daily days 1–14 Repeated every 21 days Oxaliplatin 130 mg/m² IV day 1 Capecitabine 850 mg/m² po twice daily days 1–14 Repeated every 21 days	35%–65%	6–8 mos	208–210

5FU, 5-fluorouracil; IV, intravenous; mg, milligrams; m², meter squared; mos, months; po, by mouth.

most common, although meningeal hemorrhage (n = 1) and limb ischemia (n = 1) were observed (178).

Substitutions with fluoropyrimidines other than 5-fluorouracil in combination with cisplatin have been examined. A phase II trial investigated the oral fluoropyrimidine derivative UFT, 300 mg/m² given daily with leucovorin 75 mg intravenously for 21 consecutive days, combined with cisplatin 60 mg/m² and epirubicin 50 mg/m² intravenously each on day 1 of a 28-day cycle. A response rate of 46% and median survival of 46 months were observed, with bone marrow suppression being the most frequent toxicity (190). S-1, an oral agent containing ftroafur, chlorohydroxy dihydropyridine, and oxonic acid, has been investigated with cisplatin in Western and Asian populations. One study investigated S-1 40–60 mg twice daily (dose based on body surface area) for 21 days, given with cisplatin

60 mg/m^2 intravenously on day 8, followed by 2 weeks rest, and repeated every 5 weeks. A response rate of 54% and median survival of 13 months were found, with myelosuppression and anorexia commonly seen toxicities (191). In Western populations, doses of S-1 must be modified due to genetic differences in the *CYP2A6* gene, whose protein product metabolizes S-1. Thus, a study of S-1 with cisplatin in the United States gave S-1 25 mg/m^2 twice daily for 21 days with cisplatin 75 mg/m^2 intravenously on day 1, repeated every 28 days, with a 51% overall response rate and median survival of 10.9 months. Fatigue, neutropenia, and gastrointestinal toxicities were most common (192). Neither UFT nor S-1 are available at present in the United States.

Taxane-Based Therapy

Paclitaxel-based regimens have been studied in several trials, with efficacy similar to the previously discussed fluoropyrimidine combination therapies. Paclitaxel with cisplatin, investigated in at least four trials with varying dosing schemes (Table 4), has shown response rates ranging from 25% to 49%, and median overall survivals between 7 and 17 months. Hematologic toxicity, fatigue, and neuropathy are common side effects observed in up to 45% of patients (193–195). A small study of 15 patients given paclitaxel 70–80 mg/m^2 IV day 1, cisplatin 35 mg/m^2 IV day 2, and infusional 5-FU 2,000 mg/m^2 with leucovorin 300 mg/m^2 IV over 24 hours day 2, given weekly for 2 or 3 weeks, followed by 1 week rest, yielded a 33% response rate and median overall survival of 12.5 months. Myelosuppression developed in 27% of patients, with no peripheral neuropathy (196). Paclitaxel also has been given with carboplatin, with a response rate in the 40% range, and neutropenia occurring in 52% of patients (197). A paclitaxel/cisplatin/etoposide combination showed dramatic response rates of 70% to 100%, although the studies evaluated small numbers of patients (32 and 22 patients, respectively). Despite the dramatic responses, median overall survival times were similar to the multiple previously discussed regimens (12–13 months). Furthermore, the dramatic responses were at the price of substantial hematologic toxicity (grade 3 anemia and neutropenia in 100% of patients in one study, including one death from neutropenic fever) (198,199).

Docetaxel, an agent with known activity in esophageal cancer (200), has been studied in multiple combinations with other drugs. The landmark TAX-325 trial compared the DCF regimen of docetaxel 75 mg/m^2 IV day 1, cisplatin 75 mg/m^2 IV day 1, with infusional 5-fluorouracil 750 mg/m^2/day days 1 through 5, repeated every 3 weeks, to CF (cisplatin 100 mg/m^2 IV day 1 with infusional 5-fluorouracil 1,000 mg/m^2/day days 1 through 5, repeated every 4 weeks), in patients with advanced gastric and gastroesophageal junction adenocarcinoma. DCF was significantly superior to CF for overall response rates (37 vs. 25%, $P = .01$), 2-year survival (18% vs. 9%, $P = .02$), and time to progression (5.6 vs. 3.7 months, $P < .001$). However, toxicity with DCF was greater compared to CF, with 82% of DCF patients experiencing grade 3 or 4 neutropenia, 29% of DCF patients developing complicated neutropenia, and 20% of DCF patients afflicted with grade 3 or 4 diarrhea, compared to 57%, 12% and 8% of CF treated patients, respectively (201). It may be possible to eliminate cisplatin from the DCF regimen, since a trial of docetaxel with infusional 5-fluorouracil (docetaxel 75 mg/m^2 IV day 1 plus infusional 5-fluorouracil 200 mg/m^2 day 1 through 21, repeated every 3 weeks) showed a 33% response rate, a median overall survival of 9.5 months, and median time to progression of 5.5 months (202). However, a randomized trial of DCF versus docetaxel/infusional 5-fluorouracil should be conducted before making this statement a firm conclusion. In addition, it is unknown whether DCF is clearly superior to ECF. Although a randomized phase 2 trial comparing the two regimens showed improved response rates with DCF versus ECF (37% compared with 26%) and median overall survival (10.4 vs. 8.3 months), the trial was underpowered to detect superiority of one regimen over the other (203). Finally, docetaxel and capecitabine have been combined in several studies (204–206), with promising response rates and median overall survivals as outlined in Table 4.

Oxaliplatin-Based Therapy

Oxaliplatin, in addition to use in combination with epirubicin and infusional 5-FU (EOF), and epirubicin with capecitabine (EOX), has been prescribed with infusional 5-FU and folinic acid (FUFOX), and capecitabine (CapeOX). The FUFOX regimen was investigated in 48 patients with advanced gastric and gastroesophageal junction adenocarcinoma, with a 54% response rate and 11.4 month median survival.

study. Stable disease was seen in 8 patients, with 1 partial response, after a median of 2 sunitinib cycles. Myelosuppression occurred in up to 29% of patients, with grade 3 or 4 toxicities including plantar-palmar erythema, fatigue, anorexia, and mucositis in fewer than 10% of patients (229).

Second-Line Therapy

Although treatment options exist for patients with metastatic esophageal cancer failing first-line combination chemotherapy with or without targeted agents, response rates are generally inferior to first-line chemotherapy. In addition, median survival is poor, in the range of 5 to 6 months (230–238). Two trials have reported a palliative benefit to patients' symptoms, including relief of dysphagia, reflux, nausea, and, interestingly, weight loss, in up to 75% of patients (232,233). Toxicities appear to be similar to the first-line regimens using the same drugs.

No trials have compared different combinations head-to-head in the second-line setting. Thus, treating this patient population in an evidence-based fashion is difficult, and trials of new drugs and regimens are greatly needed. Table 5 lists several regimens that have been investigated in patients with metastatic esophageal cancer, including patients refractory to cisplatin.

Systemic Therapy With Radiation For Inoperable Esophageal Cancer

Systemic therapy, in conjunction with radiation (chemoradiotherapy), is used frequently in patients with esophageal cancer who are not candidates for surgery. Such patients may be ineligible for surgery due to locally advanced, unresectable disease, or because of medical comorbidities that render surgery a high risk. This strategy is frequently used; one study identified that 56% of all esophageal cancer patients (with both squamous cell and adenocarcinoma histologies) received combined modality chemoradiotherapy as definitive treatment at 59 institutions between 1996 and 1999 (239). Chemoradiotherapy may result in long-term disease control for some patients, but at a minimum, it appears to palliate the symptoms of esophageal cancer, such as dysphagia.

Earlier studies comparing chemoradiotherapy to radiation alone for inoperable esophageal cancer investigated treatment schemes that are recognized now to be suboptimal. A trial of radiation alone (5,000 cGy) versus radiation (5,000 cGy) plus 5-fluorouracil 1,000 mg/m^2/day as a 72-hour continuous IV infusion, mitomycin C 10 mg/m^2 IV day 1 and bleomycin 15 units IM weekly for 5 weeks (thus giving only 1 cycle of chemotherapy), failed to show a difference in local response or survival (240). Other trials demonstrating improved responses and survival with chemoradiotherapy versus radiation alone gave relatively low chemotherapy and/or radiation doses, including trials with split courses of radiation (241–245). Some studies gave sequential chemotherapy followed by radiation (246–250). Despite the less effective regimens used in these older trials, a pooled analysis of seven randomized trials established a survival benefit at 1 year for chemoradiotherapy versus radiation alone (1-year mortality odds ratio 0.61, 95% CI, 0.44–0.94, $P < .00001$), and improved local control (odds ratio 0.52, 95% CI, 0.31–0.89, $P = .004$) (251).

Radiation Therapy Oncology Group (RTOG) trial 85–01 randomized patients with locally advanced esophageal cancer to receive cisplatin (75 mg/m^2 IV day 1 and day 29) and 5-fluorouracil (1,000 mg/m^2/day via 96-hour continuous IV infusion days 1–4 and days 29–33) with radiation (50.4 Gy in 2 Gy per day fractions), followed by two cycles of the same drugs every 3 weeks after radiation, versus radiation alone (64 Gy). Chemoradiotherapy improved both median survival (14 vs. 9 months) and 5-year survival (27% vs. 0%) compared with radiation alone ($P < .0001$). There were no differences in 5-year survival based on histology. Chemoradiotherapy resulted in more mucositis, esophagitis, and hematological toxicity, and more grade 3 and 4 toxicities overall (252,253). Because the protocol did not specify that patients must have unresectable tumors, it is possible that study patients had better prognoses as a group, thus limiting the applicability of the study's findings to the average patient with locally advanced, unresectable esophageal cancer. Despite these limitations, cisplatin plus 5-fluorouracil with radiation has become the standard of care for locally advanced, unresectable esophageal cancer, as recommended by the National Comprehensive Cancer Network and National Cancer Institute (186,254).

Other approaches to chemoradiotherapy as a definitive treatment for unresectable disease have

TABLE 5 Combination chemotherapy regimens for second-line treatment of metastatic esophageal cancer

Drugs	Number of Previous Regimens	Dosage	Response Rate	Stable Disease Rate	Median Overall Survival (Months)	Reference
Capecitabine + Docetaxel	1	Capecitabine 1000 mg/m^2 po BID days 1–14 Docetaxel 75 mg/m^2 IV day 1 Repeated every 3 weeks	25%	17%	6.2	230
Oxaliplatin + Infusional 5FU + Leucovorin	1 or more	Oxaliplatin 85 mg/m^2 IV day 1 Leucovorin 200 mg/m^2/day via 22-hour continuous IV infusion 5FU 400 mg/m^2 IV bolus day 1 5FU 600 mg/m^2 via 22-hour continuous IV infusion Repeated every 2 weeks	19%	31%	5.8	231
Irinotecan + Infusional 5FU + Leucovorin	1 or more	Irinotecan 180 mg/m^2 IV day 1 5FU 400 mg/m^2 IV bolus day 1 Leucovorin 125 mg/m^2 IV day 1 5FU 1200 mg/m^2 via 48-hour continuous IV infusion Repeated every 2 weeks	29%	34%	6.4	232
Irinotecan + Capecitabine	2 or fewer	Irinotecan 250 mg/m^2 IV day 1 Capecitabine 2000 mg/m^2/day po Days 1–14 Repeated every 3 weeks	17%	24%	6.5	233
Irinotecan	1 (Cisplatin refractory)	Irinotecan 100 mg/m^2 IV days 1, 8, 15[a] Repeated every 28 days	15%	23%	5	234
Irinotecan + Docetaxel	2 or fewer (Cisplatin pretreated or refractory)	Irinotecan 55 mg/m^2 IV day 1, 8, 15 Docetaxel 65 mg/m^2 IV day 1, 8, 15 Repeated every 28 days	12.5%	33.3%	6.5	235
Docetaxel + Nedaplatin	1 or more (Cisplatin refractory)	Docetaxel 30 mg/m^2 IV day 1 Nedaplatin 50 mg/m^2 IV day 1 Repeated every 2 weeks	27.1%	NR	5.9	236
Docetaxel + 5FU + Cisplatin	1 or more (Cisplatin refractory)	Docetaxel 60 mg/m^2 IV day 1 5FU 500 mg/day IV days 1–5 Cisplatin 10 mg/day days 1–5 Repeated every 3 weeks	30%	30%	8	237
Mitomycin C + Ifosfamide + Cisplatin	1	Mitomycin 6 mg/m^2 IV day 1 Ifosfamide 3 g/m^2 IV day 1 Cisplatin 50 mg/m^2 IV day 1 Repeated every 3 weeks	12.5%	37.5%	5.2	238

5FU, 5-fluorouracil; IV, intravenous; mg, milligrams; m^2, meter squared; po, by mouth.
[a]Dose escalated to 140 mg/m^2 in 20 mg/m^2 increments with each cycle for patients with grade 3 or less toxicities.
[b]59.4% of study patients were treated in second-line setting; other study patients received regimen as first-line therapy.

been examined. When FOLFOX4 (oxaliplatin 85 mg/m^2 IV day 1, leucovorin 200 mg/m^2 IV day 1, 5-fluorouracil 400 mg/m^2 IV bolus day 1, followed by 5-fluorouracil 600 mg/m^2 via 22-hour continuous IV infusion days 1–2), was given for three cycles with radiation (5,000 cGy) and three cycles after radiation, an endoscopic complete response rate of 44.7% was seen, with a median overall survival of 22.7 months. This compared favorably to patients randomized to cisplatin 75 mg/m^2 IV day 1 with 5-fluorouracil 1,000 mg/m^2/day via 96 hour continuous IV infusion for 2 cycles with radiation (5,000 cGy) and two cycles after radiation (endoscopic complete response rate of 30% and median overall survival of 14.7 months). Neutropenia and neuropathy were more frequent in the FOLFOX4-treated patients (255). In patients with locally advanced esophageal cancer who were given radiation (6,000 cGy) with paclitaxel 175 mg/m^2 IV (day 1 and once on week 5 of radiation) and cisplatin 75 mg/m^2 IV (day 1 and once on week 5 of radiation), a complete clinical response of 27% was observed, with a 45% partial response rate, and a 30% stable disease rate. Three-year overall survival was 23.2%. However, the majority of patients in this study ultimately underwent surgical resection followed by additional chemotherapy; only 10 patients in the study were deemed inoperable from the outset. Unfortunately, data on these 10 patients were not presented separately from the other patients in the report (256). Thus, these results probably do not apply specifically to patients with unresectable esophageal cancer.

Although investigators have studied induction chemotherapy (i.e., chemotherapy given prior to chemoradiotherapy) extensively, few trials of this approach have been conducted specifically for patients with inoperable esophageal cancer. Furthermore, these trials did not compare induction chemotherapy to chemoradiotherapy alone, making it unclear which of these approaches might be superior.

In one study of induction chemotherapy, 5-fluorouracil 500 mg/m^2 IV bolus days 1–3, leucovorin 300 mg/m^2 IV days 1–3, etoposide 100 mg/m^2 IV days 1–3 and cisplatin 50 mg/m^2 IV days 1–3 for 3 cycles, followed by cisplatin 50 mg/m^2 IV days 2–8 and etoposide 80 mg/m^2 IV days 3–5 with radiation (4,000 cGy), was given to 86 patients with T3–4, N0–1, M0 disease, followed by observation. This treatment was compared with 86 patients receiving the same induction chemotherapy, followed by chemoradiotherapy with 50 or 60 Gy of radiation (depending on tumor size and location) and the same chemotherapy concomitantly, followed by surgery. At 2 years, there was no significant difference in overall survival between the two groups, with a median overall survival of 35.4% in those not proceeding to surgery. Freedom from progression at 2 years was 40.7% in the group not undergoing surgery (257).

A second study of induction chemotherapy investigated 5-fluorouracil 700 mg/m^2/day via continuous IV infusion days 1 through 5, cisplatin 15 mg/m^2 days 1 through 5, paclitaxel 200 mg/m^2 via 24-hour continuous IV infusion on day 1, repeated a second time after 29 days, followed by radiation (50.4 Gy) with 5-fluorouracil 300 mg/m^2 via 96-hour continuous IV infusion weeks 1 through 5, and paclitaxel 50 mg/m^2 IV once weekly for 5 weeks. This regimen was compared to a nonfluoropyrimidine-based therapy with paclitaxel 175 mg/m^2 IV on day 1 and cisplatin 75 mg/m^2 IV on day 1, repeated once after 21 days, followed by radiation (50.4 Gy) with cisplatin 30 mg/m^2 IV days 1, 8, 15, 22, 29, and 36, and paclitaxel 60 mg/m^2 via 96-hour continuous IV infusion days 1, 8, 15, 22, 29, and 36. As one might expect, toxicities were profound, with a total rate of grade 3 or 4 toxicities of greater than 80%. Grade 3 or 4 myelosuppression occurred in 38% of patients in the fluoropyrimidine-based arm and 69% in the nonfluoropyrimidine treated arm. Median survival was 29 months in the fluoropyrimidine-based arm (56% alive at 2 years) versus 15 months in the nonfluoropyrimidine treated arm (37% alive at 2 years). The authors concluded that due to the excessive toxicity and lack of improvement in survival compared with historic controls, the regimens should not be investigated further (258).

Additional studies of novel chemotherapy regimens with radiation for treatment of unresectable esophageal cancer are needed. Until more data are available, the cisplatin plus 5-fluorouracil with radiation approach as studied in the RTOG 85–01 trial appears to be the most effective and well-tolerated regimen to use in this patient population.

■ SYSTEMIC THERAPY FOR ESOPHAGEAL CANCER IN SURGICAL CANDIDATES

Prior to a discussion of systemic therapy strategies for patients with esophageal cancer in whom surgical resection is planned or completed, a word must be said about these treatments, as they apply to the different histologies of esophageal cancer. Although squamous cell carcinomas and adenocarcinomas of the esophagus typically present in different anatomic locations, have different risk factors, and have different patterns of spread, thus probably representing different diseases, the vast majority of trials investigating systemic therapy for surgical candidates have included patients with both histologies (259,260). This confounding element in the data limits applicability to the individual patient with either squamous cell carcinoma or adenocarcinoma of the esophagus.

Some have suggested that different treatment strategies be employed for each type of esophageal cancer, such as using neoadjuvant chemoradiotherapy for squamous cell carcinomas of the esophagus and induction chemotherapy (without radiation) for esophageal adenocarcinomas (260). However, until more contemporary trials of systemic therapy strategies in surgical candidates are conducted based on histology, most patients with either locally advanced, resectable squamous cell carcinoma or adenocarcinoma of the esophagus will probably continue to be treated identically. Indeed, current national guidelines in the United States do not truly differentiate treatment strategies for locally advanced, resectable esophageal cancer based on histology, other than to suggest induction chemotherapy (rather than preoperative chemoradiotherapy) may be considered for T1b, N1 or T2-T4, N0–1, NX, or stage IVA, adenocarcinoma of the distal esophagus/gastroesophageal junction (186).

Systemic Therapy with Radiation Followed by Surgery (Neoadjuvant Chemoradiotherapy)

In an effort to improve local control and decrease rates of distant failure, chemotherapy with radiation, prior to surgical resection, has been studied. It is theorized that neoadjuvant chemoradiotherapy followed by surgical resection may improve local control by downstaging the disease, allowing a more complete resection with negative margins, with esophagectomy ensuring removal of residual microscopic local disease. The chemotherapy portion of treatment may help to control micrometastatic disease at distant sites (14).

Over 40 nonrandomized trials have investigated this approach. A complete review of the chemotherapy and radiation regimens used in each of these studies is beyond the scope of this chapter, and since evidence for or against any particular treatment from nonrandomized trials is weak, these results will not be presented in detail. In general, 5-fluorouracil and cisplatin-based chemotherapy has been given, with radiation doses ranging between 30 and 60 Gy. Median overall survival has ranged from 8 to 37 months, with 5-year survival rates of up to 71% in those patients achieving a pathological complete response (259).

Stronger evidence for an advantage to the neoadjuvant chemoradiotherapy approach comes from randomized trials and meta-analyses. Eight trials have compared preoperative chemoradiotherapy to surgery alone, as shown in Table 6. Only two of these trials have demonstrated a significant survival advantage with preoperative chemoradiotherapy over surgery alone (261,262). It should be noted that two of the seven trials (263,264) gave "sequential" chemoradiotherapy, meaning that chemotherapy was started up to 7 days before radiation, and in one trial (264) additional doses of chemotherapy were given after radiation was completed, with no significant differences in 3-year survival found. A meta-analysis of randomized trials of neoadjuvant chemoradiotherapy and surgery versus surgery alone found a significant improvement in survival at 3 years (odds ratio 0.47 for chemoradiotherapy followed by surgery vs. 0.92 for surgery alone, $P = .016$). When the analysis was restricted to chemoradiotherapy trials alone, not including "sequential" chemoradiotherapy trials, a more significant improvement in 3-year survival was noted (odds ratio 0.45, $P = .005$) (265). A second meta-analysis found lower all-cause mortality in patients receiving neoadjuvant chemoradiotherapy (hazard ratio 0.81, 95% CI 0.70–0.93, $P = .002$), with an absolute benefit in survival at 2 years of 13%. When the analysis was restricted to patients with squamous cell carcinoma, preoperative chemoradiotherapy did not appear to provide a survival advantage (hazard ratio 0.88, 95% CI 0.75–1.03, $P = .12$); but a survival advantage was shown for patients with adenocarcinoma of the esophagus (hazard ratio 0.78, 95% CI 0.64–0.95, $P = .014$) (266).

Additional studies of neoadjuvant chemoradiotherapy employing more intense systemic agents have been conducted. Although the trials are nonrandomized, they are worth mentioning for the

TABLE 6 Randomized trials of neoadjuvant chemoradiotherapy followed by surgical resection versus surgery alone for resectable esophageal cancer

No. of patients	Histology	Radiation Dose	Chemotherapy	R0 Resection%	pCR%	Survival	Local Failure %	Reference
113	100% A	40 Gy in 15 fractions over 3 weeks	5FU 15 mg/kg IV days 1–5 Cisplatin 75 mg/m^2 IV day 7	NR	25	At 3 years: 32% CRT+S 6% S $P = .001$	NR	261
100	75% A 25% SCC	45 Gy in 30 fractions over 3 weeks	Cisplatin 20 $mg/m^2/d$ IV days 1–5 and 17–21 5FU 300 $mg/m^2/d$ IV 1–21 Vinblastine 1 $mg/m^2/d$ IV days 1–4 and 17–20	90 CRT+S 90 S	28	At 3 years: 32% CRT+S 15% S $P = .15$	19 CRT+S 42 S	272
56	77% A 23% SCC	50.4 Gy in 25 fractions over 5.5 weeks	Cisplatin 100 mg/m^2 days 1 and 29 5FU 1,000 $mg/m^2/d$ via 96-hour continuous IV days 1–4 and 29–32	NR	40[a]	At 5 years: 39% CRT+S 16% S *P* NR	44 CRT+S[b] 33 S	262
282	100% SCC	37 Gy in 10 fractions over 4 weeks	Cisplatin 80 mg/m^2 IV 0–2 days before radiation	81 CRT+S 69 S	26	At 3 years: 34% CRT+S 36% S $P = .8$	NR	263
86	100% SCC	20 Gy in 10 fractions over 12 days, days 8–19	Cisplatin 100 mg/m^2 IV day 1 and 21 5FU 600 $mg/m^2/d$ via 96-hour continuous IV infusion days 2–5 and 22–25	NR	12	At 3 years: 19% CRT+S 14% *P* NR	27 CRT+S 20 S	264
257	63% A 35% SCC	35 Gy in 15 fractions over 3 weeks	Cisplatin 80 mg/m^2 IV day 1 5FU 800 $mg/m^2/d$ IV days 1–4	80 CRT+S 59 S	16	At 5 years: 16% CRT+S 15% S *P* NR	20 CRT+S 39 S	296
69	100% SCC	40 Gy in 20 fractions over 4 weeks	Cisplatin 100 mg/m^2 IV days 1 and 29 5FU 1000 $mg/m^2/d$ via 24-hour continuous IV infusion days 1–4 and 29–32	NR	20	At 3 years: 26% CRT+S 20% S $P = .4$	NR	297
123	100% SCC	45.6 Gy in 38 fractions over 4 weeks	Cisplatin 60 mg/m^2 IV day 1 5FU 1000 $mg/m^2/d$ via 96-hour continuous IV infusion days 2–5	100 CRT+S 88 S	43	At 2 years: 55% CRT+S 57% S $P = .69$	22 CRT+S 12 S	298

A, adenocarcinoma; CRT+S, chemoradiotherapy plus surgery; 5FU, 5-fluorouracil; Gy, Gray; IV, intravenous; mg, milligrams; m^2, meter squared; NR, not reported; pCR, pathologic complete response; R0, no cancer at surgical margins; S, surgery alone; SCC, squamous cell carcinoma.

[a]Only 25 patients evaluable.

[b]Only 9 patients evaluable on CRT+S arm and 12 patients evaluable on S arm.

impressive results obtained, although with substantially increased toxicity. A multi-institution phase 2 study from the Minnie Pearl Cancer Research Network investigated preoperative chemoradiotherapy in 123 patients with locally advanced esophageal cancer. Patients received paclitaxel 200 mg/m^2 IV on days 1 and 22 with carboplatin AUC 6 IV on days 1 and 22 with 5-fluorouracil 225 mg/m^2/day via 24-hour continuous IV infusion on days 1–42 with radiation (45 Gy in 1.8 Gy/day fractions), followed by surgery. The pathologic complete response rate was 38%, with a median overall survival of 22 months and a 3-year survival rate of 41%. The chemoradiotherapy strategy proved toxic, with 57% of patients requiring hospitalization for an adverse event, 73% of patients developing grade 3 or 4 leukopenia, and 43% of patients experiencing grade 3 or 4 esophagitis (267). Another phase 2 study investigated neoadjuvant chemoradiotherapy using paclitaxel 175 mg/m^2 IV on days 1 and 22 with carboplatin AUC 5 IV on days 1 and 22 with 5-fluorouracil 200 mg/m^2/day via continuous IV infusion on days 1 through 42 with radiation (45 Gy in 1.8 Gy/day fractions) followed by surgery. A 38% pathologic complete response rate and a 96% R0 resection rate was found, with a 48% estimated 5-year survival, and an estimated 3-year survival of 61% in "responders." Grade 3 neutropenia developed in 46% of patients, with all patients experiencing grade 2 or less esophagitis (268). A trial of FOLFOX-type chemotherapy with radiation (oxaliplatin 60 mg/m^2 IV and leucovorin 20 mg/m^2 IV on days 1, 8, 15, 29, 36, 43, 50, and 57, with 5-fluorouracil 200 mg/m^2/day via continuous IV infusion on days 1–22 and 29–64, given with radiation (45 Gy in 1.8 Gy/day fractions) followed by surgery, showed a 1-year overall survival of 63%, a pathologic complete response rate of 18% and R0 resections in 79% of patients. As with other trials, esophagitis and hematologic toxicity were observed (269).

There is limited experience with additional chemotherapy given after neoadjuvant chemoradiotherapy and surgery. A single institution phase 2 trial investigated adjuvant chemotherapy after neoadjuvant chemoradiotherapy and surgery. Patients were hospitalized to receive cisplatin 20 mg/m^2/day via continuous IV infusion on days 1 through 5 and 26 through 30, and received 5-fluorouracil 225 mg/m^2/day via ambulatory continuous IV infusion on days 1 through 30 with radiation (44 Gy in 2 Gy/day fractions), followed by surgery, followed by adjuvant paclitaxel 135 mg/m^2 IV on day 1 and cisplatin 75 mg/m^2 IV on day 2 repeated every 3 weeks for 3 cycles in all patients achieving an R0 resection (83% of patients). A 28% complete pathologic response rate was reported, with a 2-year survival of 91% in those achieving complete pathologic response, and 62% 2-year survival for the entire group. During neoadjuvant chemoradiotherapy, grade 3 or 4 neutropenia and grade 3 or 4 esophagitis were observed in 24% of patients each. During adjuvant chemotherapy, 69% of patients developed grade 3 or 4 neutropenia (270). Another study investigated 5-fluorouracil 200 mg/m^2/day via continuous IV infusion with cisplatin 30 mg/m^2 IV on days 3, 10, 17, and 24, with paclitaxel 45 mg/m^2 IV on days 3, 10, 17, and 24, given with radiation (45 Gy total dose), followed by surgery. Adjuvant chemotherapy consisted of two cycles of 5-fluorouracil 750 mg/m^2 IV bolus days 1 to 5, cisplatin 50 mg/m^2 IV on days 1 and 2, and paclitaxel 135 mg/m^2 IV on day 1. A pathologic complete response rate of 17% was observed with a 3-year survival of 50%. Only 40 of 60 patients completing surgery were able to complete both cycles of adjuvant chemotherapy (271).

Although each of the trials of neoadjuvant chemoradiotherapy has limitations, including small numbers of patients, inclusion of patients with both esophageal squamous cell carcinoma and adenocarcinoma, and variable chemotherapy dosing and timing, it appears that neoadjuvant chemoradiotherapy may have advantages compared to up-front surgical resection or neoadjuvant radiation alone. These advantages include downstaging of disease to achieve a margin-negative resection specimen, probable improved survival for those patients achieving a complete pathologic response (259,272–275), and possible improved local control (273). Most cancer care providers now use this approach for locally advanced, resectable esophageal cancer, especially those cancers involving the distal esophagus and gastroesophageal junction.

Induction Chemotherapy Followed by Chemoradiotherapy, Followed by Surgery

In an effort to improve the response rates and overall survival observed with neoadjuvant therapy, some trials have intensified systemic therapies by giving induction chemotherapy followed by chemoradiotherapy, and/or giving additional chemotherapy agents with radiation. A review of these trials is presented here.

Induction Therapy With Irinotecan-Based Regimens

Irinotecan has been given as a part of induction chemotherapy followed by chemoradiotherapy and surgery for locally advanced esophageal cancer. In one trial of induction chemotherapy, patients with localized esophageal squamous cell carcinoma, or adenocarcinoma were given irinotecan 70 mg/m^2 IV and cisplatin 30 mg/m^2 IV on days 1, 7, 21, and 28, repeated beginning day 42, followed by radiation (45 Gy in 1.8 Gy per fraction) with 5-fluorouracil 300 mg/m^2/day via 5-day continuous IV infusion each week of radiation and paclitaxel 45 mg/m^2 IV weekly during radiation, followed by surgery. An R0 resection was achieved in 91% of patients, with a 28% pathologic complete response rate. A median survival of 22.1 months was observed. Myelosuppression, esophagitis, gastrointestinal toxicity, and fatigue were common grade 3 or 4 toxicities (276).

A phase 1 trial gave patients with locally advanced esophageal squamous cell carcinoma and adenocarcinoma cisplatin 30 mg/m^2 IV with irinotecan 65 mg/m^2 IV weekly on weeks 1, 2, 4, and 5, followed by chemoradiotherapy with cisplatin 30 mg/m^2 IV and irinotecan (given in a dose-escalating fashion of 40, 50, 65, and 80 mg/m^2) IV on days 1, 8, 22, and 29 of radiation (50.4 Gy in 1.8 Gy per day fractions), followed by surgery. Irinotecan 65 mg/m^2 IV with radiation was recommended for a phase 2 study, as dose-limiting myelosuppression was seen in two of six patients given the 80 mg/m^2 irinotecan dose with radiation. A 27% pathologic complete response rate was observed. Myelosuppression (32% of patients had grade 3 neutropenia during induction therapy), and grade 1 or 2 gastrointestinal toxicity were the most common adverse events (277).

Induction Therapy With Paclitaxel-Based Regimens

Paclitaxel has been given as a component of induction therapy for localized esophageal cancer in 2 trials. The first of these investigated 5-fluorouracil 750 mg/m^2/day via 5-day continuous IV infusion days 1 through 5, with cisplatin 15 mg/m^2/day IV bolus days 1 through 5 and paclitaxel 200 mg/m^2 via 24-hour continuous IV infusion on day 1, repeated after 29 days, followed by radiation (45 Gy in 25 fractions) with 5-fluorouracil (300 mg/m^2/day via 5-day continuous IV infusion each week of radiation) and cisplatin 20 mg/m^2 IV days 1–5 of radiation, followed by surgery. All patients (37) achieved an R0 resection, with a pathologic complete response rate of 30%. Median survival had not been reached at a median follow-up time of 20 months. Myelosuppression and gastrointestinal toxicity were common grade 3 or 4 toxicities in up to 14% of patients during the induction phase of treatment, with esophagitis (grade 1) in 51% of patients during chemoradiotherapy (278).

Paclitaxel with induction therapy also was investigated in a phase 2 trial, in which 5-fluorouracil 750 mg/m^2/day via continuous IV infusion on days 1 to 5, cisplatin 15 mg/m^2/day IV on days 1 to 5, and paclitaxel 200 mg/m^2 IV on day 1, repeated once after 28 days, was followed by radiation (45 Gy in 1.8 Gy per day fractions) with cisplatin 15 mg/m^2/day IV on days 1 to 5 and 5-fluorouracil 300 mg/m^2/day via 5-day continuous IV infusion each week of radiation, followed by surgery. All patients achieved R0 resections. A pathologic complete response rate of 71% was reported, with a 51% disease-free and 39% overall survival at 5 years. Myelosuppression was seen in 30% of patients during induction therapy (279).

Induction Therapy With Cisplatin and 5-Fluorouracil Alone

To date, the only reported randomized trial of induction chemotherapy followed by chemoradiotherapy followed by surgery, compared with surgery alone, has come from Sweden. Ninety-one patients with esophageal cancer (50% squamous cell carcinoma and 50% adenocarcinoma) were randomized to receive one cycle of cisplatin 100 mg/m^2 IV on day 1 and 5-fluorouracil 750 mg/m^2/day via continuous 5-day IV infusion, followed by radiation (64 Gy in 32 fractions) concurrent with the same chemotherapy agents and doses repeated every 3 weeks for two additional cycles during radiation, followed by surgery, or surgery alone. Median overall survival was 12.8 months for the chemoradiotherapy-treated patients versus 15.8 months for patients receiving surgery alone, but 4-year overall survival was 29% for the chemoradiotherapy group compared to 23% for the surgery-alone group, although this was not a statistically significant difference (280).

A randomized trial of induction chemotherapy and chemoradiotherapy followed by surgery, compared to induction chemotherapy followed by surgery, showed an advantage to the combined modality preoperative approach. All patients had adenocarcinoma of the distal esophagus or gastric cardia. Induction chemotherapy consisted of 5-fluorouracil 2,000 mg/m^2 via 24-hour continuous IV infusion weekly for 6 weeks, with leucovorin 500 mg/m^2 IV weekly for 6 weeks, with cisplatin 50 mg/m^2 IV every 2 weeks for 2.5 cycles. Patients randomized to chemoradiotherapy then received cisplatin 50 mg/m^2 IV days 1 and 8 with etoposide 80 mg/m^2 IV days 3 to 5, with radiation (30 Gy in 2 Gy/day fractions), followed by surgery. Patients randomized to induction chemotherapy only proceeded to surgery 3 to 4 weeks after completing induction treatment. The trial was closed early due to poor accrual (only 126 patients enrolled out of a planned total to enroll 354 patients). A complete pathologic response rate was higher in patients receiving induction chemotherapy plus neoadjuvant chemoradiotherapy compared to induction chemotherapy alone (15.6% vs. 2.0%, $P = .03$). Survival at 3 years was also better, although not significantly different, in the group treated with induction chemotherapy plus neoadjuvant chemoradiotherapy (47.4% vs. 27.7% in those given induction chemotherapy only, $P = .07$). All 8 patients achieving a complete pathologic response (1 in the induction chemotherapy only arm vs. 7 in the arm receiving chemoradiotherapy) survived to the median follow-up time of 4.1 years. Treatments appeared to be well tolerated, with less than 5% of patients experiencing a grade 3 or 4 toxicity during the induction phase, and only 12% of patients experiencing myelosuppression during chemoradiotherapy. These results suggested that preoperative chemoradiotherapy plus induction chemotherapy improves survival compared with induction chemotherapy alone (281).

In summary, induction chemotherapy followed by chemoradiotherapy and surgery is an intriguing approach to the management of locally advanced, resectable esophageal cancer. Published trials of this approach to date show results comparable to, but unfortunately no better, than conventional neoadjuvant chemoradiotherapy followed by surgery. In the absence of trials comparing induction chemotherapy plus neoadjuvant chemoradiotherapy followed by surgery to neoadjuvant chemoradiotherapy followed by surgery, this strategy remains investigational, and probably should be employed only in the context of a clinical trial.

SYSTEMIC THERAPY FOLLOWED BY SURGERY (INDUCTION CHEMOTHERAPY)

As with neoadjuvant chemoradiotherapy, induction chemotherapy has been used in patients with locally advanced, resectable esophageal cancer in an effort to downstage disease prior to surgical resection, thus improving local control, and with a goal of increasing overall survival by treating micrometastatic disease. Induction chemotherapy has been studied in this patient population since the 1970s in multiple nonrandomized trials. This section will discuss in detail only recent (i.e., published since 1990) randomized trials of induction chemotherapy followed by esophagectomy. The results of these trials have been incongruent, with some trials suggesting a benefit to induction chemotherapy, but other trials showing no benefit in outcomes with induction chemotherapy.

Randomized Trials Demonstrating a Benefit to Induction Chemotherapy

An early randomized trial of induction chemotherapy randomized 39 patients with resectable squamous cell carcinoma of the esophagus to induction chemotherapy with cisplatin (3 mg/kg or 120 mg/m^2 IV on day 1, whichever was less), vindesine (3 mg/m^2 IV on days 1, 8, 15, and 22) and bleomycin (10 U/m^2/day via continuous IV infusion on days 4–6), followed by surgery, followed by adjuvant cisplatin and vindesine, compared with immediate surgery. A response rate of 47% was seen following induction chemotherapy, and patients who demonstrated a response to chemotherapy had a median survival of 20 months compared with 8.6 months in patients undergoing surgery alone. Overall survival at 3 years was 25% in patients receiving chemotherapy compared with 5% in surgery-only patients (282).

The United Kingdom Medical Research Council Adjuvant Gastric Infusional Chemotherapy (MAGIC) trial randomized patients with locally advanced adenocarcinoma of the distal esophagus and stomach to receive three pre- and three postoperative cycles of epirubicin (50 mg/m^2 IV on day 1), cisplatin (60 mg/m^2 IV on day 1), and 5-fluorouracil (200 mg/m^2/day via 21-day continuous IV infusion for days 1–21), followed by surgery, or surgery alone. Five-year overall survival was 36.3% in patients receiving chemotherapy compared to 23% in surgery-alone treated patients, giving a significantly higher likelihood of treated group (n = 45). The authors speculate that overall survival was not different between the two groups because 86% of patients who recurred in the surgery-only treated group went on to receive systemic therapy (292).

A report from Korea compared outcomes of 52 historical controls undergoing curative esophagectomy with 40 patients receiving adjuvant chemotherapy with three cycles of cisplatin (60 mg/m^2 IV on day 1) and 5-fluorouracil (1,000 mg/m^2/day via continuous IV infusion on days 1–4), repeated every 3 weeks. All patients had squamous cell histology. Overall survival at 3 years was significantly better in patients receiving chemotherapy (47.6%) compared with historical controls (35.6%) (P = .049). More historical controls had distant recurrences (n = 18) than in the chemotherapy-treated patients (n = 9), a difference that was not significantly different (293).

The only trial evaluating adjuvant chemotherapy for adenocarcinoma of the esophagus was conducted by the Eastern Cooperative Oncology Group in the United States. Following R0 resection, 55 patients with T2–4, node positive adenocarcinoma of the distal esophagus, gastroesophageal junction, or gastric cardia received four cycles of paclitaxel 175 mg/m^2 IV on day 1 with cisplatin 75 mg/m^2 IV on day 1, repeated every 21 days. Patients were compared with historical controls (surgery-only treated patients in the aforementioned INT 0113 trial, reference 289). At 2 years, a 60% overall survival rate was observed, compared with 38% of historical controls (P = .0008). A 3-year overall survival of 42% was reported. Myelosuppression, gastrointestinal toxicity, and peripheral neuropathy were common grade 3 or 4 adverse events in 54% of patients (294).

Adjuvant Chemoradiotherapy

Combined modality chemotherapy with radiation has been examined in the adjuvant setting, although in a limited fashion. A United States Intergroup trial (INT 0116) randomized 556 patients with adenocarcinoma of the gastroesophageal junction or stomach completing R0 resection to surgery alone or surgery followed by chemoradiotherapy with 5-fluorouracil 425 mg/m^2 IV on days 1 to 5 plus leucovorin 20 mg/m^2 IV on days 1 to 5, followed 28 days later by radiation (45 Gy in 1.8 Gy/day fractions) with concomitant 5-fluorouracil 400 mg/m^2 IV and leucovorin 20 mg/m^2 IV on the first 4 days and last 3 days of radiation. Median overall survival was 36 months in the chemoradiotherapy arm versus 27 months in the surgery-only arm, giving a hazard ratio for death of 1.35 for surgery-only compared with adjuvant chemoradiotherapy (95% CI 1.09–1.66, P = .005). Overall survival at 3 years was 50% in the chemotherapy arm versus 41% in the surgery-only arm (P value not reported). Relapse-free survival also appeared to favor adjuvant chemoradiotherapy-treated patients, with a hazard ratio for relapse in surgery-only treated patients compared with chemoradiotherapy-treated patients of 1.52 (95% CI 1.23–1.86, $P < .001$). Locoregional relapse rates were also lower in the chemoradiotherapy-treated patients (n = 101) versus patients receiving surgery alone (n = 178), but a statistical analysis of differences in relapse rates was not performed since centers were only required to document a single site of recurrence. Grade 3 or 4 hematologic toxicity (54%) and gastrointestinal toxicity (33%) were the most common adverse events in chemoradiotherapy-treated patients (295). Since only 20% of patients in this trial had cancer involving the esophagus (gastroesophageal junction), while the majority of patients had adenocarcinomas of the distal stomach, the applicability of these findings to a patient with adenocarcinoma of the gastroesophageal junction who has undergone curative resection is limited.

Taken together, these data suggest a role for adjuvant chemotherapy, and possibly adjuvant chemoradiotherapy, for selected patients with locally advanced, lymph node positive esophageal cancer who have undergone R0 resection without preoperative chemotherapy or radiation. In the modern era, such patients are likely few in number, since most patients are given neoadjuvant treatment. Thus, it does not appear that adjuvant chemotherapy will ever have much role in the treatment of patients with locally advanced esophageal cancer, except perhaps as a treatment following neoadjuvant chemoradiotherapy and surgery if further clinical trials demonstrate a benefit to such an approach.

■ CONCLUSIONS

An algorithm for esophageal cancer treatment is presented in Chapter 9, "Radiotherapy for Esophageal Cancer." However, it is important to note that the treatment of esophageal cancer is evolving. Clinical trials currently under way incorporate targeted therapies with conventional chemotherapy in the neoadjuvant, adjuvant, and metastatic treatment settings. In addition, most modern clinical trials now include patients with only one type of histology, rather than the "mixed bag" of histologies included in esophageal cancer trials of the past. Many of these trials also incorporate correlative molecular analyses of patients' tumors and treatment response, thereby gradually moving the treatment of esophageal cancer toward an ever more personalized approach.

A majority of patients with esophageal cancer now receive systemic therapy as a component of their treatment. It may be given prior to surgical resection, as with the induction chemotherapy and/or neoadjuvant chemoradiotherapy strategies, as a component of definitive therapy with radiation for unresectable disease, or as palliative treatment for metastatic disease. No longer are patients with localized esophageal cancer treated strictly in the realm of surgeons or radiation oncologists, only to be sent to the medical oncologist once relapse has occurred or distant metastases have developed. As the incidence of esophageal cancer increases over the coming years, medical oncologists can expect this disease to develop a larger presence in their practice.

It is hoped, of course, that by placing a greater emphasis on risk factor modification, and possibly by making better efforts at and developing better techniques for early detection, the predicted increase in esophageal cancer cases will be mitigated. Until that occurs, the results of trials conducted over the past three decades and the trials currently in progress will help clinicians to develop sound treatment plans for their patients with this difficult, deadly disease.

REFERENCES

1. Pera M, Manterola C, Vidal O, Grande L. Epidemiology of esophageal adenocarcinoma. *J Surg Oncol.* 2005;92(3): 151–159.
2. American Cancer Society. *Cancer Facts & Figures 2000.* Dublin, Ohio: American Cancer Society.
3. American Cancer Society. *Cancer Facts & Figures 2008.* Dublin, Ohio: American Cancer Society.
4. SEER Cancer Statistics. 2009. Available at: http://seer.cancer.gov/statistics. Accessed October 13, 2009.
5. Parkin DM, Bray F, Ferlay J, Pisani P. Global Cancer Statistics, 2002. *CA Cancer J Clin.* 2005;55:74–108.
6. Eslick, GD. Epidemiology of esophageal cancer. *Gastroenterol Clin N Am.* 2009;38:17–25.
7. Blot BJ, Devesa SS, Frauměni JF Jr. Continuing climb in rates of esophageal adenocarcinoma: An update [letter]. *JAMA.* 1993;270:1320.
8. Devesa SS, Bolt, WJ, Fraumeni JF Jr. Changing patterns in the incidence of esophageal and gastric carcinoma in the United States. *Cancer.* 1998;83:2049–2053.
9. Brown LM, Devesa SS, Chow WH. Incidence of adenocarcinoma of the esophagus among white Americans by sex, stage and age. *JNCI.* 2008;100:1184–1187.
10. Zheng T, Mayne ST, Holford TR, et al. The time trend and age-period-cohort effects on incidence of adenocarcinoma of the stomach in Connecticut from 1955–1989. *Cancer.* 1993;72:330–340.
11. Powell J, McConkey CC. Increasing incidence of adenocarcinoma of the gastric cardia and adjacent sites. *Br J Cancer.* 1990;62:440–443.
12. Baquet CR, Commiskey P, Mack K, Meltzer S, Mishra SI. Esophageal cancer epidemiology in blacks and whites: racial and gender disparities in incidence, mortality, survival rates and histology. *J Natl Med Assoc.* 2005;97:1471–1478.
13. Blot WJ, McLaughlin JK. The changing epidemiology of esophageal cancer. *Semin Oncol.* 1999;26:2–8.
14. Posner MC, Forastiere AA, et al. Cancer of the Esophagus. In: DeVita VT, Hellman S, Rosenberg SA, eds. *Cancer: Principles & Practice Of Oncology.* Philadelphia, Lippincott Williams & Wilkins; 2005:861–909.
15. Sons HU. Esophageal cancer: autopsy findings in 171 cases. *Arch Pathol Lab Med.* 1984;108:983–988.
16 Anderson LL, Lad TE. Autopsy findings in squamous cell carcinoma of the esophagus. *Cancer.* 1982;50: 1587–1590.
17. Begin LR. The Pathobiology of Esophageal Cancer in Thoracic Oncology. In: Roth JA, Ruckdeschel JC, Weisenburger TH, eds. Philadelphia, WB Saunders; 1995: 288.
18. Steiger Z, Wilson RF, Leichman L, Busuito MJ, Rosenberg JC. Primary adenocarcinoma of the esophagus. *J Surg Oncol.* 1987;36:68–70.
19. Cameron AJ, Ott BJ, Payne WS. The incidence of adenocarcinoma in columnar-lined (Barrett's) esophagus. *N Engl J Med.* 1985;313:857–859.
20. Drewitz DJ, Sampliner RE, Garewal HS. The incidence of adenocarcinoma in Barrett's esophagus: a prospective study of 170 patients followed 4.8 years. *Am J Gastroenterol.* 1997;92:212–215.
21. Haggit RC, Tryzelaar J, Ellis FH, Colcher H. Adenocarcinoma complicating columnar epithelium-lined (Barrett's) esophagus. *Am J Clin Pathol.* 1978;70:1–5.
22. Skinner DB, Walther BC, Riddell RH, et al. Barrett's esophagus. Comparison of benign and malignant cases. *Ann Surg.* 1983;198:554–565.
23. Smith RR, Hamilton SR, Boitnott JK, Rogers EL. The spectrum of carcinoma arising in Barrett's esophagus. *Am J Surg Pathol.* 1984;8:563–573.
24. Rosenberg JC, Budy H, Edwards RC, et al. Analysis of adenocarcinoma in Barrett's esophagus utilizing a staging system. *Cancer.* 1985;55:1353–1360.
25. Paraf F, Flejou JF, Pignon JP, Fékété F, Potet F. Surgical pathology of adenocarcinoma arising in Barrett's esophagus. *Am J Surg Pathol.* 1995;l19:183–191.

88. Sarbia M, Bektas N, Müller W, et al. Expression of cyclin E in dysplasia, carcinoma, and nonmalignant lesions of Barrett esophagus. *Cancer*. 1999;86:2597–2601.
89. Leckband D, Prakasam A. Mechanism and dynamics of cadherin adhesion. *Annu Rev Biomed Eng*. 2006;8: 259–287.
90. Bailey T, Biddlestone L, Shepherd N, et al. Altered cadherin and catenin complexes in the Barrett's esophagus-dysplasia-adenocarcinoma sequence: correlation with disease progression and dedifferentiation. *Am J Pathol*. 1998;152:135–144.
91. Corn PG, Heath EI, Heitmiller R, et al. Frequent hypermethylation of the 5' CpG island of E-cadherin in esophageal adenocarcinoma. *Clin Cancer Res*. 2001;7: 2765–2769.
92. Lin J, Beerm DG. Molecular biology of upper gastrointestinal malignancies. *Semin Oncol*. 2004;31:476–486.
93. Lam AK. Molecular biology of esophageal squamous cell carcinoma. *Crit Rev Oncol Hematol*. 2000;33:71–90.
94. Ozawa S, Ueda M Ando N, Shimizu N, Abe O. Prognostic significance of epidermal growth factor receptor in esophageal squamous cell carcinomas. *Cancer*. 1989; 63:2167–2173.
95. Itakura Y, Sasano H, Shiga C, et al. Epidermal growth factor receptor overexpression in esophageal carcinoma. *Cancer*. 1994;74:795–804.
96. Ikeda Y, Ozawa S, Ando N, et al. Meanings of c-erbB and int-2 amplification in superficial esophageal squamous cell carcinomas. *Ann Thorac Surg*. 1996;62:830–834.
97. Lam KY, Tin L, Ma L. c-erbB-2 protein expression in oesophageal squamous epithelium from oesophageal squamous cell carcinomas, with special reference to histological grade of carcinoma and pre-invasive lesions. *Eur J Surg Oncol*. 1998;24:431–435.
98. Miyazaki S, Sasano H, Shiga K, et al. Analysis of c-myc oncogene in human esophageal carcinoma: immunohistochemistry, in situ hybridization and Northern and Southern blot studies. *Anticancer Res*. 1992;12: 1747–1756.
99. Lyronis ID, Baritaki S, Bizakis I, Krambovitis E, Spandidos DA. K-ras mutation, HPV infection and smoking or alcohol abuse positively correlate with esophageal squamous carcinoma. *Pathol Oncol Res*. 2008;14:267–273.
100. Lam KY, Loke SI, Chen WZ, Cheung KN, Ma L. Expression of p53 in oesophageal squamous cell carcinoma in Hong Kong Chinese. *Eur J Surg Oncol*. 1995;21:242–247.
101. Casson AG, Tammemagi M, Eskandarian S, et al. p53 alterations in esophageal cancer: associated with clinicopathological features, risk factors, and survival. *J Clin Pathol Mol Pathol*. 1998;51:71–79.
102. Wagata T, Shibagaki I, Imamura M, et al. Loss of 17p mutation of the p53 gene, and overexpression of p53 protein in esophageal squamous cell carcinomas. *Cancer Res*. 1993;53:846–850.
103. Igaki H, Sasaki H, Kishi T, et al. Highly frequent homozygous deletion of the p16 gene in esophageal cancer cell lines. *Biochem Biophys Res Comm*. 1994;203: 1090–1095.
104. Tanaka H, Shimada Y, Imamura M, Shibagaki I, Ishizaki K. Multiple types of aberrations in the p16 (INK4a) and the p15 (INK4b) genes in 30 esophageal squamous cell carcinoma cell lines. *Int J Cancer*. 1997;70:437–432.
105. Jiang W, Zhang YJ, Kahn SM, et al. Altered expression of the cyclin D1 and retinoblastoma genes in human esophageal cancer. *Proc Natl Acad Sci*. 1993;90:9026–9030.
106. Chetty R, Chetty S. Cyclin D1 and retinoblastoma protein expression in oesophageal squamous cell carcinoma. *Mol Pathol*. 1997;50:257–260.
107. Boynton RF, Huang Y, Blount PL, et al. Frequent loss of heterozygosity at the retinoblastoma locus in human esophageal cancer. *Cancer Res*. 1991;51:5766–5769.
108. Boynton R, Blount PL, Yin J, et al. Loss of heterozygosity involving the APC and MCC genetic loci occurs in the majority of human esophageal cancers. *Proc Natl Acad Sci*. 1992;89:3385–3388.
109. Takashima T, Fujiwara Y, Hamaguchi M, et al. Relationship between peroxisome proliferator-activated receptor-gamma expression and differentiation of human esophageal squamous cell carcinoma. *Oncol Rep*. 2005;13: 601–606.
110. Iwaya T, Maesawa C, Ogasawara S, Tamura G. Tylosis esophageal cancer locus on chromosome 17q25.1 is commonly deleted in sporadic human esophageal cancer. *Gastroenterology*. 1998;114:1206–1210.
111. von Brevern M, Hollstein MC, Risk JM, et al. Loss of heterozygosity in sporadic oesophageal tumors in the tylosis oesophageal cancer (TOC) gene region of chromosome 17q. *Oncogene*. 1998;17:2101–2105.
112. Shibakita M, Tachibana M, Dhar DK, et al. Prognostic significance of Fas and Fas ligand expressions in human esophageal cancer. *Clin Cancer Res*. 1999;5:2464–2469.
113. Dabrowski A, Filip A, Zgodziński W, et al. Assessment of prognostic significance of cytoplasmic survivin expression in advanced esophageal cancer. *Folia Histochem Cytobiol*. 2004;42: 169–172.
114. Puglisi F, Di Loreto C, Panizzo R, et al. Expression of p53 and bcl-2 and response to preoperative chemotherapy and radiotherapy for locally advanced squamous cell carcinoma of the esophagus. *J Clin Pathol*. 1996;49: 456–459.
115. Koide N, Koike S, Adachi W, et al. Immunohistochemical expression of bcl-2 protein in squamous cell carcinoma and basaloid carcinoma of the esophagus. *Surg Today*. 1997;27:685–691.
116. Ohbu M, Saegusa M, Kobayashi N, et al. Expression of bcl-2 protein in esophageal squamous cell carcinomas and its association with lymph node metastasis. *Cancer*. 1997;79:1287–1293.
117. Naitoh H, Shibata J, Kawaguchi A, Kodama M, Hattori T. Overexpression and localization of cyclin D1 mRNA and antigen in esophageal cancer. *Am J Pathol*. 1995;146:1161–1169.
118. Gramlich TL, Fritsch CR, Maurer D, Eberle M, Gansler TS. Differential polymerase chain reaction assay of

cyclin D1 gene amplification in esophageal carcinoma. *Diagn Mol Pathol.* 1994;3:255–259.
119. Sarbi M, Stahl M, Fink U, et al. Prognostic significance of cyclin D1 in esophageal squamous cell carcinoma patients treated with surgery alone or combined therapy modalities. *Int J Cancer Pred Oncol.* 1999;84:86–91.
120. Pelucchi C, Gallus S, Garavello W, Bosetti C, La Vecchia C. Alcohol and tobacco use, and cancer risk for upper aerodigestive tract and liver. *Eur J Cancer Prev.* 2008;17:340–344.
121. Engel LS, Chow WH, Vaughan TL, et al. Population attributable risks of esophageal and gastric cancers. *J Natl Cancer Inst.* 2003;95:1404–1413.
122. Lagergren J, Bergstrom R, Lindgren A, Nyrén O. The role of tobacco, snuff and alcohol use in the aetiology of cancer of the esophagus and gastric cardia. *Int J Cancer.* 2000;85:340–346.
123. Kabat GC, Ng SK, Wynder EL. Tobacco, alcohol intake, and diet in relation to adenocarcinoma of the esophagus and gastric cardia. *Cancer Causes Control.* 1993;4:123–132.
124. Gammon MD, Schoenberb JB, Ahsan H, et al. Tobacco, alcohol, and socioeconomic status and adenocarcinomas of the esophagus and gastric cardia. *J Natl Cancer Inst.* 1997;89:1277–1284.
125. Brown LM, Hoover R, Silverman D, et al. Excess incidence of squamous cell esophageal cancer among US black men: role of social class and other risk factors. *Am J Epidemiol.* 2001;153:114–122.
126. Castellsague X, Munoz N, De Stefani E, et al. Smoking and drinking cessation and risk of esophageal cancer (Spain). *Cancer Causes Control.* 2000;11:813–818.
127. Kubo A, Levin TR, Block G, et al. Dietary antioxidant, fruits, and vegetables and the risk of Barrett's esophagus. *Am J Gastroenterol.* 2008;103:1614–1623.
128. Mayne ST, Risch HA, Dubrow R, et al. Nutrient intake and risk of subtypes of esophageal and gastric cancer. *Cancer Epidemiol Biomarkers Prev.* 2001;10:1055–1062.
129. Larsson SC, Giovannucci E, Wolk A. Folate intake, MTHFR polymorphisms, and risk of esophageal, gastric, and pancreatic cancer: a meta-analysis. *Gastroenterology.* 2006;131:1271–1283.
130. Lu SH, Montesano R, Zhang MS, et al. Relevance of N-nitrosamines to esophageal cancer in China. *J Cell Physiol Suppl.* 1986;4:51–58.
131. Yang WX. [Exposure level of N-nitrosamines in the gastric juice and its inhibition by vitamin C in high risk areas of esophageal cancer.] *Zhonghua Zhong Liu Za Zhi.* 1992;14:407–410.
132. Ghadirian P. Thermal irritation and esophageal cancer in northern Iran. *Cancer.* 1987;60:1909–1914.
133. Mark SD, Qiao YL, Dawsey SM, et al. Prospective study of serum selenium levels and incident esophageal and gastric cancers. *J Natl Cancer Inst.* 2000;92:1753–1763.
134. Abnet CC, Lai B, Qiao YL, et al. Zinc concentration in esophageal biopsy specimens measured by x-ray fluorescence and esophageal cancer risk. *J Natl Cancer Inst.* 2005;97:301–306.
135. Ashworth MT, Nash JR, Ellis A, Day DW. Abnormalities of differentiation and maturation in the oesophageal squamous epithelium of patients with tylosis: morphological features. *Histopathology.* 1991;19:303–310.
136. Stoler MH. Human papillomaviruses and cervical neoplasia: a model for carcinogenesis. *Int J Gynecol Pathol.* 2000;19:16–28.
137. Lam KY, He D, Ma L, et al. Presence of human papillomavirus in esophageal squamous cell carcinomas in Hong Kong Chinese and its relationship with p53 gene mutation. *Hum Pathol.* 1997;28:657–663.
138. Shuyama K, Castillo A, Aguayo F, et al. Human papillomavirus in high- and low-risk areas of oesophageal squamous cell carcinoma in China. *Br J Cancer.* 2007; 96:1554–1559.
139. Poljak M, Cerar A, Seme K. Human papillomavirus infection in esophageal carcinomas: a study of 121 lesions using multiple broad-spectrum polymerase chain reactions and literature review. *Hum Pathol.* 1998;29: 266–271.
140. Rugge M, Bovo D, Busatto G, et al. p53 alterations but no human papillomavirus infection in preinvasive and advanced squamous esophageal cancer in Italy. *Cancer Epidemiol Biomarkers Prev.* 1997;6:171–176.
141. Turner JR, Shen LH, Crum CP, Dean PJ, Odze RD. Low prevalence of human papillomavirus infection in squamous cell carcinomas from North America: analysis by a highly sensitive and specific polymerase chain reaction-based approach. *Hum Pathol.* 1997;28:174–178.
142. Lagergren J, Wang Z, Bergström R, Dillner J, Nyrén O. Human papillomavirus infection and esophageal cancer: a nationwide seroepidemiologic case-control study in Sweden. *J Natl Cancer Inst.* 1999;91:156–162.
143. Xia HH, Talley NJ. Helicobacter pylori infection, reflux esophagitis, and atrophic gastritis: an unexplored triangle. *Am J Gastroenterol.* 1998;93:394–400.
144. Rokkas T, Pistiolas D, Sechopoulos P, Robotis I, Margantinis G. Relationship between Helicobacter pylori infection and esophageal neoplasia: a meta-analysis. *Clin Gastroenterol Hepatol.* 2007;5:1413–1417.
145. Vicari JJ, Peek RM, Falk GW, et al. The seroprevalence of cag-A positive Helicobacter pylori strains in the spectrum of gastroesophageal reflux. *Gastroenterology.* 1998;115:50–57.
146. Chow WH, Blaser MJ, Blot WJ, et al. An inverse relationship between cagA+ strains of Helicobacter pylori infection and risk of esophageal and gastric cardia adenocarcinoma. *Cancer Res.* 1998;58:588–590.
147. Loffeld RJ, Ten Tije BJ, Arends JW. Prevalence and significance of Helicobacter pylori in patients with Barrett's esophagus. *Am J Gastroenterol.* 1992;87:1598–1600.
148. Csendes A, Smok G, Cerda G, et al. Prevalence of Helicobacter pylori infection in 190 control subjects and 236 patients with gastroesophageal reflux, erosive esophagitis or Barrett's esophagus. *Dis Esophagus.* 1997; 10:38–42.
149. Leon X, Quer M, et al. Second neoplasms in patients with head and neck cancer. *Head Neck.* 1999;21:204–210.

150. Levi F, Randimbison L, Te VC, La Vecchia C. Second primary cancers in patients with lung carcinoma. *Cancer.* 1999;86:186–190.
151. Muto M, Hironaka S, Nakane M, et al. Association of multiple Lugol-voiding lesions with synchronous and metachronous esophageal squamous cell carcinoma in patients with head and neck cancer. *Gastrointest Endosc.* 2002;56:517–521.
152. Sandler RS, Nyren O, Ekbom A, et al. The risk of esophageal cancer in patients with achalasia: A population-based study. *JAMA.* 1995;274:1359–1362.
153. Appelqvist P, Salmo M. Lye corrosion carcinoma of the esophagus: a review of 63 cases. *Cancer.* 1980;45: 2655–2658.
154. Ribeiro U, Posner MC, et al. Risk factors for squamous cell carcinoma of the esophagus. *Br J Surg.* 1996;83: 1174–1185.
155. Lagergren J, Bergstrom R, Adami HO, Nyrén O. Association between medications that relax the lower esophageal sphincter and risk for esophageal adenocarcinoma. *Ann Intern Med.* 2000;133:165–175.
156. Vaughan TL, Farrow DC, Hansten PD, et al. Risk of esophageal and gastric adenocarcinomas in relation to use of calcium channel blockers, asthma drugs, and other medications that promote gastroesophageal reflux. *Cancer Epidemiol Biomarkers Prev.* 1998;7:749–756.
157. Corley DA, Levin TR, Habel LA, Buffler PA. Barrett's esophagus and medications that relax the lower esophageal sphincter. *Am J Gastroenterol.* 2006;101:937–944.
158. Wysowski DK. Reports of esophageal cancer with oral bisphosphonate use. *N Engl J Med.* 2009;360:89–90.
159. Chow WH, Blot WJ, Vaughan TL, et al. Body mass index and risk of adenocarcinomas of the esophagus and gastric cardia. *J Natl Cancer Inst.* 1998;90:150–155.
160. Cook MB, Greenwood DC, Hardie LJ, Wild CP, Forman D. A systematic review and meta-analysis of the risk of increasing adiposity on Barrett's esophagus. *Am J Gastroenterol.* 2008;103:292–300.
161. Hampel H, Abraham NS, El-Serag HB. Meta-analysis: obesity and the risk for gastroesophageal reflux disease and its complications. *Ann Intern Med.* 2005;143:199–211.
162. Lagergren J, Bergstrom R, Lindgren A, Nyrén O. Symptomatic gastroesophageal reflux as a risk factor for esophageal adenocarcinoma. *N Engl J Med.* 1999;340: 825–831.
163. Chow WH, Finkle WD, McLaughlin JK, et al. The relation of gastroesophageal reflux disease and its treatment to adenocarcinoma of the esophagus and gastric cardia. *JAMA.* 1995;274:474–477.
164. O'Connor JB, Falk JW, et al. The incidence of adenocarcinoma and dysplasia in Barrett's esophagus: report on the Cleveland Clinic's Barrett's Esophagus Registry. *Am J Gastroenterol.* 1999;94:2037–2042.
165. Shaheen NJ, Crosby MA, Bozymski EM, Sandler RS. Is there a publication bias in the reporting of cancer risk in Barrett's esophagus? *Gastroenterology.* 2000;119:333–338.
166. Rudolph RE, Vaughan TL, Storer BE, et al. Effect of segment length on risk for neoplastic progression in patients with Barrett's esophagus. *Ann Intern Med.* 2000;132:612–620.
167. Corley DA, Kubo A, Levin TR, et al. Abdominal obesity and body mass index as risk factors for Barrett's esophagus. *Gastroenterology.* 2007;133:34–41.
168. Edelstein ZR, Farrow DC, Bronner MP, Rosen SN, Vaughan TL. Central adiposity and risk of Barrett's esophagus. *Gastroenterology.* 2007;133:403–411.
169. Csendes A, Smok G, et al. Prevalence of Barrett's esophagus by endoscopy and histology studies: a prospective evaluation of 306 control subjects and 376 patients with symptoms of gastroesophageal reflux. *Dis Esophagus.* 2000;13:5–11.
170. Belhocine K, Galmiche JP. Epidemiology of the complications of gastroesophageal reflux disease. *Dig Dis.* 2009;27:7–13.
171. Wang KK, Sampliner RE. Updated guidelines 2008 for the diagnosis, surveillance and therapy of Barrett's esophagus. *Am J Gastroenterol.* 2008;103:788–797.
172. Yagoda A, Mukherji B, Young C, et al. Bleomycin, an antitumor antibiotic. Clinical experience in 274 patients. *Ann Intern Med.* 1972;77:861–870.
173. Stephens FO. Bleomycin—a new approach in cancer chemotherapy. *Med J Aust.* 1973;1:1277–1283.
174. Ravry M, Moertel CG, Schutt AJ, Hahn RG, Reitemeier RJ. Treatment of advanced squamous cell carcinoma of the gastrointestinal tract with bleomycin (NSC-125066). *Cancer Chemother Rep.* 1973;47:493–495.
175. Ezdinli ER, Gelber R, Desai DV, et al. Chemotherapy of advanced esophageal adenocarcinoma: Eastern Cooperative Oncology Group experience. *Cancer.* 1980; 46:2149–2153.
176. Advani SH, Saikia TK, Swaroop S, et al. Anterior chemotherapy in esophageal cancer. *Cancer.* 1985;56: 1502–1506.
177. Whittington RM, Close HP. Clinical experience with mitomycin C (NSC-26980). *Cancer Chemother Rep.* 1970;54:195–198.
178. Bleiberg H, Conroy T, Paillot B, et al. Randomised phase II study of cisplatin and 5-fluorouracil (5-FU) versus cisplatin alone in advanced squamous cell oesophageal cancer. *Eur J Cancer.* 1997;33:1216–1220.
179. Beer M, Cocconi G, et al. A phase II study of cisplatin in advanced esophageal cancer. *Eur J Cancer Clin Oncol.* 1983;19:717–720.
180. Kok TC, van der Gaast A, Splinter TA. et al. 5-fluorouracil and folinic acid in advanced adenocarcinoma of the esophagus or esophago-gastric junction area. Rotterdam Esophageal Tumor Study Group. *Ann Oncol.* 1996;7: 533–534.
181. Alberts AS, Schoeman L, et al. A phase II study of 5-flurouracil and leucovorin in advanced carcinoma of the esophagus. *Am J Clin Oncol.* 1992;15:35–36.
182. Ohtsu A, Shimada Y, Shirao K, et al. Randomized phase III trial of fluorouracil alone versus fluorouracil plus cisplatin versus uracil and tegafur plus mitomycin in

patients with unresectable, advanced gastric cancer: The Japanese Clinical Oncology Group Study (JCOG9205). *J Clin Oncol.* 2003;21:54–59.
183. Koizumi W, Narahara H, Hara T, et al. S-1 plus cisplatin versus S-1 alone for first-line treatment of advanced gastric cancer (SPIRITS trial): a phase III trial. *Lancet Oncol.* 2008;9:214–221.
184. Cullinan SA, Moertel CG, Fleming TR, et al. A comparison of three chemotherapeutic regimens in the treatment of advanced pancreatic and gastric carcinoma. Fluorouracil vs fluorouracil and doxorubicin vs fluorouracil, doxorubicin, and mitomycin. *JAMA.* 1985; 253:2061–2067.
185. Wagner AD, Grothe W, Haerting J, et al. Chemotherapy in advanced gastric cancer: a systematic review and meta-analysis based on aggregate data. *J Clin Oncol.* 2006;24:2903–2909.
186. National Comprehensive Cancer Network. (2009). NCCN Clinical Practice Guidelines in Oncology. Esophageal Cancer. Available at: http://www.nccn.org. Accessed July 1, 2009.
187. Findlay M, Cunningham D, Norman A, et al. A phase II study in advanced gastro-esophageal cancer using epirubicin and cisplatin in combination with continuous infusion 5-fluorouracil (ECF). *Ann Oncol.* 1994;5:609–616.
188. Webb A, Cunningham D, Scarffe JH, et al. Randomized trial comparing epirubicin, cisplatin, and fluorouracil versus fluorouracil, doxorubicin, and methotrexate in advanced esophagogastric cancer. *J Clin Oncol.* 1997;15:261–267.
189. Cunningham D, Starling N, Rao S, et al. Capecitabine and oxaliplatin for advanced esophagogastric cancer. *N Engl J Med.* 2008;358:36–46.
190. Choi IK, Seo HY, Sung HJ, et al. Epirubicin, cisplatin, oral UFT, and leucovorin combination chemotherapy in advanced and metastatic esophageal cancer. *Med Oncol.* 2007;24:33–37.
191. Koizumi W, Narahara H, Hara T, et al. S-1 plus cisplatin versus S-1 alone for first-line treatment of advanced gastric cancer (SPIRITS trial): a phase III trial. *Lancet Oncol.* 2008;9:214–221.
192. Ajani JA, Lee FC, Singh DA, et al. Multicenter phase II trial of S-1 plus cisplatin in patients with untreated advanced gastric or gastroesophageal junction adenocarcinoma. *J Clin Oncol.* 2006;24:663–667.
193. Polee MB, Eskens FA, van der Burg ME, et al. Phase II study of bi-weekly administration of paclitaxel and cisplatin in patients with advanced oesophageal cancer. *Br J Cancer.* 2002;86:669–673.
194. Petrasch S, Welt A, Reinacher A, et al. Chemotherapy with cisplatin and paclitaxel in patients with locally advanced, recurrent or metastatic oesophageal cancer. *Br J Cancer.* 1998;511–514.
195. Ilson DH, Forastiere A, Arquette M, et al. A phase II trial of paclitaxel and cisplatin in patients with advanced carcinoma of the esophagus. *Cancer J.* 2000;6:316–323.
196. Huang T, Tsai Y, et al. Weekly paclitaxel, cisplatin, and 24-hour infusion of high-dose 5-fluorouracil plus leucovorin (weekly TP-HDFL) in patients with metastatic or recurrent esophageal cancer. (Abstract.) *J Clin Oncol.* 2007;25:647s. 197. El-Rayes BF, Shields A, Zalupski M, et al. A phase II study of carboplatin and paclitaxel in esophageal cancer. *Ann Oncol.* 2004;15: 960–965.
198. Lokich JJ, Sonneborn H, Anderson NR, et al. Combined paclitaxel, cisplatin, and etoposide for patients with previously untreated esophageal and gastroesophageal carcinomas. *Cancer.* 1999;85:2347–2351.
199. Sharma A, Raina V, Lokeshwar N, et al. Phase II study of cisplatin, etoposide and paclitaxel in locally advanced or metastatic adenocarcinoma of gastric/gastroesophageal junction. *Indian J Cancer.* 2006;43:16–19.
200. Heath EI, Urba S, Marshall J, Piantadosi S, Forastiere AA. Phase II trial of docetaxel chemotherapy in patients with incurable adenocarcinoma of the esophagus. *Invest New Drugs.* 2002;20:95–99.
201. Van Cutsem E, Moiseyenko VM, Tjulandin S, et al. Phase III study of docetaxel and cisplatin plus fluorouracil compared with cisplatin and fluorouracil as first-line therapy for advanced gastric cancer: a report of the V325 Study Group. *J Clin Oncol.* 2006;24:4991–4997.
202. Thuss-Patience PC, Kretzschmar A, Repp M, et al. Docetaxel and continuous-infusion fluorouracil versus epirubicin, cisplatin, and fluorouracil for advanced gastric adenocarcinoma: A randomized phase II study. *J Clin Oncol.* 2005;23:494–501.
203. Roth AD, Fazio N, Stupp R, et al. Docetaxel, cisplatin, and fluorouracil; docetaxel and cisplatin; and epirubicin, cisplatin, and fluorouracil as systemic treatment for advanced gastric carcinoma: a randomized phase II trial of the Swiss Group for Clinical Cancer Research. *J Clin Oncol.* 2007;25:3217–3223.
204. Giordano KF, Jatoi A, Stella PJ, et al. Docetaxel and capecitabine in patients with metastatic adenocarcinoma of the stomach and gastroesophageal junction: a phase II study from the North Central Cancer Treatment Group. *Ann Oncol.* 2006;17:652–656.
205. Kim JG, Sohn SK, Kim DH, et al. Phase II study of docetaxel and capecitabine in patients with metastatic or recurrent gastric cancer. *Oncology.* 2005;68:190–195.
206. Chun JH, Kim HK, Lee JS, et al. Weekly docetaxel in combination with capecitabine in patients with metastatic gastric cancer. *Am J Clin Oncol.* 2005;28:188–194.
207. Lordick F, Lorenzen S, Stollfuss J, et al. Phase II study of weekly oxaliplatin plus infusional fluorouracil and folinic acid (FUFOX regimen) as first-line treatment in metastatic gastric cancer. *Br J Cancer.* 2005; 93:190–194.
208. van Meerten E, Eskens FA, van Gameren EC, Doorn L, van der Gaast A. First-line treatment with oxaliplatin and capecitabine in patients with advanced or metastatic oesophageal cancer: a phase II study. *Br J Cancer.* 2007;96:1348–1352.
209. Jatoi A, Murphy BR, Foster NR, et al. Oxaliplatin and capecitabine in patients with metastatic adenocarcinoma of the esophagus, gastroesophageal junction and gastric

cardia: a phase II study from the North Central Cancer Treatment Group. *Ann Oncol.* 2006;17:29–34.
210. Park YH, Kim BS, Ryoo BY, Yang SH. A phase II study of capecitabine plus 3-weekly oxaliplatin as first-line therapy for patients with advanced gastric cancer. *Br J Cancer.* 2006;94:959–963.
211. Ilson DH. Phase II trial of weekly irinotecan/cisplatin in advanced esophageal cancer. *Oncology (Williston Park).* 2004;18:22–25.
212. Ilson D, Saltz L, Enzinger P, et al. Phase II trial of weekly irinotecan plus cisplatin in advanced esophageal cancer. *J Clin Oncol.* 1999;17:3270–3275.
213. Boku N, Ohtsu A, Shimada Y, et al. Phase II study of a combination of irinotecan and cisplatin against metastatic gastric cancer. *J Clin Oncol.* 1999;17:319–323.
214. Jatoi A, Tirona MT, Cha SS, et al. A phase II trial of docetaxel and CPT-11 in patients with metastatic adenocarcinoma of the esophagus, gastroesophageal junction, and gastric cardia. *Int J Gastrointest Cancer.* 2002;32:115–123.
215. Enzinger PC, Ryan DP, Clark JW, et al. Weekly docetaxel, cisplatin, and irinotecan (TPC): results of a multicenter phase II trial in patients with metastatic esophagogastric cancer. *Ann Oncol.* 2009;20:475–480.
216. Dank M, Zaluski J, Barone C,et al. Randomized phase III study comparing irinotecan combined with 5-fluorouracil and folinic acid to cisplatin combined with 5-fluorouracil in chemotherapy naïve patients with advanced adenocarcinoma of the stomach or esophagogastric junction. *Ann Oncol.* 2008;19:1450–1457.
217. Oh SC, Sur HY, Sung HJ, et al. A phase II study of biweekly dose-intensified oral capecitabine plus irinotecan (bXELIRI) for patients with advanced or metastatic gastric cancer. *Br J Cancer.* 2007;96:1514–1519.
218. Di Lauro L, Nunziata C, Arena MG, et al. Irinotecan, docetaxel and oxaliplatin combination in metastatic gastric or gastroesophageal junction adenocarcinoma. *Br J Cancer.* 2007;97:593–597.
219. Lorenzen S, Schuster T, Porschen R, et al. Cetuximab plus cisplatin-5-fluorouracil versus cisplatin-5-fluorouracil alone in first-line metastatic squamous cell carcinoma of the esophagus: a randomized phase II study of the Arbeitsgemeinschaft Internistische Onkologie. *Ann Oncol.* 2009;10:1667–1673.
220. Pinto C, Di Fabio F, Siena S,et al. Phase II study of cetuximab in combination with FOLFIRI in patients with untreated advanced gastric or gastroesophageal junction adenocarcinoma (FOLCETUX study). *Ann Oncol.* 2007;18:510–517.
221. Pinto C, Di Fabio F, et al. Cetuximab in combination with cisplatin and docetaxel as first-line treatment in patients with locally advanced or metastatic gastric or gastroesophageal junction (GEJ) adenocarcinoma (Italian phase II DOCETUX study) (Abstract). *J Clin Oncol.* 2008;26:231s.
222. Lordick F, Lorenzen S, et al. Cetuximab plus weekly oxaliplatin/5-FU/FA in first line metastatic gastric cancer. Final results from a multicenter phase II study of the AIO upper GI study group (abstract). *J Clin Oncol.* 2007;25:204s.
223. Gold PJ, Goldman B, et al. Cetuximab as second-line therapy in patients with metastatic esophageal cancer: a phase II Southwest Oncology Group Study (abstract). *J Clin Oncol.* 2008;26:222s.
224. Dragovich T, McCoy S, Fenoglio-Preiser CM,et al. Phase II trial of erlotinib in gastroesophageal junction and gastric adenocarcinomas: SWOG 0127. *J Clin Oncol.* 2006;24:4922–4927.
225. Janmaat ML, Gallegos-Ruiz MI, Rodriguez JA, et al. Predictive factors for outcome in a phase II study of gefitinib in second-line treatment of advanced esophageal cancer patients. *J Clin Oncol.* 2006;24:1612–1619.
226. Ferry DR, Anderson M, Beddard K, et al. A phase II study of gefitinib monotherapy in advanced esophageal adenocarcinoma: evidence of gene expression, cellular, and clinical response. *Clin Cancer Res.* 2007;13:5869–5875.
227. Fondevila C, Metges JP, Fuster J, et al. p53 and VEGF expression are independent predictors of tumor recurrence and survival following curative resection of gastric cancer. *Br J Cancer.* 2004;90:206–215.
228. Shah MA, Ramanathan RK, Ilson DH, et al. Multicenter phase II study of irinotecan, cisplatin, and bevacizumab in patients with metastatic gastric or gastroesophageal junction adenocarcinoma. *J Clin Oncol.* 2006;24:5201–5206.
229. Bang Y, Kang Y, et al. Sunitinib as second-line treatment for advanced gastric cancer: preliminary results from a phase II study (abstract). *J Clin Oncol.* 2007;25:223s.
230. Lorenzen S, Duyster J, Lersch C, et al. Capecitabine plus docetaxel every 3 weeks in first- and second-line metastatic oesophageal cancer: final results of a phase II trial. *Br J Cancer.* 2005;92:2129–2133.
231. Kim Y, Park S, et al. Oxaliplatin, 5-fluorouracil, and leucovorin (FOLFOX4) combination chemotherapy as salvage treatment in pretreated patients with advanced gastric cancer (abstract). *J Clin Oncol.* 2008;26:232s.
232. Assersohn L, Brown G, Cunningham D, et al. Phase II study of irinotecan and 5-fluorouracil/leucovorin in patients with primary refractory or relapsed advanced oesophageal and gastric carcinoma. *Ann Oncol.* 2004; 15:64–69.
233. Leary A, Assersohn L, et al. A phase II study evaluating capecitabine and irinotecan as second line treatment in patients with oesophago-gastric cancer who have progressed on, or within 3 months of platinum-based chemotherapy. *Cancer Chemother Pharmachol.* 2009;64:455–462.
234. Burkart C, Bokemeyer C, Klump B, et al. A phase II trial of weekly irinotecan in cisplatin-refractory esophageal cancer. *Anticancer Res.* 2007;27:2845–2848.
235. Lordick F, von Schilling C, Bernhard H, et al. Phase II trial of irinotecan plus docetaxel in cisplatin-pretreated relapsed or refractory oesophageal cancer. *Br J Cancer.* 2003;89:630–633.
236. Jin J, Xu X, et al. Second-line combination chemotherapy with docetaxel and nedaplatin for cisplatin-refractory

metastatic/recurrent esophageal squamous cell carcinoma. 2009 June 17. [Epub ahead of print].

237. Tanaka T, Fujita H, Sueyoshi S, et al. Second-line combination chemotherapy with docetaxel for cisplatin-pretreated refractory metastatic esophageal cancer: a preliminary report of initial experience. *Chemotherapy.* 2007;53:449–453.
238. Park BB, Im YH, et al. Salvage chemotherapy with mitomycin D, ifosfamide, and cisplatin (MIC) for previously treated metastatic or recurrent esophageal squamous cell carcinoma. *Invest New Drugs.* 2008;26: 387–392.
239. Suntharalingham M, Moughan J, Coia LR, et al. The national practice for patients receiving radiation therapy for carcinoma of the esophagus: results of the 1996–1999 patterns of care study. *Int J Radiat Oncol Biol Phys.* 2003;56:981–987.
240. Araujo C, Souhami L, Gil RA, et al. A randomized trial comparing radiation therapy versus concomitant radiation therapy and chemotherapy in carcinoma of the thoracic esophagus. *Cancer.* 1991;67:2258–2261.
241. Roussel A, Haegele B, et al. Results of the EORTC-GTCCG phase III trial of irradiation vs irradiation and CDDP in inoperable esophageal cancer (abstract). *Proc Am Soc Clin Oncol.* 1994;13:199.
242. Slabber CF, Nel JS, Schoeman L, et al. A randomized study of radiotherapy alone versus radiotherapy plus 5-fluorouracil and platinum in patients with inoperable, locally advanced squamous cell cancer of the esophagus. *Am J Clin Oncol.* 1998;21:462–465.
243. Andersen AP, Berdal P, Edsmyr F, et al. Irradiation, chemotherapy and surgery in esophageal cancer: A randomized clinical study. *Radiother Oncol.* 1984;2:179–188.
244. Kaneta T, Takai Y, Nemoto K, et al. Effect of combination chemotherapy with daily low-dose CDDP for esophageal cancer: results of a randomized trial. *Jpn J Cancer Chemother.* 1997;24:2099–2104.
245. Cooper JS, Guo MD, Herskovic A, et al. Chemoradiotherapy of locally advanced esophageal cancer: long-term follow-up of a prospective randomized trial (RTOG 85–01). *JAMA.* 1999;281:1623–1627.
246. Roussel A, Bleiberg H, Dalesio O, et al. Palliative therapy f inoperable oesophageal carcinoma with radiotherapy and methotrexate: final results of a controlled clinical trial. *Int J Radiat Oncol Biol Phys.* 1989;16:67–72.
247. Zhou JC. [Randomized trial of combined chemotherapy including high dose cisplatin, and radiotherapy for esophageal cancer (Chinese)]. *Chung Hua Chung Liu Tsa Chih.* 1991;13:291–294.
248. Hishikawa Y, Miura T, et al. A randomized prospective study of adjuvant chemotherapy after radiotherapy in unresectable esophageal carcinoma. *Dis Esophagus.* 1991;4:85–90.
249. Hatlevoll R, Hagen S, Hansen HS,et al. Bleomycin/cis-platin as neoadjuvant chemotherapy before radical radiotherapy in localized, inoperable carcinoma of the esophagus: A prospective randomized multicentre study—the second Scandinavian trial in esophageal cancer. *Radiother Oncol.* 1992;24:114–116.
250. Lu XJ, Miao RH, et al. [Combination of selective arterial infusion chemotherapy with radiotherapy in the treatment of advanced esophageal carcinoma (Chinese)]. *Chinese J Clin Oncol.* 1995;22:262–265.
251. Wong RK, Malthaner RA, Zuraw L, et al. Combined modality radiotherapy and chemotherapy in nonsurgical management of localized carcinoma of the esophagus: a practice guideline. *Int J Radiat Oncol Biol Phys.* 2003;55:930–942.
252. al-Sarraf M, Martz K, Herskovic A, et al. Progress report of combined chemoradiotherapy versus radiotherapy alone in patients with esophageal cancer: an intergroup study. *J Clin Oncol.* 1997;15:277–284.
253. Herskovic A, Martz K, al-Sarraf M, et al. Combined chemotherapy and radiotherapy compared with radiotherapy alone in patients with cancer of the esophagus. *N Engl J Med.* 1992;326:1593–1598.
254. National Cancer Institute. Esophageal Cancer Treatment PDQ. 2009. Available at: http://www.cancer.gov/cancertopics/pdq/treatment/esophageal/HealthProfessional/page9. Accessed July 13, 2009.
255. Conroy T, Yataghene Y, et al. Definitive chemoradiotherapy (CRT) with folfox 4 or 5FU-cisplatin as first line treatment for patients (pts) with inoperable esophageal cancer (IEC): final results of a randomized phase II study (abstract). *J Clin Oncol.* 2007;25:205s.
256. Kim DW, Blanke CD, Wu H, et al. Phase II study of preoperative paclitaxel/cisplatin with radiotherapy in locally advanced esophageal cancer. *Int J Radiother Oncol Biol Phys.* 2007;67:397–404.
257. Stahl M, Stuschke M, Lehmann N, et al. Chemoradiation with and without surgery in patients with locally advanced squamous cell carcinoma of the esophagus. *J Clin Oncol.* 2005;23:2310–2317.
258. Ajani JA, Winter K, Komaki R, et al. Phase II randomized trial of two nonoperative regimens of induction chemotherapy followed by chemoradiation in patients with localized carcinoma of the esophagus: RTOG 0113. *J Clin Oncol.* 2008;26:4551–4556.
259. Geh JI, Crellin AM, Glynne-Jones R. Preoperative (neoadjuvant) chemoradiotherapy in oesophageal cancer. *Br J Surg.* 2001;88:338–356.
260. Siewert JR, Ott K. Are squamous and adenocarcinomas of the esophagus the same disease? *Semin Radiat Oncol.* 2007;17:38–44.
261. Walsh TN, Noonan N, Hollywood D, et al. A comparison of multimodality therapy and surgery for esophageal adenocarcinoma. *N Engl J Med.* 1996;335: 462–467.
262. Tepper J, Krasna MJ, Niedzwiecki D, et al. Phase III trial of trimodality therapy with cisplatin, fluorouracil, radiotherapy, and surgery compared with surgery alone for esophageal cancer: CALGB 9781. *J Clin Oncol.* 2008;26:1086–1092.
263. Bosset JF, Gignoux M, Triboulet JP, et al. Chemoradiotherapy followed by surgery compared with surgery alone in squamous-cell cancer of the esophagus. *N Engl J Med.* 1997;337:161–167.

264. Le Prise E, Etienne PL, Meunier B, et al. A randomized study of chemotherapy, radiation therapy, and surgery versus surgery for localized squamous cell carcinoma of the esophagus. *Cancer.* 1994;73:1779–1784.
265. Urschel JD, Vasan H. A meta-analysis of randomized controlled trials that compared neoadjuvant chemoradiation and surgery to surgery alone for resectable esophageal cancer. *Am J Surg.* 2003;185:538–543.
266. Gebski V, Burmeister B, Smithers BM, et al. Survival benefits from neoadjuvant chemoradiotherapy or chemotherapy in oesophageal carcinoma: a meta-analysis. *Lancet Oncol.* 2007;8:226–234.
267. Meluch AA, Greco FA, Gray JR, et al. Preoperative therapy with concurrent paclitaxel/carboplatin/infusional 5-FU and radiation therapy in locoregional esophageal cancer: final results of a Minnie Pearl Cancer Research Network phase II trial. *Cancer J.* 2003;9:251–260.
268. van de Schoot L, Romme EA, van der Sangen MJ, et al. A highly active and tolerable neoadjuvant regimen combining paclitaxel, carboplatin, 5-FU and radiation therapy in patients with stage II and III esophageal cancer. *Ann Surg Oncol.* 2008;15:88–95.
269. Chiarion-Sileni V, Innocente R, Cavina R, et al. Multi-center phase II trial of chemo-radiotherapy with 5-fluorouracil, leucovorin and oxaliplatin in locally advanced esophageal cancer. *Cancer Chemother Pharmacol.* 2009;16:191–199.
270. Heath ET, Burtness BA, Heitmiller RF, et al. Phase II evaluation of preoperative chemoradiation and postoperative adjuvant chemotherapy for squamous cell and adenocarcinoma of the esophagus. *J Clin Oncol.* 2000;18:868–876.
271. Urba S, Hayman J, et al. Preoperative chemoradiotherapy with cisplatin, 5-FU and paclitaxel followed by surgery and adjuvant chemotherapy, for loco-regional esophageal carcinoma (Abstract). *Proc Am Soc Clin Oncol.* 2004;23:319a.
272. Urba SG, Orringer MB, Turrisi A, et al. Randomized trial of preoperative chemoradiation versus surgery alone in patients with locoregional esophageal carcinoma. *J Clin Oncol.* 2001;19:305–313.
273. Rohatgi PR, Swisher SG, Correa AM, et al. Failure of patterns correlate with the proportion of residual carcinoma after preoperative chemoradiotherapy for carcinoma of the esophagus. *Cancer.* 2005;104:1349–1355.
274. Kleinberg L, Knisely JP, Heitmiller R, et al. Mature survival results with preoperative cisplatin, protracted infusion 5-fluorouracil, and 44-Gy radiotherapy for esophageal cancer. *Int J Radiat Oncol Biol Phys.* 2003;56:328–334.
275. Berger AC, Farma J, Scott WJ, et al. Complete response to neoadjuvant chemoradiotherapy in esophageal carcinoma is associated with significantly improved survival. *J Clin Oncol.* 2005;23:4330–4337.
276. Ajani JA, Walsh G, Komaki R, et al. Preoperative induction of CPT-11 and cisplatin chemotherapy followed by chemoradiotherapy in patients with locoregional carcinoma of the esophagus or gastroesophageal junction. *Cancer.* 2004;100:2347–2354.
277. Ilson DH, Bains M, Kelsen DP, et al. Phase I trial of escalating-dose irinotecan given weekly with cisplatin and concurrent radiotherapy in locally advanced esophageal cancer. *J Clin Oncol.* 2003;21:2926–2932.
278. Ajani JA, Komaki R, Putnam JB, et al. A three-step strategy of induction chemotherapy then chemoradiation followed by surgery in patients with potentially resectable carcinoma of the esophagus or gastroesophageal junction. *Cancer.* 2001;92:279–286.
279. Swisher SG, Ajani JA, Komaki R, et al. Long-term outcome of phase II trial evaluating chemotherapy, chemoradiotherapy, and surgery for locoregionally advanced esophageal cancer. *Int J Radiat Oncol Biol Phys.* 2003;57:120–127.
280. Carstens H, Albertsson M, et al. A randomized trial of chemoradiotherapy versus surgery alone in patients with resectable esophageal cancer. (Abstract.) *J Clin Oncol.* 2007;25:205s.
281. Stahl M, Walz MK, Stuschke M, et al. Phase III comparison of preoperative chemotherapy compared with chemoradiotherapy in patients with locally advanced adenocarcinoma of the esophagogastric junction. *J Clin Oncol.* 2009;27:851–856.
282. Roth JA, Pass HI, Flanagan MM, et al. Randomized clinical trial of preoperative and postoperative adjuvant chemotherapy with cisplatin, vindesine, and bleomycin for carcinoma of the esophagus. *J Thorac Cardiovasc Surg.* 1988;96:242–288.
283. Cunningham D, Allum WH, Stenning SP, et al. Perioperative chemotherapy versus surgery alone for resectable gastroesophageal cancer. *N Engl J Med.* 2006; 355:11–20.
284. Boige V, Pignon J, et al. Final results of a randomized trial comparing preoperative 5-fluorouracil/cisplatin to surgery alone in adenocarcinoma of the stomach and lower esophagus (ASLE): FNLCC ACCORD07-FFCD 9703 (Abstract.) *J Clin Oncol.* 2007;25:200s.
285. Bancewicz J, Clark PI, et al. Surgical resection with or without preoperative chemotherapy in oesophageal cancer: a randomized controlled trial. *Lancet.* 2002; 359:1727–1733.
286. Nygaard K, Hagen S, Hansen HS, et al. Pre-operative radiotherapy prolongs survival in operable esophageal carcinoma: a randomized, multicenter study of preoperative radiotherapy and chemotherapy. The second Scandinavian trial in esophageal cancer. *World J Surg.* 1992;16:1104–1109.
287. Schlag PM. Randomized trial of preoperative chemotherapy for squamous cell cancer of the esophagus. *Arch Surg.* 1992;127:1446–1550.
288. Ancona E, Ruol A, Santi S, et al. Only pathologic complete response to neoadjuvant chemotherapy improves significantly the long term survival of patients with resectable esophageal squamous cell carcinoma: final report of a randomized, controlled trial of preoperative chemotherapy versus surgery alone. *Cancer.* 2001;91:2165–2174.
289. Kelsen DP, Ginsberg R, Pajak TF, et al. Chemotherapy followed by surgery compared with surgery alone

for localized esophageal cancer. *N Engl J Med.* 1998; 339:1979–1984.
290. Japanese Esophageal Oncology Group. A comparison of chemotherapy and radiotherapy as adjuvant treatment to surgery for esophageal carcinoma. *Chest.* 1993;104:203–207.
291. Ando N, Iizuka T, Kakegawa T, et al. A randomized trial of surgery with and without chemotherapy for localized squamous cell carcinoma of the thoracic esophagus: a Japan Clinical Oncology Group Study. *J Thorac Cardiovasc Surg.* 1997;114:205–209.
292. Ando N, Iizuka T, Ide H, et al. Surgery plus chemotherapy compared with surgery alone for localized squamous cell carcinoma of the thoracic esophagus: a Japan Clinical Oncology Group study—JCOG9204. *J Clin Oncol.* 2003;21:4592–4596.
293. Lee J, Kyoung-Eun L, Im YH, et al. Adjuvant chemotherapy with 5-fluorouracil and cisplatin in lymph node-positive thoracic esophageal squamous cell carcinoma. *Ann Thorac Surg.* 2005;80:1170–1175.
294. Armanios M, Xu R, Forastiere AA, et al. Adjuvant chemotherapy for resected adenocarcinoma of the esophagus, gastro-esophageal junction, and cardia: phase II trial (E8296) of the Eastern Cooperative Oncology Group. *J Clin Oncol.* 2004;22:4495–4499.
295. Macdonald JS, Smalley SR, Benedetti J, et al. Chemoradiotherapy after surgery compared with surgery alone for adenocarcinoma of the stomach or gastroesophageal junction. *N Engl J Med.* 2001; 345:725–730.
296. Burmeister BH, Smithers BM, Gebski V, et al. Surgery alone versus chemoradiotherapy followed by surgery for resectable cancer of the oesophagus: a randomized controlled phase III trial. *Lancet Oncol.* 2005;6:659–668.
297. Apinop C, Puttisak P, Preecha N. A prospective study of combined therapy in esophageal cancer. *Hepatogastroenterology.* 1994;41:391–393.
298. Lee J, Park S, Kim SB, et al. A single institutional phase III trial of preoperative chemotherapy with hyperfractionation radiotherapy plus surgery versus alone for resectable esophageal squamous cell carcinoma. *Ann Oncol.* 2004;15:947–954.
299. Louvet C, Andre T, Tigaud JM, et al. Phase II study of oxaliplatin, fluorouracil, and folinic acid in locally advanced or metastatic gastric cancer patients. *J Clin Oncol.* 2002;20:4543–4548.
300. Al-Batran SE, Atmaca A, Hegewisch-Becker S, et al. Phase II trial of biweekly infusional fluorouracil, folinic acid, and oxaliplatin in patients with advanced gastric cancer. *J Clin Oncol.* 2004;22:658–663.

demos MEDICAL

RADIATION MEDICINE ROUNDS

Thymomas

Sandra C. Tomaszek and Dennis A. Wigle*
Mayo Clinic, Rochester, MN

ABSTRACT

Thymomas are rare neoplasms arising from tissue elements of the thymus and developing in the anterior mediastinum. Despite a low annual incidence of only 0.15 cases per 100,000 person-years, thymomas represent the most frequent tumors of the anterior mediastinum.

Thymomas are derived from thymic epithelium and typically occur in middle-aged adults. They are slow growing and infrequently metastasize. Thymomas can be associated with various systemic autoimmune disorders, such as red cell aplasia, hypogammaglobulinemia, inflammatory bowel disease, systemic lupus erythematosus, and in 30% of patients, with myasthenia gravis. For clinical evaluation of a mediastinal mass, radiographic imaging is obtained, usually by means of computed tomography. Differential diagnoses of an enlarging thymus include thymic hyperplasia, thymic cyst, and lymphoma. Tissue diagnosis prior to surgery is not routinely obtained but may be considered as an option to exclude the differential diagnosis of lymphoma, as treatment approaches are dramatically different in these two diseases.

The most frequently used classification systems are the Masaoka staging system and the World Health Organization (WHO) classification system, as they have prognostic significance.

Surgery is the primary therapy of most thymomas. This is typically accomplished by means of median sternotomy with complete thymectomy.

Postoperative radiotherapy is currently not considered for completely resected Masaoka stage I thymomas, as no additional benefit on survival has been observed. Incompletely resected or invasive thymomas (Masaoka stages II and III) may benefit from adjuvant radiotherapy. Thymomas are generally considered chemotherapy-sensitive tumors, and therefore, chemotherapy is used in select patients with inoperable or gross residual disease after local treatment. This is mainly for Masaoka stages III or IV thymomas. In advanced or primarily unresectable tumors, multimodality treatment is adopted for management.

INTRODUCTION

Thymomas are among the rarest human neoplasms arising from tissue elements of the thymus and developing in the anterior mediastinum (1). Despite a very low annual incidence of only 0.15 cases per 100,000 person-years (2), thymomas represent the most frequent tumor of the anterior mediastinum (3). Generally, they present as an incidental radiographic finding without any symptoms. They may, however, become symptomatic as part of a systemic or autoimmune disorder, such as myasthenia gravis, pure red

*Corresponding author, Division of General Thoracic Surgery, Mayo Clinic, 200 1st St. SW, Rochester, MN 55905
E-mail address: wigle.dennis@mayo.edu

Radiation Medicine Rounds 1 (2010) 211–224.

DOI: 10.5003/2151–4208.1.1.211

cell aplasia, pancytopenia, collagen-vascular disease, hypogammaglobulinemia, inflammatory bowel disease, or systemic lupus erythematosus (4–8).

Structure and Function of the Thymus

Thymus (Latin) is derived from the Greek word θύμός, thyme. Galen of Pergamum (AD 129–200) applied this term to a glandular formation found in the chest of young animals, thus the thymus gland. The first accurate description of the thymus followed by Berengarius of Capri (1480–1550) in 1524 (9).

Its anatomic location is in the upper anterior mediastinum. The thymus may extend from the inferior aspects of the thyroid glands to the level of the fourth costal cartilage or below. Furthermore, extracapsular or ectopic thymic tissue can be present elsewhere in the mediastinum (10).

The thymus is a two-lobed encapsulated organ. It is highly vascular, with lymphatic vessels that drain into the mediastinal lymph nodes. As a primary lymphoid organ, its main function is T-lymphocyte maturation (11). At birth, the gland has a weight of 10 to 15 g, which increases to its maximum in puberty before undergoing involution (fatty replacement) to less than 15% of its maximum weight (11). Thus it is usually a nondetectable structure on chest radiograph, unless there is involvement of a disease process (4).

Histopathological Classification Systems and Staging

Various classification systems for thymomas have been developed and described historically. However, clinical, pathological, and surgical classification of thymomas is very complex due to the various classification schemes being in clinical use and remains controversial. A major factor guiding this debate is the histomorphologic variability and the heterogeneity of cells within thymomas (12–15).

In clinical practice the most widely used staging system is that defined by Masaoka and colleagues (16), acknowledging the presence of invasion and anatomic extent of involvement, both clinically and histopathologically (Table 1). The classification system is regarded as a good predictor of prognosis and has been verified as the most significant independent prognostic parameter for survival in the literature.

TABLE 1 Modified Masaoka stage

Stage I	Tumor completely encapsulated, grossly and microscopically; nontransmural capsular invasion
Stage II	Complete transmural (transcapsular) invasion
IIA	microscopic invasion only
IIB	macroscopic invasion into extracapsular soft tissue, or tumor grossly adherent to mediastinal pleura or pericardium without invasion through these structures
Stage III	Macroscopic invasion into neighboring organs
IIIA	invasion spares the great vessels
IIIB	invasion includes the great vessels
Stage IV	Locally advanced thoracic disease or metastasis
IVA	pleural or pericardial dissemination
IVB	lymphovascular metastasis

Source: From Ref. 16.

Kaplan-Meyer survival statistics are illustrated in Figure 1.

Another frequently used thymoma classification system is the WHO histologic typing of tumors of the thymus (1999), based on cytologic similarities between normal thymic epithelial cells and neoplastic cells (17). The definitions of the WHO types A, AB, B1-B3, and C are illustrated in detail in Table 2. Similar to the Masaoka staging system, the WHO classification is a statistically significant predictor of prognosis. Survival statistics are illustrated in Figure 2.

The WHO classification system has been built upon the histologic classification system originally described by Marino and Müller-Hermelink (1985), which is based on the *presumed* origin of the malignant thymoma cells and includes five subtypes as derivatives of the medullary and cortical cells typically seen in the different types of thymomas: medullary, mixed, predominantly cortical, and cortical thymomas, and well-differentiated thymic carcinomas (19) (Table 2).

In 1999, Suster and Moran (20) suggested a schema condensing thymic epithelial tumor into three histologic groups based on morphology and epithelial cytology: thymoma, atypical thymoma, and thymic carcinoma (Table 2).

Other existing classification schemes are listed subsequently in chronological order. Bernatz (21) described thymomas in 1961 according to their dominant cell type as predominantly spindle cell,

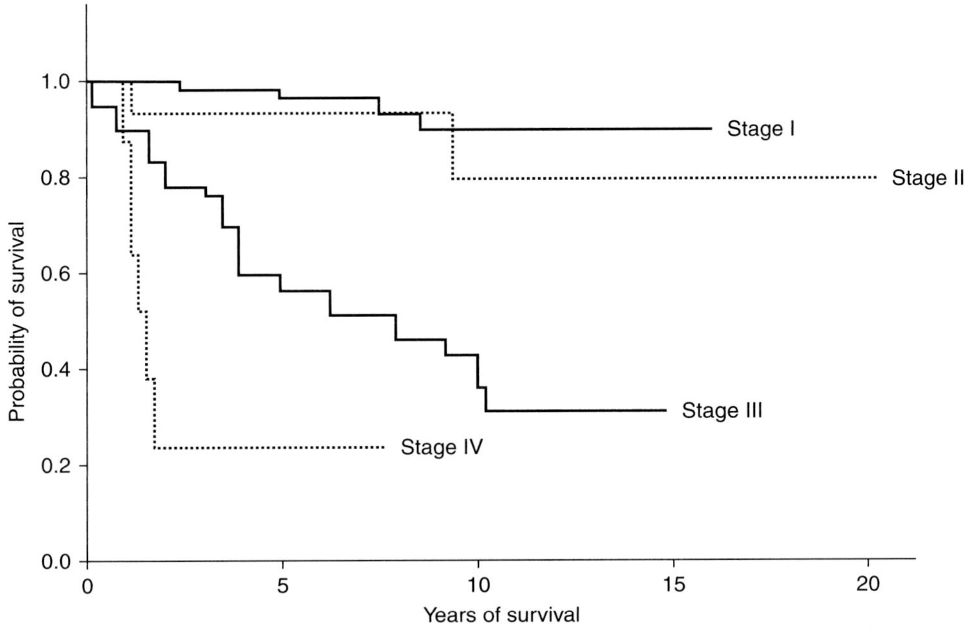

FIGURE 1 Kaplan-Meier survival statistic for thymomas according to Masaoka tumor stage. Adapted from Ref. 17.

TABLE 2 Correspondence of different histologic classification systems

WHO		Müller-Hermelink	Suster-Moran
A	Bland spindle/oval epithelial tumor cells, recapitulating the involuted thymus with few or no lymphocytes	Medullary	Thymoma
AB	Mixture of a lymphocyte-poor type A thymoma component and a more lymphocyte-rich type B–like component	Mixed	
B1	Histological appearance of normal thymus composed predominantly of areas resembling cortex with epithelial cells scattered in a predominant population of immature lymphocytes, and areas of medullary differentiation (synonym: "lymphocyte-rich")	Predominantly cortical	
B2	Large, polygonal tumor cells that are arranged in a loose network and exhibit large vesicular nuclei with prominent large nucleoli; relative proportion of epithelial cells is increased compared with type B1 Synonym: "mixed lymphoepithelial"	Cortical	
B3	Increased numbers of large, round, or polygonal cells with fewer lymphocytes compared with types B1 or B2. Epithelial cells present in large clusters, with mild nuclear irregularities, if any Synonym: "epithelial-rich"	Differentiated thymic carcinoma	Atypical thymoma
C	Heterogeneous group of thymic carcinomas.		Thymic carcinoma

Source: From Ref. 18.

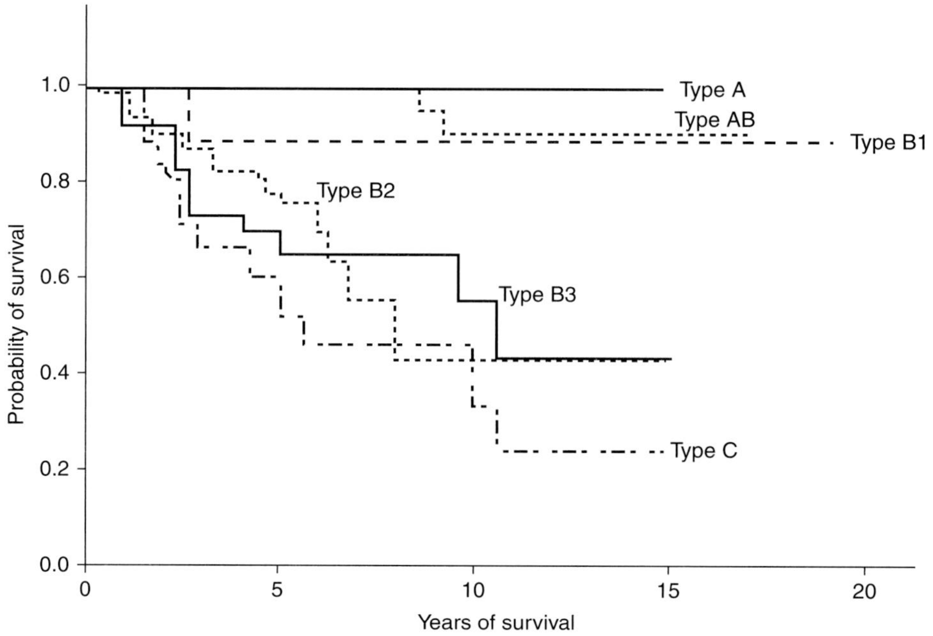

FIGURE 2 Kaplan-Meier survival statistic for thymomas according to World Health Organization classification. Adapted from Ref. 17.

predominantly lymphocytic, predominantly mixed, or predominantly epithelial thymomas.

Levine and Rosai (22) emphasized the importance of presence or absence of invasiveness by classifying thymomas into (a) benign encapsulated thymomas, (b) type 1 malignant thymomas (invasive thymomas), and (c) type 2 malignant thymomas (thymic carcinomas).

Derived from Masaoka, the French Study Group on Thymic Tumors (GETT) developed the GETT classification system of thymomas in 1991, relating extent of surgical resection to tumor histopathology (23). However, this classification is rarely used in clinical practice.

Finally, several approaches have been undertaken to adopt a TNM-based classification system for thymomas because it is commonly used for other malignancies. Yamakawa and colleagues (24) developed a TNM-classification system in 1994, which the authors adopted to 207 patients with thymoma or thymic carcinoma. However, this classification system has neither been widely used nor officially recognized by WHO (24,25). In 2005, Bedini and colleagues published a novel TNM-based staging system called INT ("Istituto Nazionale Tumori," the Italian National Cancer Institute) (26). The authors have developed this system as a clinically applicable staging system to update the Masaoka system. Further assessment of the INT system in larger multicenter series will be required to justify its clinical implementation.

DIAGNOSIS OF THYMOMA

Noninvasive Diagnostic Tools

Radiologic Imaging

Computed tomography (CT) is the current gold standard to characterize a mediastinal mass with regard to its anatomy, potential invasion of neighboring structures, and distant metastases, as chest radiographs may show merely a nonspecific broadened mediastinum (27). It is therefore an essential tool for clinical staging and surgical planning. Furthermore, CT imaging may be useful to distinguish thymomas from benign mediastinal lesions or lymphoma in the case of multiple mediastinal abnormalities (28).

Magnetic resonance imaging (MRI) resembles an additional, yet not routinely implemented, technique in the radiologic diagnostic workup of patients (29). The value of MRI is the verification of potential invasion into surrounding structures such as great vessels or the heart for surgical planning, rather than as a primary diagnostic tool. Reports suggesting that MRI findings correlate with the WHO classification need to be studied further (30,31).

The Role of Nuclear Medicine in the Diagnosis of Thymomas

Recently, fluorodeoxyglucose positron emission tomography (FDG-PET) scanning has been used in addition to computed tomography (CT) to diagnose thymomas. Data suggest that maximal standardized uptake values (SUVs) of thymic carcinomas are significantly higher than those of high- or low-risk thymomas (32,33). Moreover, a higher proportion of thymic carcinoma patients show homogeneous 18F-FDG uptake than low- or high-risk thymoma patients. The authors concluded from their data that PET might be a useful tool for predicting the grade of malignancy in thymic epithelial tumors.

^{11}C-Acetate-PET has recently been described as a novel PET modality in the diagnosis of thymomas in addition to 18F-FDG-PET imaging. Shibata and coworkers (34) found in their recent study of 40 patients that the SUV can be applied to predict the histologic type of thymoma: an SUV of <6.3 in FDG-PET and of >5.7 in ^{11}C-Acetate-PET were predictive of a WHO A/AB thymoma. Larger controlled studies are needed to confirm these findings, as they may have consequences in regard with prognosis and management of thymomas.

PET imaging might also be a decision-facilitating tool to help the clinician in choosing patients for which a preoperative biopsy should be obtained. In a recent study of 19 patients by Luzzi and colleagues (35), the authors recommend obtaining a preoperative biopsy of mediastinal lesions with an SUV_{max} of >5, as they have a higher probability of lymphoma or thymic carcinoma.

Further clinical investigation is needed to determine whether PET scanning should play a specific role in preoperative staging of thymomas, for early detection of recurrent disease during follow-up, as well as in restaging of mediastinal tumors after neoadjuvant therapy.

Another potentially useful modality not routinely used in the diagnosis of thymomas is scintigraphy. Its adoption seems to be useful in patients with

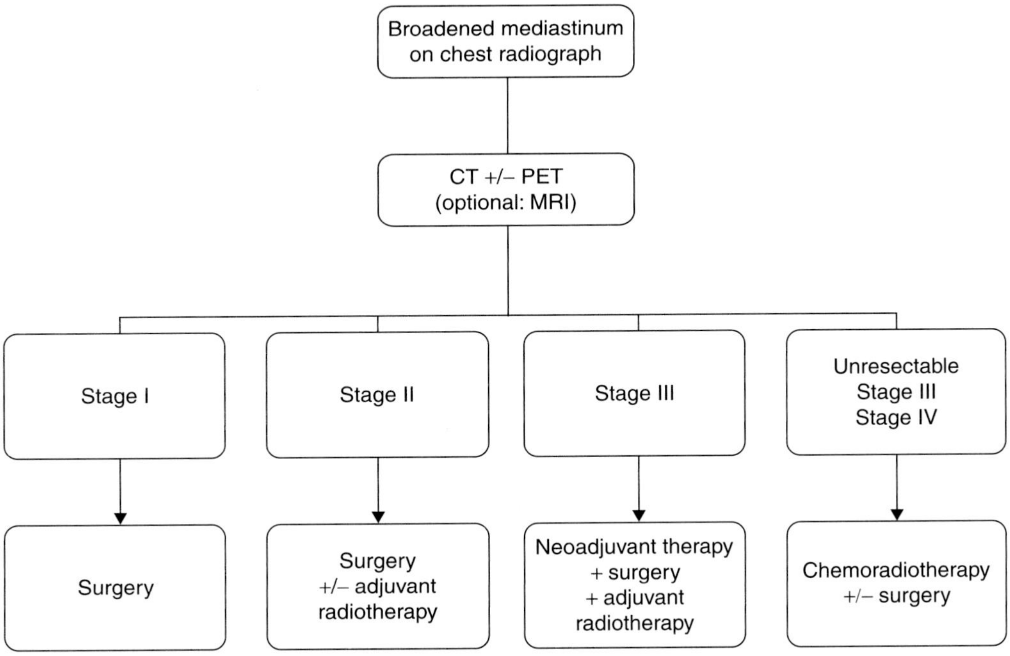

FIGURE 3 Algorithm for diagnosis and treatment of thymomas.

myasthenia gravis, as thallium 201 single photon emission computed tomography can help to differentiate normal thymic tissue from hyperplastic tissue or thymoma (36).

Invasive Diagnostic Tools

Patients with an anterior mediastinal mass suspicious of thymoma without any B-symptoms typically do not need invasive preoperative tissue diagnosis. Its diagnostic role is to exclude potential differential diagnoses where surgical resection is not the primary treatment modality, such as lymphomas.

Fine needle aspiration (FNA) biopsy is an accepted and feasible method to differentiate mediastinal lesions and to diagnose or classify thymomas histopathologically (37–39). However, as in other malignant tumors, needle track malignant cell seeding is feared, and therefore, many programs do not routinely perform FNA biopsy in tumors suspicious of thymoma. In addition, FNA biopsy is not suitable to assess capsular or neighboring organ invasion (40). New approaches such as the implementation of ultrasonically guided core needle biopsy rather than percutaneous needle biopsies have been adopted to obtain larger specimens for histological examination. Annessi and colleagues (41) were able to establish a diagnosis in all patients who had undergone anterior mediastinal core needle biopsy by ultrasound guidance (n = 47) with a sensitivity and specificity of 100%. They evaluated the procedure as superior to FNA because surgical diagnostic procedures can be reduced and repetition of unsuccessful FNA is avoided. For the same reason, endoscopic ultrasound-guided fine needle aspiration (EUS-FNA) has been increasingly applied to obtain cytologic specimens from mediastinal lesions (42,43). As histological examination allows superior differentiation of malignant lesions, Larghi and colleagues have implemented an altered EUS-FNA technique in a pilot study of 27 patients using continuous high negative pressure suction for core tissue acquisition and compared this technique with standard EUS-FNA. To apply high negative pressure suction, the authors attached an inflation system to the proximal end of the FNA needle and applied suctioning at 35 mL of a 60-mL syringe. This value was arbitrarily chosen by the authors. The diagnostic accuracy for both methods was 76.9%, and when combined, a correct diagnosis was achieved in 84.6% of the patients (43). No superiority over standard EUS-FNA could be shown in this study.

Percutaneous image-guided FNA biopsy of a mediastinal mass is diagnostic in up to 82% of cases (44). However, histological differentiation between thymomas, lymphomas, and thymic hyperplasia can be problematic for this form of biopsy.

In our clinical practice we do not routinely obtain an invasive tissue diagnosis if thymoma is the presumed diagnosis based on imaging, clinical examination, and medical history. In patients reporting B-symptoms or in those with radiographic imaging findings suggestive of lymphoma, we will obtain a core biopsy to be able to exclude lymphoma as a potential differential diagnosis, as the treatment approaches for thymoma and lymphoma differ substantially.

■ THERAPY

Surgery

Surgery is the primary therapy for most thymomas. The first thymic operation was performed in transcervical fashion at the end of the 19th century by Ludwig Rehn on a patient with a symptomatically enlarged thymus (45). This operative technique remained the preferred approach until the 1930s, when Alfred Blalock performed the first transsternal thymectomy in a patient with myasthenia gravis (MG) and an anterior mediastinal tumor in 1936 (45,46). Complete and partial median sternotomy with complete thymectomy evolved from this technique and remains the operative approach of choice for the resection of thymomas (47–53). In advanced tumors, especially if the lung or pleural space is invaded, the extension of a sternotomy to a hemiclamshell incision or a full clamshell incision can be suitable. To reduce morbidity and mortality associated with this procedure, minimally invasive techniques have been developed in the past years. We do not routinely use the minimally invasive approach for the resection of thymomas given concern regarding oncologic equivalence with open approaches.

Minimally Invasive Techniques

Minimally invasive approaches such as transcervical, video-assisted thoracoscopic (VATS), or robotic-assisted thymectomy are being intensely studied for thymomas (54–57). As with any other minimally invasive approach, video-assisted thymectomy is associated with significantly lower morbidity resulting in a significantly shorter hospital length of stay as well as a comparable relief of symptoms from MG when compared with transsternal thymectomy (56,58). Another benefit is the better cosmetic result of minimally invasive surgery. Advantages of robot-assisted surgery are seen in the ease of dissection in the narrow mediastinum and neck due to 3-dimensional visualization (57). No data are currently available on the influence of this advanced minimally invasive technique on morbidity and mortality when compared with VATS thymectomy.

In thymomas, however, these approaches are generally viewed as contraindicated (54,55) due to concern regarding oncologic equivalence with the open approach. Despite the lack of controlled long-term clinical trials evaluating the oncologic equivalence, some investigators consider minimal invasive thymectomy to be an effective alternative procedure for noninvasive thymomas if performed carefully in experienced hands (59–61). Pennathur and colleagues (62) compared their results of VATS thymectomy with the results of an open resection in a total of 38 patients with stages I (n = 14) and II (n = 24) thymomas with a median follow-up time of 34.8 months. The study showed oncologic equivalence of the two approaches, yet further studies evaluating the long-term outcome of these patients are required to evaluate these approaches in the therapy of thymomas.

Transcervical Thymectomy

For this approach, a transverse 5-cm cervical incision is made approximately 2 cm above the sternal notch without splitting the sternum. Visualization is achieved via a 5-mm thoracoscopic camera inserted through the cervical incision. This approach is prominent for thymectomy in the treatment of myasthenia gravis, but concerns remain about its oncologic efficacy for removal of thymomas.

VATS Thymectomy

This technique typically uses three ports, placed anterior to the midaxillary line, two of which function as utility ports, while through a third the camera is introduced. After dissection, the mobilized thymus is removed from the thoracic cavity through the most anterior port, which may be extended to a 3- to 5-cm utility incision to facilitate retraction of the specimen. Although an adequate thymectomy for either the right- or left-hand side can be performed through this approach, it is difficult, if not impossible, to see across the midline to adequately dissect on the side opposite to that of entry into the chest. As a consequence, oncologic concerns have inhibited the wide adoption of this approach, even for fully encapsulated stage I thymomas.

Robotic-Assisted Thymectomy

The ports for the arms of the robotic device are inserted in a similar manner as that described above for the VATS technique, with the consideration of somewhat broader spacing for adequate room for arm movement. The camera offers 3-dimensional visualization for the surgeon, who is performing the surgery from a console in the operating room, while the assistant surgeon is operating at the patient's side. Despite enhanced operative visualization compared with the VATS approach, similar concerns regarding oncologic efficacy remain.

Clinical Outcomes After Surgical Resection

For patients with completely resected Masaoka stage I thymoma, 10-year survival rates of approximately 80% have been reported (63). According to a multicenter study on 1,320 patients by Kondo and colleagues, total resection is the most important prognostic factor for survival: the 5-year survival rate of Masaoka stages III and IV thymomas is 92.9% after total resection versus 64.4% ($P < .001$) after subtotal resection versus 35.6% if inoperable (64). Rea and colleagues confirmed these findings; however, they found no statistical difference in survival between patients who underwent incomplete resection (debulking) versus biopsy only (49).

Recurrence rates after complete resection vary between 11% and 19% (50,65) and correlate with stage: WHO tumor type A and AB 0%, B1 and B2 8%, B3 27%, and C 50%, as shown by Wright and associates (65). Haniuda and colleagues (50) followed 126 patients after complete resection and identified 24 recurrences (19%) with 83% of relapses in Masaoka stage IVa thymomas and no recurrences in Masaoka stage I thymomas, which once again indicates that the recurrence rate increases with stage. As reported by Cowen and associates (1), metastatic spread is significantly ($P < .02$) more often seen in patients who were not treated (biopsy only: 27%) or underwent subtotal resection (23%) than in patients who underwent complete resection (7.9%).

With completeness of resection being an important prognostic factor for local control of the disease and hence survival, it has to be aimed for whenever feasible (1,47–49,51,53,64,66,67).

Radiation Therapy

Postoperative radiotherapy is currently not recommended for completely resected Masaoka stage I thymomas, as no additional benefit on survival has been observed (67). However, in incompletely resected or invasive thymomas (Masaoka stages II and III), adjuvant radiotherapy is frequently applied with the option of irradiating either the tumor bed or the entire mediastinum and/or the supraclavicular fossae (53,68). The applied radiation dose ranges from 40 to 60 Gy based on the extent of disease, pathologic factors, and completeness of resection (1,53,64,68).

Adjuvant radiation therapy for completely resected Masaoka stage II thymomas remains controversial but is recommended in the current National Comprehensive Cancer Network (NCCN) guidelines. Some authors suggest that an R0-resection alone is adequate in the treatment of Masaoka stages I and II thymomas (69). Yet, particularly in Masaoka stage II tumors of a high-risk WHO category such as B2, B3, or C, adjuvant radiotherapy should be considered because a significantly increased 5-year survival rate of 86% compared with 48% without adjuvant therapy has been reported ($P < .002$) (3,68). Recurrences and metastatic disease after resection of WHO B2 and B3 thymomas reflect their malignant behavior and suggest potential benefit for intensified treatment (51,64,66).

Several studies have shown that neither increases of the irradiation dose nor extension of the radiation field (thymic bed vs. entire mediastinum) seems to improve the outcome after resection (1,53,68). As reported by Zhu and coworkers (53), the 5-year local control rate after irradiation of the tumor bed of 68% is comparable to that after extension of radiotherapy fields (67%). Comparing different radiation doses (≤50 vs. >50 Gy), no significant differences on local control or survival were observed. A report by Kondo and colleagues suggests that the recurrence rate of completely resected Masaoka stages II and III thymomas is not significantly decreased by postoperative radiotherapy. Recurrence rates of Masaoka stages II and III thymomas were 5% and 23% in patients with postoperative radiotherapy and 4% and 26% in patients without radiotherapy, respectively (64). According to this study, even in patients after complete resection of Masaoka stages III and IV thymomas, there is no significant difference in survival rates seen between surgery alone and surgery with postoperative radiotherapy (5- and 10-year survival of 100% and 95% vs. 93% and 78%, respectively). Furthermore, the use of routine adjuvant irradiation after complete resection of Masaoka stage III thymomas does not seem to prevent pleural recurrences and therefore needs to be readdressed according to Mangi and coworkers (70). However, other studies clearly find adjuvant radiotherapy as an effective treatment in advanced thymomas (Masaoka stages III and IV) by inducing long-term complete or partial remissions, especially in Masaoka stage III thymomas (15,71–73). Postoperative radiotherapy is recommended in the current NCCN guidelines for resected Masaoka stage III patients.

Onuki and colleagues (74) reported successful tumor size reduction in Masaoka stage III thymomas after preoperatively applied radiotherapy but observed statistically significant differences based on the underlying WHO thymoma type because the treatment was more effective in B1 and B2 thymomas than in B3 thymomas. These promising results need to be confirmed by further controlled studies because neoadjuvant radiotherapy may offer the opportunity in patients with previously unresectable tumors to be amenable to definitive curative surgical resection.

Chemotherapy

Thymomas are often chemotherapy-sensitive tumors, and therefore chemotherapy is adopted in select patients with inoperable or gross residual disease after local treatment, mainly for Masaoka stages III or IV thymomas (53,65,75). Chemotherapy is not considered as treatment of choice in localized, surgically resectable thymomas (76).

Frequently applied agents in the reviewed studies are cisplatin-based protocols consisting of doxorubicin, cyclophosphamide, cisplatin, vincristine, or cisplatin with etoposide and ifosfamide (47,48). Currently, however, no standardized regimen for chemotherapy in thymoma therapy exists.

Rea and colleagues adopted the ADOC regimen (cisplatin, doxorubicin, vincristine, and cyclophosphamide) in a neoadjuvant setting for unresectable stages III or IVa thymomas, showing an improved resectability after neoadjuvant chemotherapy of 75% versus 58% if no neoadjuvant therapy was applied (49). These positive effects have been confirmed by Berruti and coworkers (77).

In a study by Cowen and colleagues (1) reviewing patients with nonmetastatic thymoma who received radiation therapy, the use of chemotherapy strongly correlated with Masaoka stages III and IVa thymomas ($P < .01$) and mediastinal compression on presentation ($P < .01$). The adjuvant platinum-based CAP regimen (cyclophosphamide, doxorubicin or adriamycin, cisplatin or carboplatin) was associated with disease-free survival at 5 years of approximately 55% versus 20% if no chemotherapy was applied ($P = .02$).

Small prospective studies focusing on the use of chemotherapy also suggest a positive effect for the combination of cisplatin and etoposide (76,78). Loehrer and colleagues (76) concluded from their prospective study of 28 patients treated with the VIP regimen (cisplatin, iphosphamide, and etoposide) that objective response rates and prolonged survival are achievable in patients with metastatic or locally progressive recurrent disease. In 32.1%, partial remission was achieved, though no patient experienced complete remission, and 7.1% developed progressive disease, whereas 60.1% of patients had stable disease. One- and two-year survival rates were 89% and 70%, respectively. In a phase 2 study conducted by Giaccone and colleagues (78), 16 patients with recurrent or metastatic thymoma were treated with a combination of cisplatin and etoposide, achieving a response rate in 56% of patients, of which 31% were complete responses with a median response duration of 3.4 years (median survival: 4.3 years; median progression-free survival: 2.2 years).

In summary, a number of studies have shown potential benefit for multiple chemotherapeutic regimens in the treatment of thymoma. The lack of prospective trials, however, with consistent regimens makes comparison across studies difficult. Therefore, larger controlled studies are clearly required for validation (64).

Multimodality Treatment

Multimodality treatment is an approach to manage primarily unresectable tumors (79,80). Bretti and colleagues (79) reported increased radical resection rates after neoadjuvant treatment from 46% to 65% in Masaoka stage III patients and from 0% to 20% in those with Masaoka stage IVa disease, respectively. A total irradiation dose of 30 Gy was administered over 3 weeks, and two chemotherapy regimens were adopted: four cycles of ADOC or CDDP+VP16 (cisplatin and etoposide). Therefore, induction chemoradiotherapy can be regarded as an attempt to potentially downstage thymomas to improve surgical resectability and consequently improve survival (79,81,82).

Lucchi and colleagues (83) reported reasonable long-term results in Masaoka stages III and IVa thymomas, applying neoadjuvant chemotherapy, surgery, and postoperative radiotherapy or primary surgery followed by adjuvant chemotherapy and/or radiation therapy. The neoadjuvant or adjuvant chemotherapy regimen consisted of three courses of cisplatin, epidoxorubicin, and etoposide every 3 weeks. Adjuvant irradiation consisted of 45 Gy for complete and 60 Gy for incomplete resections. Again, according to their data, neoadjuvant chemotherapy improved the resectability rate and survival. Kim and colleagues (84) confirmed these findings in a prospective study of 22 patients treated with induction chemotherapy (cyclophosphamide, doxorubicin, cisplatin, and prednisone), surgery, and radiotherapy plus consolidation chemotherapy. In all, 18 of 19 patients who completed the multidisciplinary regimen were disease-free at a median follow-up of 50.3 months. The overall survival rate was 95% at 5 years and 79% at 7 years with a progression-free survival rate of 77% at 5 and 7 years. Low morbidity with promising long-term survival rates have been reported, supporting a multimodality approach in a select group of thymoma patients with advanced tumors (52,85,86). However, prospective multi-institutional studies are needed for further verification (52).

■ PROGNOSTIC FACTORS IN THYMOMAS

Masaoka stage, WHO classification, and radical surgical resection are considered significant independent prognostic factors for long-term disease-free survival (3,48,49,53,64,65,67,68,72).

It is not clear whether tumor size is an independent prognostic factor for outcome in thymoma patients, although it has been suggested by various studies. Nakagawa and colleagues (67) evaluated factors limiting the prognosis of thymomas and rated tumor size as a significant predictor of outcome ($P = .001$). These results were supported by a single-center study of 179 patients by Wright and coworkers (65), finding a critical tumor size of ≥8 cm to be an independent predictor for recurrence.

The prognostic value of MG in thymomas is controversial in the reviewed literature. Kondo and colleagues (87) found in a multicenter study of 1,089 patients that thymomas associated with MG seem to behave less aggressive because thymomas associated with MG are diagnosed at an earlier stage and have lower recurrence rates (47,72,87). As a consequence, MG can be regarded as a positive prognostic factor for the outcome of thymomas.

FUTURE RESEARCH

To improve the outcome in patients who are not amenable to surgical resection, more investigation needs to be conducted to elucidate the molecular pathways involved in the pathogenesis of thymomas to be able to offer targeted therapies based on molecular understanding of the disease.

Sasaki and colleagues (88) have shown that gene expression analysis of thymomas may provide a novel and promising approach for classifying thymomas biologically. This idea has been further investigated by Lee and colleagues (89) observing genome-wide chromosomal aberrations in thymomas with correlation of specific alterations to thymoma subgroups. Recently Kaira and coworkers (90) described that expression of L-type amino acid transporter 1 might function as an immunohistochemical marker for thymic carcinomas, being able to distinguish these from thymomas.

The clinical impact of these findings is yet unknown but may offer potential opportunities for complementing the current standard classification systems and improving prognosis and clinical outcomes for thymoma patients in the future. Novel research approaches might improve the understanding of the disease further and lead to new tools for diagnosis and treatment of thymomas.

SUMMARY

The Masaoka staging system seems to be the current state of the art in thymoma diagnostics and therapy. As illustrated in Figure 3, CT is the diagnostic tool of choice to image the mediastinal lesion and its anatomical extent. For histopathological diagnosis, particularly if the lesion is invading neighboring structures, a preoperative specimen acquisition by FNA should be considered, especially if neoadjuvant therapy is considered.

Median sternotomy is the surgical approach of choice for complete surgical resection. It is effective for stage I thymomas without any further treatment. After surgical resection of stage II thymomas, adjuvant radiotherapy should be considered. Stage III thymomas may benefit from neoadjuvant therapy to achieve complete surgical resectability and minimize the risk of recurrent disease. Postoperative radiotherapy may also be useful for stage III thymomas, especially if complete resection is not feasible. Patients with stage IV thymomas and unresectable stage III thymomas may benefit from a multimodality approach including radio- and chemotherapy, and potentially surgery if significant downstaging occurs. Therapy for advanced thymomas infiltrating neighboring structures with pericardial or pleural dissemination remains controversial. Acquiring reliable data in prospective long-term studies to verify these findings is challenging and only feasible in multicenter trials given the overall low incidence of thymoma.

REFERENCES

1. Cowen D, Richaud P, Mornex F, et al. Thymoma: results of a multicentric retrospective series of 149 non-metastatic irradiated patients and review of the literature. FNCLCC trialists. Fédération Nationale des Centres de Lutte Contre le Cancer. *Radiother Oncol.* 1995;34(1):9–16.
2. Engels EA, Pfeiffer RM. Malignant thymoma in the United States: demographic patterns in incidence and associations with subsequent malignancies. *Int J Cancer.* 2003;105(4):546–551.
3. Chen G, Marx A, Wen-Hu C, et al. New WHO histologic classification predicts prognosis of thymic epithelial tumors: a clinicopathologic study of 200 thymoma cases from China. *Cancer.* 2002;95(2):420–429.
4. Benson MK. Mediastinal tumors and cysts. In: Ledingham JGG, Warrell DA, eds. *Concise Oxford Textbook of Medicine.* Oxford, U.K.: Oxford University Press; 2000:488–489.
5. Hon C, Chui WH, Cheng LC, Shek TW, Jones BM, Au WY. Thymoma associated with keratoconjunctivitis, lichen planus, hypogammaglobinemia, and absent circulating B cells. *J Clin Oncol.* 2006;24(18):2960–2961.
6. Miyakis S, Pefanis A, Passam FH, Christodulakis GR, Roussou PA, Mountokalakis TD. Thymoma with immunodeficiency (Good's syndrome): review of the literature apropos three cases. *Scand J Infect Dis.* 2006;38(4):314–319.

7. Murakawa T, Nakajima J, Sato H, Tanaka M, Takamoto S, Fukayama M. Thymoma associated with pure red-cell aplasia: clinical features and prognosis. *Asian Cardiovasc Thorac Ann.* 2002;10(2):150–154.
8. Skeie GO, Apostolski S, Evoli A, et al. Guidelines for the treatment of autoimmune neuromuscular transmission disorders. *Eur J Neurol.* 2006;13(7):691–699.
9. Skinner HA. *The Origin of Medical Terms.* Baltimore, MD: Williams & Wilkins Company; 1961:403–404.
10. Colborn GL, Skandalakis JE, Mirilas P, et al. Mediastinum. In: Skandalakis GL, Colborn GL, Weidman TA, et al., eds. *Surgical Anatomy.* Athens, Greece: Paschalidis Medical Publications Ltd.; 2004:197.
11. Sawyer Sommers M. Response of the body to immunologic challenge. In: Price SA, McCarty Wilson L, eds. Pathophysiology—Clinical Concepts of Disease Processes. St. Louis, MO: Mosby Inc.; 2003:67.
12. Harris NL, Müller-Hermelink HK. Thymoma classification. A siren's song of simplicity. *Am J Clin Pathol.* 1999;112(3):299–303.
13. Kornstein MJ. Thymoma classification: my opinion. *Am J Clin Pathol.* 1999;112(3):304–307.
14. Suster S, Moran CA. Thymoma classification. The ride of the valkyries? *Am J Clin Pathol.* 1999;112(3):308–310.
15. Kuo TT. Classification of thymic epithelial neoplasms: a controversial issue coming to an end? *J Cell Mol Med.* 2001;5(4):442–448.
16. Masaoka A, Monden Y, Nakahara K, Tanioka T. Follow-up study of thymomas with special reference to their clinical stages. *Cancer.* 1981;48(11):2485–2492.
17. Müller-Hermelink HK, Engel P, Kuo TT, et al. Tumours of the thymus. In: Travis WD, Brambilla E, Müller-Hermelink HK, Harris CC, eds. Tumours of the Lung, Pleura, Thymus and Heart. Lyon, France: IARC Press; 2004:145–198.
18. Weydert JA, De Young BR, Leslie KO; Association of Directors of Anatomic and Surgical Pathology. Recommendations for the reporting of surgically resected thymic epithelial tumors. *Hum Pathol.* 2009;40(7):918–923.
19. Marino M, Müller-Hermelink HK. Thymoma and thymic carcinoma: relation of thymoma epithelial cells to the cortical and medullary differentiation of thymus. *Virchows Arch A Pathol Anat Histopathol.* 1985;407(2):119–149.
20. Suster S, Moran CA. Thymoma, atypical thymoma, and thymic carcinoma. A novel conceptual approach to the classification of thymic epithelial neoplasms. *Am J Clin Pathol.* 1999;111(6):826–833.
21. Bernatz PE, Harrison EG, Clagett OT. Thymoma: a clinicopathologic study. *J Thorac Cardiovasc Surg.* 1961;42:424–444.
22. Rosai J, Levine GD. *Tumors of the Thymus.* Washington, DC: Armed Forces Institute of Pathology; 1976. Atlas of Tumor Pathology 2nd series, fascicle 13.
23. Gamondès JP, Balawi A, Greenland T, et al. Seventeen years of surgical treatment of thymoma: factors influencing survival. *Eur J Cardiothorac Surg.* 1991;5(3):124–131.
24. Yamakawa Y, Masaoka A, Hashimoto T, et al. A tentative tumor-node-metastasis classification of thymoma. *Cancer.* 1991;68(9):1984–1987.
25. Tsuchiya R, Koga K, Matsuno Y, Mukai K, Shimosato Y. Thymic carcinoma: proposal for pathological TNM and staging. *Pathol Int.* 1994;44(7):505–512.
26. Bedini AV, Andreani SM, Tavecchio L, et al. Proposal of a novel system for the staging of thymic epithelial tumors. *Ann Thorac Surg.* 2005;80(6):1994–2000.
27. Yang WT, Lei KI, Metreweli C. Plain radiography and computed tomography of invasive thymomas: clinico-radiologic-pathologic correlation. *Australas Radiol.* 1997;41(2):118–124.
28. Maher MM, Shepard JA. Imaging of thymoma. *Semin Thorac Cardiovasc Surg.* 2005;17(1):12–19.
29. Tomiyama N, Honda O, Tsubamoto M, et al. Anterior mediastinal tumors: diagnostic accuracy of CT and MRI. *Eur J Radiol.* 2009;69(2):280–288.
30. Han J, Lee KS, Yi CA, et al. Thymic epithelial tumors classified according to a newly established WHO scheme: CT and MR findings. *Korean J Radiol.* 2003;4(1):46–53.
31. Inoue A, Tomiyama N, Fujimoto K, et al. MR imaging of thymic epithelial tumors: correlation with World Health Organization classification. *Radiat Med.* 2006;24(3):171–181.
32. Endo M, Nakagawa K, Ohde Y, et al. Utility of 18FDG-PET for differentiating the grade of malignancy in thymic epithelial tumors. *Lung Cancer.* 2008;61(3):350–355.
33. Sung YM, Lee KS, Kim BT, Choi JY, Shim YM, Yi CA. 18F-FDG PET/CT of thymic epithelial tumors: usefulness for distinguishing and staging tumor subgroups. *J Nucl Med.* 2006;47(10):1628–1634.
34. Shibata H, Nomori H, Uno K, et al. 18F-fluorodeoxyglucose and 11C-acetate positron emission tomography are useful modalities for diagnosing the histologic type of thymoma. *Cancer.* 2009;115(11):2531–2538.
35. Luzzi L, Campione A, Gorla A, et al. Role of fluorine-flurodeoxyglucose positron emission tomography/computed tomography in preoperative assessment of anterior mediastinal masses. *Eur J Cardiothorac Surg.* 2009;36:475–479.
36. Higuchi T, Taki J, Kinuya S, et al. Thymic lesions in patients with myasthenia gravis: characterization with thallium 201 scintigraphy. *Radiology.* 2001;221(1):201–206.
37. Ali SZ, Erozan YS. Thymoma. Cytopathologic features and differential diagnosis on fine needle aspiration. *Acta Cytol.* 1998;42(4):845–854.
38. Chhieng DC, Rose D, Ludwig ME, Zakowski MF. Cytology of thymomas: emphasis on morphology and correlation with histologic subtypes. *Cancer.* 2000;90(1):24–32.
39. Shin HJ, Katz RL. Thymic neoplasia as represented by fine needle aspiration biopsy of anterior mediastinal masses. A practical approach to the differential diagnosis. *Acta Cytol.* 1998;42(4):855–864.
40. Wakely PE Jr. Fine needle aspiration in the diagnosis of thymic epithelial neoplasms. *Hematol Oncol Clin North Am.* 2008;22(3):433–442.

41. Annessi V, Paci M, De Franco S, et al. Diagnosis of anterior mediastinal masses with ultrasonically guided core needle biopsy. *Chir Ital.* 2003;55(3):379–384.
42. Kramer H, Sanders J, Post WJ, Groen HJ, Suurmeijer AJ. Analysis of cytological specimens from mediastinal lesions obtained by endoscopic ultrasound-guided fine-needle aspiration. *Cancer.* 2006;108(4):206–211.
43. Larghi A, Noffsinger A, Dye CE, Hart J, Waxman I. EUS-guided fine needle tissue acquisition by using high negative pressure suction for the evaluation of solid masses: a pilot study. *Gastrointest Endosc.* 2005;62(5):768–774.
44. Assaad MW, Pantanowitz L, Otis CN. Diagnostic accuracy of image-guided percutaneous fine needle aspiration biopsy of the mediastinum. *Diagn Cytopathol.* 2007; 35(11):705–709.
45. Mason D. Radical transsternal thymectomy. Operative techniques in thoracic and cardiovascular surgery. *Elsevier.* 2005;10(3):231–243.
46. Blalock A, Mason MF, Morgan HJ, et al. Myasthenia gravis and tumors of the thymic region. *Ann Surg.* 1939;110:544–561.
47. Evoli A, Minisci C, Di Schino C, et al. Thymoma in patients with MG: characteristics and long-term outcome. *Neurology.* 2002;59(12):1844–1850.
48. Kim DJ, Yang WI, Choi SS, Kim KD, Chung KY. Prognostic and clinical relevance of the World Health Organization schema for the classification of thymic epithelial tumors: a clinicopathologic study of 108 patients and literature review. *Chest.* 2005;127(3):755–761.
49. Rea F, Marulli G, Girardi R, et al. Long-term survival and prognostic factors in thymic epithelial tumours. *Eur J Cardiothorac Surg.* 2004;26(2):412–418.
50. Haniuda M, Kondo R, Numanami H, Makiuchi A, Machida E, Amano J. Recurrence of thymoma: clinicopathological features, re-operation, and outcome. *J Surg Oncol.* 2001;78(3):183–188.
51. Regnard JF, Magdeleinat P, Dromer C, et al. Prognostic factors and long-term results after thymoma resection: a series of 307 patients. *J Thorac Cardiovasc Surg.* 1996; 112(2):376–384.
52. Wright CD, Choi NC, Wain JC, Mathisen DJ, Lynch TJ, Fidias P. Induction chemotherapy followed by resection for locally advanced Masaoka stage III and IVa thymic tumors. *Ann Thorac Surg.* 2008;85(2):385–389.
53. Zhu G, He S, Fu X, Jiang G, Liu T. Radiotherapy and prognostic factors for thymoma: a retrospective study of 175 patients. *Int J Radiat Oncol Biol Phys.* 2004; 60(4):1113–1119.
54. Aubert A, Chaffanjon P, Brichon PY. Video-assisted extended thymectomy in patients with thymoma by lifting the sternum: is it safe? *Ann Thorac Surg.* 2004; 77(5):1878.
55. Ferguson MK. Transcervical thymectomy. *Semin Thorac Cardiovasc Surg.* 1999;11(1):59–64.
56. Augustin F, Schmid T, Sieb M, Lucciarini P, Bodner J. Video-assisted thoracoscopic surgery versus robotic-assisted thoracoscopic surgery thymectomy. *Ann Thorac Surg.* 2008;85(2):S768–S771.
57. Rückert JC, Ismail M, Swierzy M, et al. Thoracoscopic thymectomy with the da Vinci robotic system for myasthenia gravis. *Ann N Y Acad Sci.* 2008;1132:329–335.
58. Meyer DM, Herbert MA, Sobhani NC, et al. Comparative clinical outcomes of thymectomy for myasthenia gravis performed by extended transsternal and minimally invasive approaches. *Ann Thorac Surg.* 2009;97(2):385–390.
59. Cheng YJ, Kao EL, Chou SH. Videothoracoscopic resection of stage II thymoma: prospective comparison of the results between thoracoscopy and open methods. *Chest.* 2005;128(4):3010–3012.
60. Iablonskiĭ PK, Pishchik VG, Nuraliev SM. Comparative assessment of the effectiveness of traditional and videothoracoscopic thymectomies in complex treatment of myasthenic thymomas. *Vestn Khir Im I I Grek.* 2005; 164(3):38–42.
61. Sakamaki Y, Kido T, Yasukawa M. Alternative choices of total and partial thymectomy in video-assisted resection of noninvasive thymomas. *Surg Endosc.* 2008;22(5): 1272–1277.
62. Pennathur A, Qureshi I, Schuchert M, et al. Minimally invasive resection of stage 1 and stage 2 thymoma: comparison with open resection. Paper presented at: American Association for Thoracic Surgery 89th Annual Meeting; May 9–13, 2009; Boston, MA.
63. Venuta F, Anile M, Diso D, et al. Thymoma and thymic carcinoma. *Eur J Cardiothorac Surg.* 2009. [Epub ahead of print]
64. Kondo K, Monden Y. Therapy for thymic epithelial tumors: a clinical study of 1,320 patients from Japan. *Ann Thorac Surg.* 2003;76(3):878–884.
65. Wright CD, Wain JC, Wong DR, et al. Predictors of recurrence in thymic tumors: importance of invasion, World Health Organization histology, and size. *J Thorac Cardiovasc Surg.* 2005;130(5):1413–1421.
66. Okumura M, Ohta M, Tateyama H, et al. The World Health Organization histologic classification system reflects the oncologic behavior of thymoma: a clinical study of 273 patients. *Cancer.* 2002;94(3):624–632.
67. Nakagawa K, Asamura H, Matsuno Y, et al. Thymoma: a clinicopathologic study based on the new World Health Organization classification. *J Thorac Cardiovasc Surg.* 2003;126(4):1134–1140.
68. Ogawa K, Uno T, Toita T, et al. Postoperative radiotherapy for patients with completely resected thymoma. A multi-institutional, retrospective review of 103 patients. *Cancer.* 2002;94(5):1405–1413.
69. Singhal S, Shrager JB, Rosenthal DI, LiVolsi VA, Kaiser LR. Comparison of stages I-II thymoma treated by complete resection with or without adjuvant radiation. *Ann Thorac Surg.* 2003;76(5):1635–1641.
70. Mangi AA, Wain JC, Donahue DM, Grillo HC, Mathisen DJ, Wright CD. Adjuvant radiation of stage III thymoma: is it necessary? *Ann Thorac Surg.* 2005; 79(6):1834–1839.
71. Cesaretti JA. Adjuvant radiation with modern techniques is the standard of care for stage III thymoma. *Ann Thorac Surg.* 2006;81(3):1180–1181.

72. Ströbel P, Bauer A, Puppe B, et al. Tumor recurrence and survival in patients treated for thymomas and thymic squamous cell carcinomas: a retrospective analysis. *J Clin Oncol.* 2004;22(8):1501–1509.
73. Sugie C, Shibamoto Y, Ikeya-Hashizume C, et al. Invasive thymoma: postoperative mediastinal irradiation, and low-dose entire hemithorax irradiation in patients with pleural dissemination. *J Thorac Oncol.* 2008;3(1):75–81.
74. Onuki T, Ishikawa S, Yamamoto T. Pathologic radioresponse of preoperatively irradiated invasive thymoma. *J Thorac Oncol.* 2008;3(3):270–276.
75. Rena O, Papalia E, Maggi G, et al. World Health Organization histologic classification: an independent prognostic factor in resected thymomas. *Lung Cancer.* 2005;50(1):59–66.
76. Loehrer PJ Sr., Jiroutek M, Aisner S, et al. Combined etoposide, ifosfamide, and cisplatin in the treatment of patients with advanced thymoma and thymic carcinoma: an intergroup trial. *Cancer.* 2001;91(11):2010–2015.
77. Berruti A, Borasio P, Gerbino A, et al. Primary chemotherapy with adriamycin, cisplatin, vincristine and cyclophosphamide in locally advanced thymomas: a single institution experience. *Br J Cancer.* 1999;81(5):841–845.
78. Giaccone G, Ardizzoni A, Kirkpatrick A, Clerico M, Sahmoud T, van Zandwijk N. Cisplatin and etoposide combination chemotherapy for locally advanced or metastatic thymoma: a phase II study of the European Organization for Research and Treatment of Cancer Lung Cancer Cooperative Group. *J Clin Oncol.* 1996; 14(3):814–820.
79. Bretti S, Berruti A, Loddo C, et al. Multimodal management of stages III-IVa malignant thymoma. *Lung Cancer.* 2004;44(1):69–77.
80. Shin DM, Walsh GL, Komaki R, et al. A multidisciplinary approach to therapy for unresectable malignant thymoma. *Ann Intern Med.* 1998;129(2):100–104.
81. Jacot W, Quantin X, Valette S, Khial F, Pujol JL. Multimodality treatment program in invasive thymic epithelial tumor. *Am J Clin Oncol.* 2005;28(1):5–7.
82. Venuta F, Rendina EA, Pescarmona EO, et al. Multimodality treatment of thymoma: a prospective study. *Ann Thorac Surg.* 1997;64(6):1585–1591.
83. Lucchi M, Ambrogi MC, Duranti L, et al. Advanced stage thymomas and thymic carcinomas: results of multimodality treatments. *Ann Thorac Surg.* 2005;79(6):1840–1844.
84. Kim ES, Putnam JB, Komaki R, et al. Phase II study of multidisciplinary approach with induction chemotherapy, followed by surgical resection, radiation therapy, and consolidation chemotherapy for unresectable malignant thymomas: final report. *Lung Cancer.* 2004;44(3):369–379.
85. Huang J, Riely GJ, Rosenzweig KE, Rusch VW. Multimodality therapy for locally advanced thymomas: state of the art or investigational therapy? *Ann Thorac Surg.* 2008;85(2):365–367.
86. Huang J, Rizk NP, Travis WD, et al. Feasibility of multimodality therapy including extended resections in stage IVA thymoma. *J Thorac Cardiovasc Surg.* 2007; 134(6):1477–1483.
87. Kondo K, Monden Y. Thymoma and myasthenia gravis: a clinical study of 1,089 patients from Japan. *Ann Thorac Surg.* 2005;79(1):219–224.
88. Sasaki H, Ide N, Fukai I, Kiriyama M, Yamakawa Y, Fujii Y. Gene expression analysis of human thymoma correlates with tumor stage. *Int J Cancer.* 2002;101(4):342–347.
89. Lee GY, Yang WI, Jeung HC, et al. Genome-wide genetic aberrations of thymoma using cDNA microarray based comparative genomic hybridization. *BMC Genomics.* 2007;8:305.
90. Kaira K, Oriuchi N, Imai H, et al. L-type amino acid transporter 1 (LAT1) is frequently expressed in thymic carcinomas but is absent in thymomas. *J Surg Oncol.* 2009;99(7):433–438.

demos MEDICAL

RADIATION MEDICINE ROUNDS

Normal Tissue Toxicity

Sujay A. Vora*
Mayo Clinic, Phoenix, AZ

ABSTRACT

The roles of external beam radiation, chemotherapy, surgery, and combined modality treatment are well established in the treatment of thoracic malignancies (1–4). However, each treatment modality carries risks of both acute and chronic toxicities affecting normal tissues. Normal tissues potentially at risk include the esophagus, lungs, nerve tissue (brachial plexus/spinal cord), and heart. The purpose of this overview is to discuss natural history, predictive factors, and management of normal tissue toxicity.

ESOPHAGUS

The esophagus is commonly included within the treatment volume in patients receiving radiation therapy due to location of the primary tumor, involved lymph nodes, and draining lymphatics. Toxicity is usually described as acute or late toxicity. Acute toxicity occurs during and immediately after treatment. Acute symptoms of dysphagia and odynophagia generally develop after 2 to 3 weeks of daily radiation therapy. These symptoms can lead to dehydration, weight loss, and fatigue. Pathophysiologic findings include initial mucosal hyperemia and erythema, followed by epithelial denudation, erosion, and submucosal edema (5). Chronic toxicity can occur months to years after treatment. This occurs from subepithelial damage of the lumen wall, causing submucosal and muscle wall fibrosis, lumen narrowing, and mucous gland atrophy (6). These toxicities can include esophageal stricture and, rarely, perforation/ulceration or fistula formation. Patients with collagen vascular disease (especially systemic lupus and scleroderma), Bloom syndrome, and ataxia telangiectasia are particularly at risk of late esophageal injury (7).

Toxicity scales commonly used include the Radiation Therapy Oncology Group (RTOG)/European Organization for Research and Treatment of Cancer (EORTC) late toxicity scale and National Cancer Institute Common Toxicity Criteria for Adverse Events (NCI-CTCAE) acute toxicity scale (Table 1).

Risk factors for developing esophagitis include treatment-related factors and radiation dosimetry. Patient-related factors, including age, performance status, gender, body mass index, have generally been not consistently predictive of esophageal toxicity (8–10).

Corresponding author, Department of Radiation Oncology, Mayo Clinic, 5777 E. Mayo Blvd., Phoenix, AZ 85054
E-mail address: vora.sujay@mayo.edu

Radiation Medicine Rounds 1 (2010) 225–238.

DOI: 10.5003/2151-4208.1.1.225

TABLE 1 Toxicity scales for esophagitis

RTOG/EORTC	
Grade 0	None.
Grade 1	Mild fibrosis, slight difficulty in swallowing solids; no pain on swallowing.
Grade 2	Unable to take solid food normally; swallowing semisolid food, dilation may be indicated.
Grade 3	Severe fibrosis; able to swallow only liquids; may have pain on swallowing; dilation required.
Grade 4	Necrosis/perforation; fistula.
Grade 5	Death.
NCI-CTCAE v.3	
Grade 0	No symptoms.
Grade 1	Asymptomatic pathologic, radiographic, or endoscopic findings only.
Grade 2	Symptomatic; altered eating/swallowing (e.g. altered dietary habits, oral supplements); IV fluids indicated <24 h.
Grade 3	Symptomatic; severely altered eating/swallowing (e.g. inadequate oral caloric or fluid intake); IV fluids, tube feedings, or TPN indicated ≥24 h.
Grade 4	Life-threatening consequences.
Grade 5	Death.

EORTC, European Organization for Research and Treatment of Cancer; RTOG, Radiation Therapy Oncology Group.

Treatment-related factors include use of twice-daily radiation, higher radiation doses, addition of chemotherapy, and sequencing of chemotherapy. With 3-dimensional treatment planning, calculation of dose (dosimetry) to the esophagus is now possible. Numerous studies have now studied how dose-volume interactions correlate with esophageal toxicity.

Ahn et al. (11) evaluated the clinical and 3-dimensional dosimetric parameters associated with esophageal injury after radiotherapy for non–small cell lung cancer (NSCLC). Acute toxicity occurred in 199 (78%) of 254 patients. For acute toxicity of grade 2 or worse, twice-daily radiotherapy, age, nodal stage of N2/3, and most dosimetric parameters were predictive. Late toxicity occurred in 17 (7%) of 238 patients. The median and maximal time to the onset of late toxicity was 5 and 40 months after radiotherapy, respectively. For late toxicity, the severity of acute toxicity was most predictive.

Werner-Wasik et al. (10) identified in a multivariate analysis treatment-related factors predisposing patients with lung cancer to acute esophagitis, expressed as a severity grade or esophagitis index (EI). Esophagitis grades for each time point were verified by review of weekly physician and nursing treatment notes, hospital discharge summaries, and referring physician notes and then plotted on graph against time. The area under the curve (AUC) was calculated for each patient's graph and was defined as an EI. Univariate and multivariate analyses of several factors potentially influencing the maximum esophagitis grade, as well as EI, were performed. Concurrent chemotherapy and twice-daily radiotherapy, especially when combined, were associated with the highest acute maximum esophagitis grade and EI. The duration of acute esophagitis was also longest in the concurrent chemotherapy plus twice-daily radiotherapy group. The increasing length of esophagus in the radiation field did not predict for the severity of acute esophagitis.

Takeda et al. (12) evaluated the factors associated with acute esophagitis in lung cancer patients treated with thoracic radiotherapy. Median dose was 60 Gy. Eighty-six percent received concurrent chemotherapy. The most significant correlation was between esophagitis and percentage of esophageal volume receiving >35 Gy on both univariate (P = .002) and multivariate (P = .018) analyses.

Bradley et al. (13) analyzed whether the irradiated esophageal surface area (A) and/or esophageal volume (V) are predictive of acute esophagitis in relation to other clinical and treatment-related factors. All patients were treated to median dose 70 Gy. The esophageal surface area receiving ≥55 Gy, the esophageal volume receiving ≥60 Gy, and the use of concurrent chemotherapy were the most statistically significant predictive factors for early esophagitis. Age, stage, performance status, and preradiotherapy chemotherapy had no statistically significant influence on the incidence of acute esophagitis.

Belderbos et al. (14) correlated acute esophageal toxicity (AET) with dosimetric and clinical parameters for NSCLC patients treated with radiotherapy alone or with chemoradiotherapy (CRT). They analyzed the data of 156 patients with medically inoperable or locally advanced NSCLC. Seventy-four patients were irradiated with high-dose radiotherapy only, 45 patients with sequential CRT (gemcitabine/cisplatin), and 37 patients with concurrent CRT (cisplatin daily 6 mg/m^2). The radiation dose delivered ranged from

49.5 to 94.5 Gy (2.25–2.75 Gy per fraction) with an overall treatment time of 5 to 6 weeks. Grade 2 AET or higher occurred in 27% of the patient population of which nine patients developed grade 3 toxicity and one patient grade 4. All 10 patients with grade ≥3 esophageal toxicity received concurrent CRT. At multivariable analysis, the most significant clinical parameter to predict AET was the concurrent use of CRT. The most significant dosimetric parameter was the esophagus volume that received at least 35 Gy.

Kim et al. (15) retrospectively evaluated which dose-volumetric parameters are associated with the risk of grade 3 or higher AET in lung cancer patients treated with 3-dimensional conformal radiotherapy (3D-CRT). The parameters analyzed included sex, age, Karnofsky performance score, weight loss, surgery, concurrent chemotherapy, dose-volume parameters, the percent and absolute length of the esophagus irradiated, the maximum and mean dose to the esophagus, and normal tissue complication probability. In univariate and multivariate logistic regression analyses, concurrent chemotherapy and the volume of esophagus receiving 60 Gy (V60) were significantly associated with the development of severe (grade 3 or higher) AET ($P < .05$). The authors concluded that for patients being treated with concurrent chemotherapy, V60 is considered to be a useful parameter predicting the risk of severe AET after conventionally fractionated 3D-CRT for lung cancer.

Maguire et al. (8) evaluated the incidence, severity, and clinical/dosimetric predictors of acute and chronic esophageal toxicities in patients with NSCLC treated with high-dose conformal thoracic radiation treatment parameters included: median corrected dose 78.8 Gy (range 64.2–85.6); twice-daily fractionation 58 (64%); chemotherapy 43 (47%). At each axial level, the percentage of the esophageal circumference at each dose level was calculated. The length of circumferential esophagus and the maximum circumference treated to doses >50 Gy were assessed. On univariate analyses, the effects of percent organ volume treated >50 Gy (P = .05), percent surface area treated >50 Gy (P = .05), length of 100% circumference treated >50 Gy (P = .04), and maximum percent of circumference treated >80 Gy (P = .01) significantly predicted for late toxicity of all grades. On multivariate analysis, percent organ volume treated >50 Gy (P = .02) and maximum percent of circumference treated >80 Gy (P = .02) predicted for late toxicity.

Singh et al. (9) evaluated the incidence and clinical/dosimetric predictors of acute and late RTOG grades 3 to 5 esophageal toxicity in patients with NSCLC treated with definitive 3D-CRT. The following patient and treatment parameters were studied: age, gender, race, performance status, sequential chemotherapy, concurrent chemotherapy, presence of subcarinal nodes, pretreatment weight loss, mean dose to the entire esophagus, maximal point dose to the esophagus, and percentage of volume of esophagus receiving >55 Gy. The median prescription dose was 70 Gy. They found that concurrent chemotherapy and the maximal esophageal point dose were significantly associated with a risk of grades 3 to 5 esophageal toxicity. In patients who received concurrent chemotherapy, the threshold maximal esophageal point dose for grades 3 to 5 esophageal toxicity was 58 Gy. An insufficient number of patients developed grades 3 to 5 esophageal toxicity in the absence of chemotherapy to allow a valid statistical analysis of the relationship between the maximal esophageal point dose and esophagitis.

Rose et al. (16) assessed published dosimetric parameters and toxicity data systematically looking at all published literature to define reproducible predictors of esophagitis. Eighteen published studies were suitable for analysis. Eleven of these assessed acute esophagitis, whereas the remainder assessed both acute and chronic esophagitis together. Heterogeneity of esophageal contouring practices, individual differences in information reporting, and variability of esophagitis outcome definitions were assessed. They found the esophageal volumes receiving 35 and 60 Gy and area receiving 55 Gy to be the most common factors predicting for esophagitis. To summarize, in addition to the dosimetric factors outlined by Rose (16), use of concurrent chemotherapy, increased radiation dose, and twice-daily radiation correlate with increased risk of acute and chronic esophagitis.

Management and Prevention of Toxicity

Symptom management of acute esophagitis include pain medication, empiric treatment for Candida, mucosal anesthetics, nutritional supplements, and if needed, feeding tubes. Sucralfate, a basic albumin salt of sucrose octasulfate used in treatment of duodenal ulcers, has been studied to see if it could also reduce esophagitis. McGinnis et al. (17) performed a placebo-controlled double-blinded prospective randomized study. Unfortunately, there was substantially increased incidence of gastrointestinal toxicity (58% of sucralfate patients vs. 14% of placebo patients; $P > .0001$). Thus, no substantial benefit from the sucralfate was observed.

Amifostine (AM), a radioprotector, has also been studied with conflicting results (18,19). With some promising phase 2 data, RTOG 9801 (20) was initiated for locally advanced NSCLC patients receiving hyperfractionated radiation with concurrent chemotherapy. In all, 243 patients with stage II to IIIA/B NSCLC received induction paclitaxel 225 mg/m^2 intravenously (IV) days 1 and 22 and carboplatin AUC days 1 and 22, followed by concurrent weekly paclitaxel (50 mg/m^2 IV) and carboplatin (AUC 2), and hyperfractionated radiation therapy (69.6 Gy at 1.2 Gy twice daily). Patients were randomly assigned to AM 500 mg IV four times per week or no AM during CRT. AM was associated with higher rates of acute nausea ($P = .03$), vomiting ($P = .007$), cardiovascular toxicity ($P = .0001$), and infection or febrile neutropenia ($P = .03$). The rate of grade ≥ 3 esophagitis was 30% with AM versus 34% without AM ($P = .9$). Patient diaries demonstrated lower swallowing dysfunction AUC with AM ($P = .025$). Quality of life assessment was not significantly different between the two arms, except for pain, which showed more clinically meaningful improvement and less deterioration at 6 weeks follow-up (vs. pretreatment) in the AM arm ($P = .003$). The study concluded that AM did not significantly reduce esophagitis grade 3 or worse in patients receiving hyperfractionated radiation and chemotherapy.

Chronic toxicities can include esophageal stricture, perforation, or fistula formation. These are quite rare. Strictures are usually circular or nearly circular (21). They are usually managed by esophageal dilation using fluroscopic guidance. These procedures carry 0.3% risk of perforation, hemorrhage, and bacteremia. Since these tend to recur, repeat dilation or placement of stent is sometimes necessary. Esophageal perforation or fistula formation is a serious complication and is generally fatal. Stent placement, surgery, bowel rest, and IV antibiotics have been used with limited success.

Advances in treatment planning has also helped to reduce esophageal doses and, in turn, toxicity. Furthermore, omitting elective nodal irradiation (ENI) in lung cancer patients has helped to reduce field sizes and, in turn, reducing irradiated esophageal volumes (22,23). With the use of 4-dimensional treatment planning, intensity-modulated radiation therapy (IMRT) (Figure 1), and image-guided radiation therapy, treatment plans have improved with increasing data that it helps to reduce toxicity. Grills et al. (24) systematically evaluated four different techniques of radiation therapy including IMRT, optimized 3D-CRT using multiple beam angles, limited 3D-CRT using only 2 to 3 beams, and traditional radiotherapy using ENI to treat the mediastinum. They found that IMRT was associated with a greater degree of heterogeneity within the target and, correspondingly, higher mean doses and tumor control probabilities, 7% to 8% greater than 3D-CRT, and 14% to 16% greater than ENI. They found the highest risks of pulmonary and esophageal toxicity with ENI. For node-positive cases, especially where the gross tumor volume was close to the esophagus, IMRT reduced the mean esophagus dose by 40% (vs. 3D-CRT) and by 145% (vs. ENI). They concluded that both omitting ENI and use of IMRT for node-positive, central tumors helped to decrease esophageal doses and toxicity.

Pulmonary

Thoracic radiation carries risk of injury to the normal lung. Histopathology suggests a three-step process (25). The first precedes clinical manifestation of radiation pneumonitis (RP) and is characterized by cell death with sloughing of type I pneumocytes and endothelial cells, release of surfactant, fibrin exudation in alveoli, decrease in macrophage counts, and occurrence of interstitial edema. The second step marks acute RP and is characterized by tissue reaction and inflammation with hyperplasia of type II pneumocytes; increase in leukocyte, macrophage, and fibroblast counts; obstruction of endothelia; and increase in collagen and elastin connective tissue fibers. Finally, generalized fibrosis with loss of capillaries, thickening of alveolar septa, and narrowing of alveoli is seen. The mechanism of late injury is not completely understood. These toxicities are felt to be potentially related to cascade of cytokines and other factors, including TGF-β, IL-1α, IL-6, VEGF, and hypoxia, leading to progressive fibrosis (26–28).

Clinically, pulmonary toxicity can be divided into acute and chronic phases. Acute toxicity generally occurs between 6 weeks and 6 months after radiation. The incidence varies between 5% and 20% (29–31). Symptoms of fever, shortness of breath, pleuritic pain, and cough are reported. Chest radiographs or computerized tomography may show an infiltrate. It generally responds well to corticosteroids given over several weeks. Antibiotics are often added

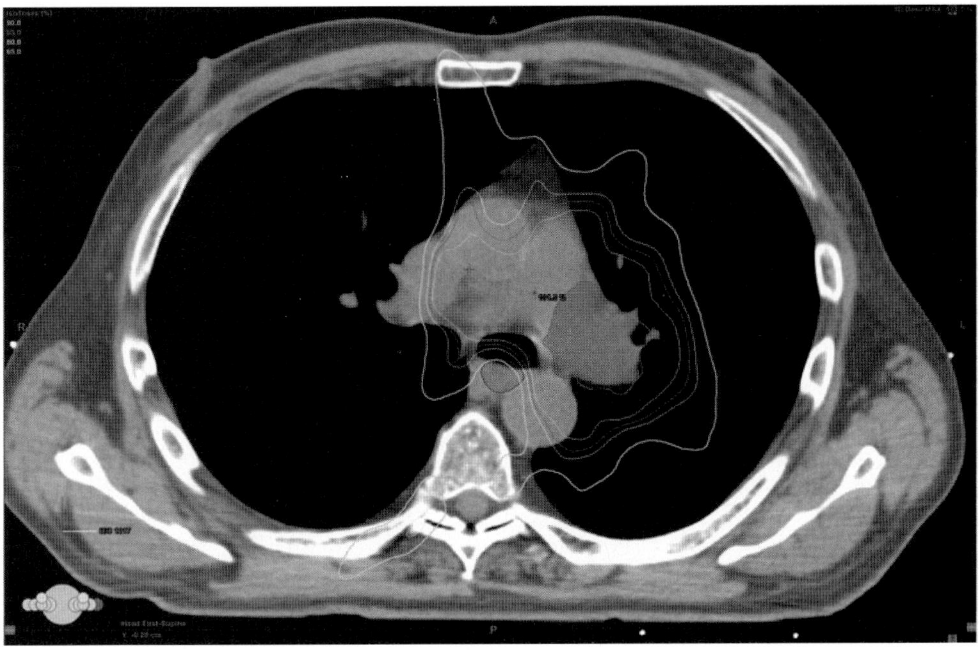

FIGURE 1 Intensity-modulated radiation therapy treatment planning to reduce esophageal dose.

if fever develops. Chronic or late toxicity can occur months to years after treatment. This is caused by progressive radiation fibrosis and loss of lung function. Dyspnea and cough can occur. Often, corticosteroids and supplemental oxygen are required. Other rare late side effects, generally linked to high-dose radiation or stereotactic body radiation therapy (SBRT) (32) include bronchial stenosis/obstruction, recurrent laryngeal nerve injury, and bronchomalacia. Toxicity scales used include the NCI-CTCAE and RTOG/EORTC (Table 2).

Patients should undergo pretreatment evaluation including history and physical, imaging, and pulmonary function testing. Imaging can include computerized tomography, chest radiograph, positron emission tomography, and ventilation/perfusion scans. The forced expiratory volume in 1 second (FEV1), forced vital capacity, and diffusion capacity are most commonly used parameters.

As opposed to surgical resection, radiation effects on pulmonary function are less predictable due to multiple factors. While surgical resection is anatomical, radiation fields and its effects are not. Changes that occur in the lung are often gradual, exacerbated by other medical conditions including continued smoking or worsening chronic obstructive lung disease. Lung function often improves if the tumor is obstructing an airway. If tumors are not controlled, continued tumor growth can also lead to pulmonary function loss. For these reasons, many medically inoperable patients with suboptimal lung function are often offered radiotherapy. Thus, there are no absolute contraindications to radiotherapy.

Numerous studies have analyzed risk factors for developing pulmonary toxicity (Table 3). Risk factors can be divided into pretreatment patient factors and treatment-related factors. Patient-related factors include performance status, age, tumor location, gender, and pretreatment pulmonary function tests. Robnett et al. (33) identified factors that may predict for severe RP. Of 144 evaluable patients, 12 (8.3%) experienced severe RP. The most significant factor predicting for severe RP was performance status (PS) ($P < .003$). The risk of severe RP was 16% for PS-1 patients versus 2% for PS-0 patients. Women were significantly more likely to develop severe RP than men ($P = .01$). FEV1 was also significant ($P = .03$). No patient suffering severe RP had a pretreatment FEV1 > 2.0 L. The size and location of tumor is also important in determining risk. Treatment-related

TABLE 2 Pulmonary toxicity scales

Adverse Effect	**1**	**2**	**3**	**4**	**5**
Cough	Symptomatic, no narcotics	Symptomatic, narcotics needed	Symptomatic	Interferes with ADL	
Dyspnea	On exertion, 1 flight of stairs OK	On exertion, unable to walk 1 flight of stairs	Dyspnea with ADL	Dyspnea at rest intubation indicated	Death
Airway obstruction	Asymptomatic on exam, radiograph or endoscopy	Symptomatic, causing no distress-medical management indicated	Interfering w/ADL endoscopic intervention indicated	Life-threatening death airway compromise	Death
Pneumonitis	Asymptomatic, Radiographic findings only	Symptomatic, not interfering with ADL	Symptomatic, interferes with ADL; oxygen indicated	Life-Threatening; ventilatory support indicated	Death
Pulmonary fibrosis	Minimal radiographic Changes; <25% lung volume	Patchy or bibasilar changes; 25 to <50% of total lung volume	Dense, widespread infiltrates; 50%–75%	>75% of total lung volume; honeycombing	Death
RTOG/EORTC Late Toxicity Scale					
Grade					
0	**1**	**2**	**3**	**4**	**5**
None	Asymptomatic or mild symptoms (dry cough); slight radiographic change	Moderate symptomatic fibrosis or pneumonitis (severe cough); low-grade fever; patchy radiographic change	Severe symptomatic fibrosis or pneumonitis; dense radiographic changes	Severe respiratory insufficiency/ continuous O_2 assisted ventilation effects	Death directly related to radiation

EORTC, European Organization for Research and Treatment of Cancer; RTOG, Radiation Therapy Oncology Group.

factors include use of chemotherapy, tumor location, mediastinal involvement, radiation dose, and radiation planning dosimetry.

There are many chemotherapeutic agents that carry increased risk of pulmonary toxicity (34). These include bleomycin, cyclophosphamide, docetaxel, etoposide, gemcitabine, and paclitaxel. Combining chemotherapy with radiation (either sequentially or concurrently) can also increase risk. Arrieta et al. (35) reported on the efficacy and safety of gemcitabine concurrent with radiotherapy after induction chemotherapy with gemcitabine plus carboplatin for locally advanced NSCLC. Patients received carboplatin (AUC of 2.5) and gemcitabine (800 mg/m^2), followed by conventional fractioned thoracic radiotherapy and concomitant weekly gemcitabine 200 mg/m, and followed by consolidation chemotherapy. High rates of grade 3–5 RP (6 of 19 patients, 31.6%) were observed, including one treatment-related death. This particular combination was found too toxic to be considered safe.

However, many studies have not shown increased pulmonary toxicity with platinum-based regimens. Sause et al. (36) conducted a phase 3 trial for stage III NSCLC comparing the following regimens: (a) standard radiation therapy, (b) induction

TABLE 3 Radiation dosimetry and risks of radiation pneumonitis

		V Dose		Mean Lung Dose	
Reference	Lung Injury Endpoint	Subgroup	Rate (%)	Subgroup (Gy)	Rate (%)
Oetzel et al. (74)	All grades			≤15	0
				17.5–20	13
				22.5–25	21
				≥27.5	43
Graham et al. (75)	Grade ≥ 2	V20 Gy < 22%	0	<10	0
		V20 Gy 22–31%	0	11–20	9
		V20 Gy 32–40%	13	21–30	24
		V20 Gy > 40%	36	>30	25
Kwa et al. (76)	Grade > 2			0–8	5
				8–16	11
				16–24	18
				24–36	43
Hernando et al. (29)	All grades	V30 Gy ≤ 18%	6	<10	10
		V30 Gy > 18%	24	10–20	16
				21–30	27
				>30	44
Tsujino et al. (77)	Grade ≥ 2 (hyperfractionated)	V20 Gy < 20%	0		
		V20 Gy 21–25%	7.1		
		V20 Gy 26–30%	25		
		V20 Gy > 31%	42.9		
Tsujino et al. (78)	Grade ≥ 2 (once a day radiation)	V20 Gy < 20%	8.7		
		V20 Gy 21–25%	18.3		
		V20 Gy 26–30%	51		
		V20 Gy > 31%	85		
Schallenkamp et al. (38)	Grade ≥ 2	V10 Gy<32%	5		
		V10 Gy 32–42%	15		
		V10 Gy 43–64%	45		
Fay et al. (39)	Grade ≥ 2	V30 Gy < 22%	10		
		V30 Gy ≥ 22%	18		

chemotherapy followed by standard radiation therapy, and (c) twice-daily radiation therapy. The pneumonitis rates were similar between treatment arms. Schaake-Koning et al. (37) randomly assigned 331 patients with nonmetastatic inoperable NSCLC to one of three treatments: radiotherapy for 2 weeks (3 Gy given 10 times, in 5 fractions a week), followed by a 3-week rest period and then radiotherapy for 2 more weeks (2.5 Gy given 10 times, 5 fractions a week); radiotherapy on the same schedule, combined with 30 mg of cisplatin per square meter of body-surface area, given on the first day of each treatment week; or radiotherapy on the same schedule, combined with 6 mg of cisplatin per square meter, given daily before radiotherapy. No increased rate of pulmonary toxicity was observed.

Tumor-related factors and radiation planning/dosimetry are intertwined risk factors. Tumor-related factors include tumor size, tumor location, and mediastinal involvement. The greater the size of the radiation field required to encompass all disease, the higher the risk of affecting lung function. With the advent of 3-dimensional radiation treatment planning, radiation doses can be compared with lung volumes. The dose volume histogram (DVH) created from the treatment plan allows physicians to determine how much of the lung is receiving a certain dose of radiation. Numerous studies have been able to take this information and translate it to symptomatic pneumonitis (Table 3).

Schallenkamp et al. (38) analyzed dosimetric parameters that correlated with the risk of clinically relevant RP after thoracic radiotherapy. DVHs using total lung volume (TL) and TL minus gross tumor volume (TL-G) were created with and without heterogeneity corrections. Mean lung dose (MLD), effective lung volume (V[eff]), and percentage of TL or TL-G receiving greater than or equal to 10, 13, 15, 20, and 30 Gy (V10–V30, respectively) were analyzed by logistic regression. They determined V10 and V13 as the best predictors of RP risk. They concluded that treatment planning should attempt to reduce the volumes that receive 10 to 15 Gy.

Fay et al. (39) also did a similar analysis in patients undergoing radical radiotherapy for primary lung cancer. The records of 156 patients with lung cancer who had been treated with radical radiotherapy (≥45 Gy) and for whom DVH data were available were reviewed. The incidence of symptomatic RP was correlated with a variety of parameters derived from the DVH data, including the volume of lung receiving 10 Gy (V [10]) through 50 Gy (V [50]) and the MLD. They concluded that V (30) and MLD can be used to predict the risk of RP in lung cancer patients undergoing radical radiotherapy.

SBRT has had increased use in the treatment of stage I/II NSCLC and in metastatic setting. This involves delivery of three to five sessions of 10 to 20 Gy. The combination of central tumor location and high radiation doses can also lead to increased toxicity. Timmerman et al. (32) reported that in a cohort of SBRT patients receiving 60 Gy in 3 fractions, patients treated for tumors in the peripheral lung had 2-year freedom from severe toxicity of 83% compared with only 54% for patients with central tumors. Song et al. (40) also found similar results. Doses of 10 to 20 Gy per fraction were delivered to the planning target volume (PTV) up to a total dose of 40 to 60 Gy with 3 to 4 fractions on consecutive days. Of nine patients with centrally located tumors, three (33%) experienced grades 3 to 5 pulmonary toxicities. Eight patients showed partial or complete bronchial stricture and secondary loss of normal lung volume. Median time to bronchial stricture was 20.5 months. They concluded that SBRT should not be given to central lung tumors because it can cause the late major airway toxicities in some patients.

To help minimize toxicity, a number of strategies have been used. This includes improving tumor definition with 4-dimensional treatment planning and PET/CT. Different techniques have also been used to improve the radiation treatment planning and delivery. This includes incorporation of IMRT, particle beam radiation therapy, image-guided radiation delivery, and respiratory gating. In lung cancer, eliminating ENI to subclinical sites has also greatly enhanced the ability to deliver higher doses of radiation while reducing radiation doses to normal tissues including lung.

Grills et al. (24) systematically evaluated four different techniques of radiation therapy used to treat NSCLC and to determine their efficacy in meeting multiple normal-tissue constraints while maximizing tumor coverage and achieving dose escalation. He compared IMRT, optimized 3D-CRT using multiple beam angles, limited 3D-CRT using only 2 to 3 beams, and traditional radiotherapy using ENI to treat the mediastinum. In node-positive cases, IMRT reduced the lung volume receiving 20 Gy (V20) and mean dose by approximately 15% and lung normal tissue complication probability by 30%, compared with 3D-CRT. The reductions were even greater as compared with patients treated with ENI. They found IMRT is of limited additional value (compared with 3D-CRT) in node-negative cases. When meeting all normal-tissue constraints in node-positive patients, IMRT can deliver radiotherapy doses 25% to 30% greater than 3D-CRT and 130% to 140% greater than standard therapy with ENI.

Vlachaki et al. (41) reported on the dosimetric impact of gated CT plans on tumor and surrounding normal tissues in patients with primary thoracic malignancies. Ten patients underwent treatment planning with gated and nongated CT at Wayne State University. Gated CT images were obtained at full inspiration, expiration, and at the 25th, 50th, and 75th percentile of respiratory effort. PTV margin for nongated and gated plans was 1.5 cm and 0.5 cm, respectively. The tumor prescription dose was 60 to 70 Gy at 2 Gy per fraction. They found that the average PTV was 292.68 mL for gated and 575.17 mL for nongated plans. Gated plans resulted in higher minimum PTV doses and comparable mean and maximum doses when compared with nongated plans.

Volumes of lung receiving doses of 20 and 10 Gy or above were 26.26% and 30.96% for gated plans and 34.82% and 40.16% for nongated plans ($P < .0001$). Gated plans resulted in lower mean lung, esophageal, and heart doses compared with nongated plans ($P \leq .003$). They concluded that 4-dimensional computed tomography (4D-CT) respiratory gating significantly decreases target volumes and normal tissue dosing. With the emerging image-guided radiation therapy technology, 4D-CT treatment planning may be used for radiation dose escalation with tighter radiation fields and has the potential for improving outcomes in patients with thoracic malignancies.

Chang et al. (42) compared DVHs in patients with NSCLC treated by photon or proton radiotherapy. DVHs were compared between photon, including 3D-CRT, IMRT, and proton plans at doses of 66 or 87.5 Gy in stage I (n = 10) and 60–63 or 74 Gy in stage III (n = 15). For stage I, the mean total lung V5, V10, and V20 were 31.8%, 24.6%, and 15.8%, respectively, for photon 3D-CRT with 66 Gy, whereas they were 13.4%, 12.3%, and 10.9%, respectively, with proton with dose escalation to 87.5 cobalt Gray equivalents (CGE) ($P = .002$). For stage III, the mean total lung V5, V10, and V20 were 54.1%, 46.9%, and 34.8%, respectively, for photon 3D-CRT with 63 Gy, whereas they were 39.7%, 36.6%, and 31.6%, respectively, for proton with dose escalation to 74 CGE ($P = .002$). In all cases, the doses to lung, spinal cord, heart, esophagus, and integral dose were lower with proton therapy even compared with IMRT. These authors concluded that proton treatment appears to reduce dose to normal tissues significantly, even with dose escalation, compared with standard-dose photon therapy, either 3D-CRT or IMRT.

Spinal Cord

Radiation-induced myelopathy is fortunately an extremely rare complication from radiation therapy. Signs and symptoms are generally subtle and progressive occurring months after treatment. Early symptoms can include Lhermitte sign, paresthesias, numbness, loss of coordination, and diminished proprioception. Late symptoms include progressive weakness, hemiparesis, pain, and spasticity. Physical exam reveals hyperreflexia, decreased sensation, weakness, and positive Babinski sign. Toxicity scores (Table 4) are based on the National Cancer Institute Common Terminology Criteria for Adverse Events version 3.0 (NCI-CTC v.3.0) and LENT-SOMA scales (43). Typically half of the patients develop symptoms within 20 months and 75% within 30 months (43). Pathologically, demyelination, white matter necrosis, and corticospinal malacia are observed, presumably due to microvascular injury and loss of oligodendrocyte cells (44).

TABLE 4 Myelitis toxicity scales

NCI-CTC v.3.0	
Grade 1	asymptomatic, mild signs (Babinski or Lhermittes sign).
Grade 2	Symptomatic (weakness or sensory loss), not interfering with activities of daily living (ADL).
Grade 3	Symptomatic (weakness or sensory loss), interfering with activities of daily living (ADL).
Grade 4	Disabling.
Grade 5	Death.
LENT-SOMA	
Grade 1	mild sensory deficits, no pain.
Grade 2	moderate sensory deficits, tolerable pain, mild weakness.
Grade 3	continuous paresthesia, incomplete motor paresis, pain medication required.
Grade 4:	Complete motor paresis, intractable pain, muscle atrophy.

Diagnosis is usually made once other factors are excluded. Other potential causes include local tumor progression, new metastasis, or trauma. Workup can include magnetic resonance imaging (MRI), nerve conduction studies, and cerebral spinal fluid examination. Wang et al. (45) reported on seven patients who developed myelopathy. The first MRI study was performed 1 to 4 months after the initial clinical manifestations of myelopathy and follow-up MRI 2 to 22 months after the onset of symptoms. On the first study, all patients showed low signal intensity in a long segment of the spinal cord on T1-weighted images, high signal on T2*-weighted images, and focal contrast enhancement. Seventy-one percent of patients also had swelling of the spinal cord. The site of eccentric focal contrast enhancement correlated with the clinical manifestations. Follow-up imaging less than 10 months after the onset of symptoms showed no significant changes in signal intensity. Atrophy of the spinal cord without abnormal signal and with faint contrast enhancement was revealed as early as 10 months after the onset of symptoms, but the contrast enhancement disappeared by 22 months. There was no correlation between clinical manifestations and spinal cord atrophy on MRI. Cerebral spinal fluid examination is generally normal, though increase in protein and white blood cells can be observed. Spinal nerve conduction velocities are reduced (46).

Doses of 45 to 50.4 Gy delivered over 25 to 28 treatments have generally been accepted to be safe with myelopathy risks of <1% (43,47,48). Schultheiss et al. (43) estimated the 5-year 5% incidence of myelopathy to be 57 to 61 Gy and 5-year 50% incidence to be 68 to 73 Gy. The length of cord irradiated was not prognostic. Factors that can increase risk of developing myelopathy include the concurrent use of chemotherapy, larger fraction sizes, and use of multiple fractions per day (43,49–51).

Survival is dependent on the location of the lesion and the length of latent period between treatment and onset of symptoms. Schultheiss et al. (52) reported that patients with cervical lesions had lower survival rates as compared with thoracic locations. They found mortality rates of 55% at 18 months for cervical lesions and 25% at 18 months for thoracic lesions. The degree of transaction is also prognosis with complete transaction faring worse (53). Patients with a shorter latent period also did worse. Unfortunately, there are no effective treatments for reversing radiation myelitis. High-dose corticosteroids can give temporary relief by treating spinal cord edema. Hyperbaric oxygen and anticoagulation has been examined with limited success (54,55).

Brachial Plexus

Brachial plexopathy has been reported as a result of treatment for breast cancer, lymphoma, head and neck cancer, and lung cancer. It is generally a late complication from radiation. Damage may be due to either direct effects on the nerve or radiation-induced fibrosis causing compression of the nerves (56,57). Differentiating tumor growth versus radiation-induced plexopathy (RIP) can be difficult. Kori et al. (58) reported on 100 cases of plexopathy to determine which clinical criteria helped differentiate tumor from radiation injury. Severe pain occurred in 80% of tumor patients but in only 19% of patients with radiation injury. The lower trunk (C7–8, T1) was involved in 72% of the tumors, and 32% also had epidural tumors. Seventy-eight percent of the radiation injuries affected the upper plexus (C5–6). Horner syndrome was more common in tumor, and lymphedema in radiation injury. They concluded that painless upper trunk lesions with lymphedema suggest radiation injury, and painful lower trunk lesions with Horner syndrome imply tumor infiltration. The upper plexus vulnerability to radiation is possibly due to a longer length of nerve exposed during radiation and lesser amount of tissue within the occipital triangle. The lower trunk has a shorter course and is protected by the clavicle (59).

The time interval between radiation exposure and development of RIP is generally >12 months with reported neuropathies occurring 5 to 15 years posttreatment (60,61). Symptoms can include paresthesias, muscular atrophy, hyporeflexia, pain, and weakness. Toxicity scales used include CTCAE v.3.0 and LENT-SOMA (Table 5).

Workup includes history and physical, electromyography (EMG), CT and MRI. EMG generally reveals a reduction conduction velocity and amplitude with an increase in latency (56,59). Imaging is generally performed to rule out tumor recurrence or progression. Hoeller et al. (57) investigated MRI features of RIP and radiation-induced fibrosis frequently associated with RIP. They identified seven patients with late radiation sequelae in the supraclavicular region were examined with MRI after a median interval of 7 years following radiotherapy and 4 to 7 years after the onset of RIP. All patients were relapse-free at the time of MRI. Fibrosis and RIP were scored clinically (RTOG classification).

TABLE 5 Brachial plexopathy toxicity scale

CTCAE v.3.0	
Grade 1	Asymptomatic.
Grade 2	Symptomatic, not interfering with activities of daily living.
Grade 3	Symptomatic, interfering with activities of daily living.
Grade 4	Disabling.
Grade 5	Death.
LENT-SOMA	
Grade 1	Mild sensory deficits, no pain
Grade 2	Moderate sensory deficits, tolerable pain, mild weakness
Grade 3	Continuous paresthesia, incomplete motor paresis, pain medication required
Grade 4	Complete motor paresis, intractable pain, muscle atrophy

Fibrosis of the supraclavicular and/or axillary region was marked in three and mild in two patients. RIP was mild, marked, and severe in two patients each. The brachial plexus appeared normal in all patients, but subtle changes of adjoining tissue (slight, linear signal intensity in T2-weighted images or contrast enhancement surrounding the plexus) were detected in patients with RIP (n = 4/6) and the patient without RIP (n = 1). However, alterations of the soft tissue (marked signal intensity in T2-weighted sequences) correlated well with the clinical degree of fibrosis and were restricted to areas of marked to severe fibrosis (n = 3/3). The authors concluded that reliable MRI signs of RIP could not be identified. The severity of fibrosis closely corresponded to MRI features. Therefore, the key role of MRI in the diagnostic workup of RIP is to exclude tumor relapse.

High radiation doses, dose per fraction, overlapping radiation fields, increased dose to the axilla in thinner patients, and use of concurrent chemotherapy are all risk factors for developing plexopathy. Emami et al. found the TD 5/5 (tolerance dose causing injury to 5% of patients in 5 years) to be 60 Gy delivered in conventional fractionation (1.8/2 Gy/day) (47). Forquer et al. reported (62) on frequency of brachial plexopathy in early-stage apical NSCLC treated with stereotactic body radiotherapy. Two-year Kaplan-Meier risk of brachial plexopathy for maximum brachial plexus dose greater than 26 Gy was 46% vs. 8% for doses 26 Gy (P = .04 for likelihood ratio test). They concluded that stereotactic body radiotherapy for apical lesions carries a risk of brachial plexopathy. Brachial plexus maximum dose should be kept <26 Gy in 3 or 4 fractions.

Higher doses per fraction to the axilla were also found to put the brachial plexus at risk. Powell et al. (63) examined 449 breast cancer patients treated with postoperative radiotherapy to the breast and lymph nodes between 1982 and 1984 have been followed for 3 to 5.5 years. Two different fractionation schedules were used. The calculated dose to the brachial plexus was 45 Gy in 15 fractions or 54 Gy in 30 fractions. These schedules are equivalent doses using the standard NSD formula. The diagnosis of a brachial plexus injury was made clinically and CT was used to distinguish radiation injury from recurrent disease. The actuarial incidence of a radiation-induced brachial plexus injury for the whole group was 4.9% at 5.5 years. No cases were seen in the first 10 months following radiotherapy. The incidence rises between 1 and 4 years and then starts to plateau. When the large fraction size group is compared with the small fraction size group the incidence at 5.5 years is 5.9% and 1.0%, respectively (P = .09). The authors concluded that using large doses per fraction are less well tolerated by the brachial plexus than small doses per fraction; a commonly used fractionation schedule such as 45 Gy in 15 fractions may give unacceptably high brachial plexus morbidity; and the use of small doses per fraction or avoiding lymphatic irradiation is advocated.

Unfortunately, if plexopathy develops, there are limited effective treatment options available. This first step is to rule out disease progression as the cause of symptoms. If there is evidence of tumor relapse, palliative radiation may be of benefit. However, if the clinical and radiographic appearances are consistent with radiation-induced brachial plexopathy, therapy is limited to symptomatic management. Hyperbaric oxygen and surgical nerve transfer have been attempted with minimal success (64,65).

Cardiovascular Disease

Due to advances in chemotherapy, radiation, and surgery, survival rates for many thoracic malignancies are improving. However, with improving survival, increased risks of cardiovascular disease are observed. This is mostly seen in patients with long natural history such as Hodgkin disease and breast cancer. Toxicities including coronary artery disease, myocardial fibrosis, valvular disease, arrhythmias, congestive heart failure, and pericarditis have been reported (66–69). The risks due to cancer therapy are also further compounded by additional factors including hypercholesterolemia, smoking, obesity, hypertension, and increasing age.

Radiation-related side effects generally occur late, months to years after treatment. Emami et al. (47) found the TD 5/5 (tolerance dose causing injury to 5% of patients in 5 years) to be 60 Gy to 1/3 of heart, 45 Gy to 2/3 of heart and 40 Gy to the whole heart delivered in conventional fractionation (1.8/2 Gy/day). Most of the available data comes from treatment of breast cancer and Hodgkin disease where long survival rates are observed. It should be noted that much of the available data on toxicity comes from patients treated with older radiation techniques, older chemotherapies, and with larger treatment fields than used today. Demirci et al. (67) looked at newer and older breast radiation trials. The trials were defined as "older" (patient accrual start year before 1980) and "modern" (patient accrual start year in or after 1980) to segregate the trials and assess the treatment era effect. A 10-year follow-up duration was used as a cutoff to segregate and analyze trials with varying lengths of follow-up. They analyzed 19 published reports of patients treated between 1968 and 2002 (5 randomized controlled trials, 5 single- or multi-institutional studies, and 9 national cancer registry database reviews). In the reviewed trials, all the older trials reported excess cardiac toxicity, typically with a median of >10 to 15 years of follow-up. However, the vast majority of modern radiotherapy trials had shorter median follow-up durations, typically ≤10 years and did not report an excess toxicity risk. The modern studies lacked longer follow-up. They concluded that additional follow-up is needed to ensure that modern methods effectively reduce cardiac toxicity.

Chemotherapy causing cardiac toxicity has also been extensively studied, particularly of anthracyclines. Toxicity is dose dependent and cumulative. Lefrak et al. (70) reported a 30% incidence of congestive heart failure in 399 patients receiving more than 550 mg/m^2. Other chemotherapies associated with increased risks of cardiac toxicity include mitoxantrone, cyclophosphamide, paclitaxel, 5-flurouracil, and trastuzumab (66,71–73).

Most treatment strategies focus on prevention. Calculations of DVHs give the radiation oncologist a better understanding of doses to the heart. Staying below accepted limits for chemotherapy doses also helps to minimize toxicity. Reducing other risk factors such as smoking, exercise, and nutrition also are helpful.

■ CONCLUSION

Cancer treatment for thoracic malignancies has improved in recent years. The incorporation of improved chemotherapies, radiation treatment planning/delivery, and surgical techniques has given patients a chance at improved survival. However, they have also introduced new challenges in managing toxicities from treatment. A better understanding of radiation and chemotherapy effects has allowed treating physicians to focus on strategies to prevent toxicity.

■ REFERENCES

1. Falkson CB, Bezjak A, Darling G, et al. The management of thymoma: a systematic review and practice guideline. *J Thorac Oncol.* 2009;4:911–919.
2. Liao Z, Zhang Z, Jin J, et al. Esophagectomy after concurrent chemoradiotherapy improves locoregional control in clinical stage II or III esophageal cancer patients. *Int J Radiat Oncol Biol Phys.* 2004;60:1484–1493.
3. Socinski MA, Zhang C, Herndon JE II, et al. Combined modality trials of the Cancer and Leukemia Group B in stage III non-small-cell lung cancer: analysis of factors influencing survival and toxicity. *Ann Oncol.* 2004;15:1033–1041.
4. Venuta F, Rendina EA, Coloni GF. Multimodality treatment of thymic tumors. *Thorac Surg Clin.* 2009;19:71–81.
5. Chowhan NM. Injurious effects of radiation on the esophagus. *Am J Gastroenterol.* 1990;85:115–120.
6. Berthrong M, Fajardo LF. Radiation injury in surgical pathology. Part II. Alimentary tract. *Am J Surg Pathol.* 1981;5:153–178.
7. Coia LR, Myerson RJ, Tepper JE. Late effects of radiation therapy on the gastrointestinal tract. *Int J Radiat Oncol Biol Phys.* 1995;31:1213–1236.
8. Maguire PD, Sibley GS, Zhou SM, et al. Clinical and dosimetric predictors of radiation-induced esophageal toxicity. *Int J Radiat Oncol Biol Phys.* 1999;45:97–103.
9. Singh AK, Lockett MA, Bradley JD. Predictors of radiation-induced esophageal toxicity in patients with non-small-cell lung cancer treated with three-dimensional conformal radiotherapy. *Int J Radiat Oncol Biol Phys.* 2003;55:337–341.
10. Werner-Wasik M, Pequignot E, Leeper D, Hauck W, Curran W. Predictors of severe esophagitis include use of concurrent chemotherapy, but not the length of irradiated esophagus: a multivariate analysis of patients with lung cancer treated with nonoperative therapy. *Int J Radiat Oncol Biol Phys.* 2000;48:689–696.
11. Ahn SJ, Kahn D, Zhou S, et al. Dosimetric and clinical predictors for radiation-induced esophageal injury. *Int J Radiat Oncol Biol Phys.* 2005;61:335–347.
12. Takeda K, Nemoto K, Saito H, Ogawa Y, Takai Y, Yamada S. Dosimetric correlations of acute esophagitis in lung cancer patients treated with radiotherapy. *Int J Radiat Oncol Biol Phys.* 2005;62:626–629.
13. Bradley J, Deasy JO, Bentzen S, El-Naqa I. Dosimetric correlates for acute esophagitis in patients treated with radiotherapy for lung carcinoma. *Int J Radiat Oncol Biol Phys.* 2004;58:1106–1113.
14. Belderbos J, Heemsbergen W, Hoogeman M, Pengel K, Rossi M, Lebesque J. Acute esophageal toxicity in non-small cell lung cancer patients after high dose conformal radiotherapy. *Radiother Oncol.* 2005;75:157–164.
15. Kim TH, Cho KH, Pyo HR, et al. Dose-volumetric parameters of acute esophageal toxicity in patients with lung cancer treated with three-dimensional conformal radiotherapy. *Int J Radiat Oncol Biol Phys.* 2005;62:995–1002.
16. Rose J, Rodrigues G, Yaremko B, Lock M, D'Souza D. Systematic review of dose-volume parameters in the prediction of esophagitis in thoracic radiotherapy. *Radiother Oncol.* 2009;91:282–287.

17. McGinnis WL, Loprinzi CL, Buskirk SJ, et al. Placebo-controlled trial of sucralfate for inhibiting radiation-induced esophagitis. *J Clin Oncol.* 1997;15:1239–1243.
18. Komaki R, Lee JS, Kaplan B, et al. Randomized phase III study of chemoradiation with or without amifostine for patients with favorable performance status inoperable stage II-III non-small cell lung cancer: preliminary results. *Semin Radiat Oncol.* 2002;12:46–49.
19. Leong SS, Tan EH, Fong KW, et al. Randomized double-blind trial of combined modality treatment with or without amifostine in unresectable stage III non-small-cell lung cancer. *J Clin Oncol.* 2003;21:1767–1774.
20. Movsas B, Scott C, Langer C, et al. Randomized trial of amifostine in locally advanced non-small-cell lung cancer patients receiving chemotherapy and hyperfractionated radiation: Radiation Therapy Oncology Group Trial 98–01. *J Clin Oncol.* 2005;23:2145–2154.
21. Siersema PD. Treatment options for esophageal strictures. *Nat Clin Pract Gastroenterol Hepatol.* 2008;5:142–152.
22. Kepka L, Bujko K, Zolciak-Siwinska A. Risk of isolated nodal failure for non-small cell lung cancer (NSCLC) treated with the elective nodal irradiation (ENI) using 3D-conformal radiotherapy (3D-CRT) techniques—a retrospective analysis. *Acta Oncol.* 2008;47:95–103.
23. Sulman EP, Komaki R, Klopp AH, Cox JD, Chang JY. Exclusion of elective nodal irradiation is associated with minimal elective nodal failure in non-small cell lung cancer. *Radiat Oncol.* 2009;4:5.
24. Grills IS, Yan D, Martinez AA, Vicini FA, Wong JW, Kestin LL. Potential for reduced toxicity and dose escalation in the treatment of inoperable non-small-cell lung cancer: a comparison of intensity-modulated radiation therapy (IMRT), 3D conformal radiation, and elective nodal irradiation. *Int J Radiat Oncol Biol Phys.* 2003; 57:875–890.
25. Madani I, De Ruyck K, Goeminne H, De Neve W, Thierens H, Van Meerbeeck J. Predicting risk of radiation-induced lung injury. *J Thorac Oncol.* 2007;2:864–874.
26. Anscher MS, Kong FM, Andrews K, et al. Plasma transforming growth factor beta1 as a predictor of radiation pneumonitis. *Int J Radiat Oncol Biol Phys.* 1998;41: 1029–1035.
27. Anscher MS, Murase T, Prescott DM, et al. Changes in plasma TGF beta levels during pulmonary radiotherapy as a predictor of the risk of developing radiation pneumonitis. *Int J Radiat Oncol Biol Phys.* 1994;30:671–676.
28. Miller KL, Shafman TD, Marks LB. A practical approach to pulmonary risk assessment in the radiotherapy of lung cancer. *Semin Radiat Oncol.* 2004;14:298–307.
29. Hernando ML, Marks LB, Bentel GC, et al. Radiation-induced pulmonary toxicity: a dose-volume histogram analysis in 201 patients with lung cancer. *Int J Radiat Oncol Biol Phys.* 2001;51:650–659.
30. Makimoto T, Tsuchiya S, Hayakawa K, Saitoh R, Mori M. Risk factors for severe radiation pneumonitis in lung cancer. *Jpn J Clin Oncol.* 1999;29:192–197.
31. Werner-Wasik M, Yu X, Marks LB, Schultheiss TE. Normal-tissue toxicities of thoracic radiation therapy: esophagus, lung, and spinal cord as organs at risk. *Hematol Oncol Clin North Am.* 2004;18:131–160, x–xi.
32. Timmerman R, McGarry R, Yiannoutsos C, et al. Excessive toxicity when treating central tumors in a phase II study of stereotactic body radiation therapy for medically inoperable early-stage lung cancer. *J Clin Oncol.* 2006;24:4833–4839.
33. Robnett TJ, Machtay M, Vines EF, McKenna MG, Algazy KM, McKenna WG. Factors predicting severe radiation pneumonitis in patients receiving definitive chemoradiation for lung cancer. *Int J Radiat Oncol Biol Phys.* 2000;48:89–94.
34. Carver JR, Shapiro CL, Ng A, et al. American Society of Clinical Oncology clinical evidence review on the ongoing care of adult cancer survivors: cardiac and pulmonary late effects. *J Clin Oncol.* 2007;25:3991–4008.
35. Arrieta O, Gallardo-Rincon D, Villarreal-Garza C, et al. High frequency of radiation pneumonitis in patients with locally advanced non-small cell lung cancer treated with concurrent radiotherapy and gemcitabine after induction with gemcitabine and carboplatin. *J Thorac Oncol.* 2009;4:845–852.
36. Sause WT, Scott C, Taylor S, et al. Radiation Therapy Oncology Group (RTOG) 88–08 and Eastern Cooperative Oncology Group (ECOG) 4588: preliminary results of a phase III trial in regionally advanced, unresectable non-small-cell lung cancer. *J Natl Cancer Inst.* 1995;87:198–205.
37. Schaake-Koning C, van den Bogaert W, Dalesio O, et al. Effects of concomitant cisplatin and radiotherapy on inoperable non-small-cell lung cancer. *N Engl J Med.* 1992;326:524–530.
38. Schallenkamp JM, Miller RC, Brinkmann DH, Foote T, Garces YI. Incidence of radiation pneumonitis after thoracic irradiation: dose-volume correlates. *Int J Radiat Oncol Biol Phys.* 2007;67:410–416.
39. Fay M, Tan A, Fisher R, Mac Manus M, Wirth A, Ball D. Dose-volume histogram analysis as predictor of radiation pneumonitis in primary lung cancer patients treated with radiotherapy. *Int J Radiat Oncol Biol Phys.* 2005;61:1355–1363.
40. Song SY, Choi W, Shin SS, et al. Fractionated stereotactic body radiation therapy for medically inoperable stage I lung cancer adjacent to central large bronchus. *Lung Cancer.* 2009;66:89–93.
41. Vlachaki M, Castellon I, Leite C, Perkins T, Ahmad S. Impact of respiratory gating using 4-dimensional computed tomography on the dosimetry of tumor and normal tissues in patients with thoracic malignancies. *Am J Clin Oncol.* 2009;32:262–268.
42. Chang JY, Zhang X, Wang X, et al. Significant reduction of normal tissue dose by proton radiotherapy compared with three-dimensional conformal or intensity-modulated radiation therapy in stage I or stage III non-small-cell lung cancer. *Int J Radiat Oncol Biol Phys.* 2006;65:1087–1096.
43. Schultheiss TE, Kun LE, Ang KK, Stephens LC. Radiation response of the central nervous system. *Int J Radiat Oncol Biol Phys.* 1995;31:1093–1112.

44. Schultheiss TE, Stephens LC, Maor MH. Analysis of the histopathology of radiation myelopathy. *Int J Radiat Oncol Biol Phys.* 1988;14:27–32.
45. Wang PY, Shen WC, Jan JS. Serial MRI changes in radiation myelopathy. *Neuroradiology.* 1995;37:374–377.
46. Snooks SJ, Swash M. Motor conduction velocity in the human spinal cord: slowed conduction in multiple sclerosis and radiation myelopathy. *J Neurol Neurosurg Psychiatry.* 1985;48:1135–1139.
47. Emami B, Lyman J, Brown A, et al. Tolerance of normal tissue to therapeutic irradiation. *Int J Radiat Oncol Biol Phys.* 1991;21:109–122.
48. Marcus RB Jr, Million RR. The incidence of myelitis after irradiation of the cervical spinal cord. *Int J Radiat Oncol Biol Phys.* 1990;19:3–8.
49. Dische S. Accelerated treatment and radiation myelitis. *Radiother Oncol.* 1991;20:1–2.
50. Dische S, Saunders MI. Continuous, hyperfractionated, accelerated radiotherapy (CHART): an interim report upon late morbidity. *Radiother Oncol.* 1989;16:65–72.
51. Wong CS, Van Dyk J, Simpson WJ. Myelopathy following hyperfractionated accelerated radiotherapy for anaplastic thyroid carcinoma. *Radiother Oncol.* 1991;20:3–9.
52. Schultheiss TE, Stephens LC, Peters LJ. Survival in radiation myelopathy. *Int J Radiat Oncol Biol Phys.* 1986; 12:1765–1769.
53. Holdorff B. Dose effect relationships in cervical and thoracic radiation myelopathies. *Acta Radiologica.* 1980; 19:271–277.
54. Calabro F, Jinkins JR. MRI of radiation myelitis: a report of a case treated with hyperbaric oxygen. *Eur Radiol.* 2000;10:1079–1084.
55. Liu CY, Yim BT, Wozniak AJ. Anticoagulation therapy for radiation-induced myelopathy. *Ann Pharmacother.* 2001;35:188–191.
56. Wadd NJ, Lucraft HH. Brachial plexus neuropathy following mantle radiotherapy. *Clin Oncol (R Coll Radiol).* 1998;10:399–400.
57. Hoeller U, Bonacker M, Bajrovic A, Alberti W, Adam G. Radiation-induced plexopathy and fibrosis. Is magnetic resonance imaging the adequate diagnostic tool? *Strahlenther Onkol.* 2004;180:650–654.
58. Kori SH, Foley KM, Posner JB. Brachial plexus lesions in patients with cancer: 100 cases. *Neurology.* 1981; 31:45–50.
59. Brennan MJ. Breast cancer recurrence in a patient with a previous history of radiation injury of the brachial plexus: a case report. *Arch Phys Med Rehabil.* 1995;76:974–976.
60. Johansson S, Svensson H, Larsson LG, Denekamp J. Brachial plexopathy after postoperative radiotherapy of breast cancer patients—a long-term follow-up. *Acta Oncol.* 2000;39:373–382.
61. Gillette EL, Mahler PA, Powers BE, Gillette SM, Vujaskovic Z. Late radiation injury to muscle and peripheral nerves. *Int J Radiat Oncol Biol Phys.* 1995;31: 1309–1318.
62. Forquer JA, Fakiris AJ, Timmerman RD, et al. Brachial plexopathy from stereotactic body radiotherapy in early-stage NSCLC: dose-limiting toxicity in apical tumor sites. *Radiother Oncol.* 2009;93:408–413.
63. Powell S, Cooke J, Parsons C. Radiation-induced brachial plexus injury: follow-up of two different fractionation schedules. *Radiother Oncol.* 1990;18:213–220.
64. Pritchard J, Anand P, Broome J, et al. Double-blind randomized phase II study of hyperbaric oxygen in patients with radiation-induced brachial plexopathy. *Radiother Oncol.* 2001;58:279–286.
65. Wong M, Tang AL, Umapathi T. Partial ulnar nerve transfer to the nerve to the biceps for the treatment of brachial plexopathy in metastatic breast carcinoma: case report. *J Hand Surg.* 2009;34:79–82.
66. Anderson B, Sawyer DB. Predicting and preventing the cardiotoxicity of cancer therapy. *Expert Rev Cardiovasc Ther.* 2008;6:1023–1033.
67. Demirci S, Nam J, Hubbs JL, Nguyen T, Marks LB. Radiation-induced cardiac toxicity after therapy for breast cancer: interaction between treatment era and follow-up duration. *Int J Radiat Oncol Biol Phys.* 2009;73:980–987.
68. Prosnitz RG, Chen YH, Marks LB. Cardiac toxicity following thoracic radiation. *Semin Oncol.* 2005;32:S71–S80.
69. Senkus-Konefka E, Jassem J. Complications of breast-cancer radiotherapy. *Clin Oncol (R Coll Radiol).* 2006;18:229–235.
70. Lefrak EA, Pitha J, Rosenheim S, Gottlieb JA. A clinicopathologic analysis of adriamycin cardiotoxicity. *Cancer.* 1973;32:302–314.
71. Bird BR, Swain SM. Cardiac toxicity in breast cancer survivors: review of potential cardiac problems. *Clin Cancer Res.* 2008;14:14–24.
72. Broder H, Gottlieb RA, Lepor NE. Chemotherapy and cardiotoxicity. *Rev Cardiovasc Med.* 2008;9:75–83.
73. de Azambuja E, Bedard PL, Suter T, Piccart-Gebhart M. Cardiac toxicity with anti-HER-2 therapies: what have we learned so far? *Target Oncol.* 2009;4:77–88.
74. Oetzel D, Schraube P, Hensley F, Sroka-Perez G, Menke M, Flentje M. Estimation of pneumonitis risk in three-dimensional treatment planning using dose-volume histogram analysis. *Int J Radiat Oncol Biol Phys.* 1995;33:455–460.
75. Graham MV, Purdy JA, Emami B, et al. Clinical dose-volume histogram analysis for pneumonitis after 3D treatment for non-small cell lung cancer (NSCLC). *Int J Radiat Oncol Biol Phys.* 1999;45:323–329.
76. Kwa SL, Lebesque JV, Theuws JC, et al. Radiation pneumonitis as a function of mean lung dose: an analysis of pooled data of 540 patients. *Int J Radiat Oncol Biol Phys.* 1998;42:1–9.
77. Tsujino K, Hirota S, Kotani Y, et al. Radiation pneumonitis following concurrent accelerated hyperfractionated radiotherapy and chemotherapy for limited-stage small-cell lung cancer: dose-volume histogram analysis and comparison with conventional chemoradiation. *Int J Radiat Oncol Biol Phys.* 2006;64:1100–1105.
78. Tsujino K, Hirota S, Endo M, et al. Predictive value of dose-volume histogram parameters for predicting radiation pneumonitis after concurrent chemoradiation for lung cancer. *Int J Radiat Oncol Biol Phys.* 2003;55:110–115.

Index

Note: Page number followed by "f" and "t" refers to figures and tables, respectively.